COVID-19 and Public Health

COVID-19 and Public Health

Global Responses to the Pandemic

Edited by Caroline Kingori

ATHENS

OHIO UNIVERSITY PRESS

Ohio University Press, Athens, Ohio 45701
ohioswallow.com
© 2024 by Ohio University Press
All rights reserved

Printed in the United States of America
Ohio University Press books are printed on acid-free paper ∞ ™

Library of Congress Cataloging-in-Publication Data
Names: Kingori, Caroline M., editor.
Title: COVID-19 and public health : global responses to the pandemic / edited by Caroline Kingori.
Description: Athens : Ohio University Press, [2024] | Includes bibliographical references and index.
Identifiers: LCCN 2023043738 (print) | LCCN 2023043739 (ebook) | ISBN 9780821425329 (paperback ; alk. paper) | ISBN 9780821425336 (pdf)
Subjects: MESH: COVID-19 | Social Determinants of Health | Public Health | Vulnerable Populations
Classification: LCC RA644.C67 (print) | LCC RA644.C67 (ebook) | NLM WC 506.7 | DDC 362.1962/4144—dc23/eng/20240301
LC record available at https://lccn.loc.gov/2023043738
LC ebook record available at https://lccn.loc.gov/2023043739

Contents

v

Illustrations

vii

Preface

As 2019 was winding down and getting ready to usher in 2020, I started hearing rumors of an infectious disease outbreak in China. I was overseas as the year ended, and when I returned to the United States mid-January, I went about my business. Little did I know I had dodged the travel-mayhem bullet that ensued a few months later. Moments like this came often as the pandemic continued, and, as a public health professional, I wasn't alone in grappling with them.

COVID-19 and Public Health: Global Responses to the Pandemic was born from various conversations my public health colleagues and I had in 2020–21. The writing collected here addresses the complex interplay between COVID-19 and public health and attempts to identify contributing factors to the pandemic, missed prevention opportunities, behavioral perspectives, health disparities, and lessons learned to inform future strategies. My colleagues and I wanted to contribute our public health expertise to the ongoing pandemic discourse, given the confusion and missteps that have occurred in the past.

I am a global and public health professional with extensive experience in reproductive and sexual health research, particularly HIV/AIDS. My passion for enriching communities globally to reduce health disparities motivated the development of this book.

I would like to thank all the people who submitted abstracts and chapters during the formative stages of developing this text. For the final chapters included in this book, I recognize the effort that went into improving previous drafts. I would also like to recognize the contribution of my mentors Drs. Michael Reece and Tania Basta, who helped brainstorm the overall objective of the book. Additional gratitude to Dr. Michele Morrone for her support and guidance while putting together this project and to Dr. Peter Memiah for his insight on the book structure and chapter topics. Finally, a huge thank you to my family and friends for their ongoing support with my academic and research endeavors.

Introduction

Social Determinants of COVID-19

CAROLINE KINGORI

> In fighting COVID-19 we must commit to leaving no-one behind, to
> ensuring equitable access to vaccines, therapeutics, and diagnostics
> from the start. We cannot repeat the mistakes we made with HIV, or for
> that matter, TB. In combating these pandemics, the world left the fights
> unfinished, leaving "residual pandemics" that continued to kill the poor
> and vulnerable long after the public health threats had been largely
> removed from high income countries.
>
> —Peter Sands and Mark Vermeulen, "Without Equity, We
> Cannot End COVID-19, HIV or Any Other Pandemic"

The earliest COVID-19 infection reportedly occurred in Wuhan Province, China, sometime between December 2019 and early January 2020 (Worobey 2021; Benavides 2020). Also known as severe acute respiratory syndrome coronavirus 2 (SARS-CoV-2), COVID-19 was declared a pandemic in March 2020 due to the fast-growing number of infections globally (Cucinotta and Vanelli 2020). Collectively, the virus is a zoonotic disease transmitted from an animal host, and it mutates when it transfers to a human host (World Health Organization 2021b). Transmission among humans is associated with exposure to infectious respiratory fluids (Centers for Disease Control and Prevention 2021b).

COVID-19 has left in its wake a catastrophic impact on the quality of life globally, as evidenced by high rates of disease incidence and prevalence, hospitalization, and death. As of March 2023, there were an estimated 759 million confirmed cases and 6.8 million deaths globally. In the United States, which has the highest number of COVID-19 confirmed cases globally, there have been an estimated 102 million confirmed cases and 1 million deaths (World Health Organization, n.d.). Further, the virus challenged global public health even in countries that were historically deemed to have strong public health systems, such as Spain and Italy (Benavides 2020). Primary preventive behaviors include wearing a mask, social distancing, washing/sanitizing hands, and getting vaccinated. Other prevention strategies include avoiding congregating in poorly ventilated spaces, covering coughs and sneezes with a tissue or inside an elbow, and monitoring one's health. Adherence to the preventive strategies dictates the extent to which the virus spreads (Centers for Disease Control and Prevention 2021a).

Even though mortality rates have gone down since the pandemic was declared (Horwitz et al. 2020; Liang et al. 2021), the majority of those at risk for COVID-19 include people of advanced age, those with underlying health conditions, the unvaccinated, and people from underserved communities, with the majority representing historically minoritized communities, e.g., African American, Latinx, and Native American communities (Jordan, Adab, and Cheng 2020; Tai et al. 2021). The disparities associated with COVID-19 incidence, prevalence, and mortality rates in historically minoritized communities include a lack of access to adequate healthcare services, subpar working and living conditions, and chronic medical issues stemming from the influence of structural and social factors (Tai et al. 2021). However, the demographic factors associated with those infected with COVID-19 slowly changed to include young people (Horwitz et al. 2020; Ward et al. 2022).

Vaccines have largely contributed to the reduction in mortality rates, transmission, and severity of the disease (Thompson et al. 2021). Unfortunately, global vaccine distribution has been disparate, especially in Africa, where only 6% of the populace were vaccinated initially by 2021 (World Health Organization 2021a). When COVID-19 was first declared a pandemic in 2020, Africa was spared the catastrophic mayhem of the spread that was seen in the United Kingdom and the US (Nordling 2020). However, with the mutation of the virus into variants such as Alpha-B.1.1.7, Delta-B.1.617.2, and Omicron-B.1.1.529 (Katella 2021), the second and third waves of the transmission took a toll on the already broken health systems in the continent (Loembé and Nkengasong 2021). The result was a continuing shortage of first responders such as healthcare workers and reallocations of limited resources from other chronic diseases such as tuberculosis, HIV, malaria, diabetes, and cardiovascular disease, which were sidelined to address COVID-19 (Loembé and Nkengasong 2021).

Between 2021 and 2022, morbidity and mortality rates in Africa became increasingly concerning, largely due to the inconsistent supply of vaccines from Western nations (Lucero-Prisno et al. 2021). The inequitable access to such lifesaving vaccines significantly contributed to spread of the Omicron-B.1.1.529 virus, which prompted Western nations to discriminately impose travel bans on many African nations, even though research shows that travel bans aren't that effective, but instead perpetuate stigma (Yu and Keralis 2020). Such social injustice continues to impact Africa's success in eliminating diseases, improving health outcomes, and economies of scale (Casaglia 2021).

The COVID-19 pandemic had a huge impact on economies worldwide. For instance, the US saw a major drop of 8.9% in its gross domestic product (GDP) in the second quarter of 2020, the largest in over seventy years. Similarly, other big economies, like those of the UK, Europe, Canada, and Mexico, also had significant GDP declines. The recovery, however, varied widely, with the US rebounding faster, surpassing prepandemic GDP levels by the second quarter of 2021, thanks to government support and economic adaptability (Executive Office of the President Council of Economic Advisers 2022). Furthermore, in resource-limited countries, the costs of providing COVID-19 healthcare every month rose to a whopping US$52 billion (US$8.60 per person) (Kaye et al. 2021). Given the burden of already existing health issues and diseases in such regions, COVID-19 set resource-limited countries back many years, and financial recovery will be slow given their dependence on loans, financial aid, and remittances from immigrants/migrants to their home countries.

We cannot forget the negative impact of COVID-19 on the environment. On one hand, limited movement during lockdowns brought environmental benefits due to decreased transportation; on the other hand, disposal mechanisms for medical waste (masks, wipes, gloves, and sanitizers) led to increased environmental pollution (Bashir, Ma, and Shahzad 2020). Furthermore, challenges in decontamination protocols were experienced due to the novel virus and compliance with existing health guidelines (Phan and Ching 2020). Due to the necessity of their exposure to public spaces, cleaning staff, trash collectors, and medical workers were placed at an increased risk of acquiring COVID-19 and other pathogens, such as meningitis and hepatitis B (Bashir, Ma, and Shahzad 2020).

Given that COVID-19 wreaked havoc globally, it is necessary to scrutinize the contribution of national policies and politics in addressing the virus. Since the pandemic was declared, there have been varying political and policy responses globally. Such responses have led to varying partisanship and political trust among the populace (Gadarian, Goodman, and Pepinsky 2021; Altiparmakis et al. 2021). The expediency with which governments in various nations responded to the pandemic—by instituting quarantines, school closures, or travel bans, as well as in the distribution of vaccines—played a key role in controlling the pandemic (Bel, Gasulla, and Mazaira-Font 2021). In the US, the delayed response in acknowledging the novel virus and instituting public health measures to limit further transmission contributed to a catastrophic increase in morbidity and mortality rates in the country (Béland et al. 2021). On the other hand, in Africa, as soon as the virus was declared a pandemic, various governments instituted lockdowns and travel bans that largely mitigated high rates of illness and deaths (Antwi-Boasiako et al. 2021).

The other significant political and policy issue is the distribution of vaccines across the world. Toward mid-2020, Western nations, particularly the US, worked expeditiously to authorize and approve the development of the Pfizer-BioNTech, Moderna, and Johnson & Johnson's Janssen vaccines (US Food and Drug Administration 2020). Other approved vaccines globally include Oxford/AstraZeneca, Serum Institute of India, Bharat Biotech, Sinopharm (Beijing), and Sinovac (COVID-19 Vaccine Tracker 2021). While these are commendable achievements, policies were slow in ensuring adequate distribution of vaccines in underserved communities and resource-limited countries (Lei 2021; Singh and Chattu 2021). Due to the lag in adequate distribution, resource-limited countries reported high morbidity and mortality rates, whereas there was a decrease in such rates in high-income countries (Loembé and Nkengasong 2021).

This book seeks to contribute to the public health and COVID-19 prevention discourse in the following ways. First, by examining the impact that COVID-19 has had on underserved and resource-limited communities, it addresses a continued challenge in public health in ensuring equitable access to adequate healthcare services. Contextually relevant initiatives that recognize injustices, stigma, racism, and discrimination are needed to support the public health system. Second, by arguing that despite policies in high-income countries leading to the approval and authorization of lifesaving vaccines, without a concerted effort in ensuring equal distribution of COVID-19 vaccines, the efforts to curtail further transmission globally are futile. Third, by assessing the environmental impact of COVID-19 due to medical waste as an emerging issue that should not be glossed over with short-term solutions. Given the increase in viral mutations, strategies to address medical waste like sanitizers, masks, gloves, and other products should be included in national policy to protect the populace and first responders.

The nature of the information provided is an opportunity for the book to serve as an introductory text in a public health course or other related courses such as health policy, health disparities, cross-cultural issues, or health behavior. One challenge with this topic is that COVID-19 is a moving target, as the pandemic is ever-evolving. However, this book takes a retrospective approach, examining lessons learned at the end of each chapter. Chapters also include discussion questions for reflecting on what worked, what did not, and what to do moving forward.

COVID-19 and Public Health is divided into six parts. The three chapters in part 1, "Community Engagement," explore how to successfully address COVID-19 from a public health perspective. Without the buy-in of the community, prevention strategies will not be sustainable. In chapter 1, Timnit Berhane Ghebretinsae and colleagues discuss how they adapted to the new public health guidelines that negatively impacted physical interaction in their community-engaged research. To enhance community engagement, the authors utilized validated virtual tools and platforms for ongoing community-based participatory research. They highlight examples of virtual activities that they engaged in to keep the community partnership thriving. In chapter 2, Kobi Ajayi and colleagues advocate for "gender-responsive frameworks for infection control measures." In essence, they highlight the need for a concerted effort in addressing gender disparities within COVID-19 preventive strategies, particularly among males, who were reported to have high mortality rates compared to women. Since men typically do not seek healthcare services while women have more interaction with the health system, it is important to recognize and develop sustainable strategies that increase males' involvement with the healthcare system. Nevertheless, the authors discuss the importance of addressing unmet needs in women as well, especially in historically minoritized communities. In chapter 3, Jaih Craddock and colleagues explore the extent to which social network methods can be enhanced to comprehend the social determinants of the disparities associated with COVID-19 in communities. They examine COVID-19 as a socially transmitted infection that stems from people's interactions within their social networks and how to utilize such networks to minimize the spread of COVID-19.

Messaging is a critical component in promoting behavioral changes. Given the misconceptions and misunderstandings of COVID-19, contributors to part 2, "Risk Communication," address how best to effectively communicate risk and rally communities to uptake new behaviors. Notably, adequate communication that considers heterogeneity across various communities is essential in sustainable community engagement. In chapter 4, Aggrey Otieno and colleagues examine risk communication strategies via social media content posted by the COVID-19 office at a large midwestern university and informed by online Risk Communication and Community Engagement strategies. To better communicate and engage communities, messages need to resonate with their realities and actively involve members who have influence. In chapter 5, Katherine Tossas and colleagues examine misinformation and mistrust within faith-based communities in underserved communities. They highlight the importance of examining the intersection of the pandemic with injustice, systematic racism, inadequate access to healthcare, and previous public health missteps. Involving trusted establishments like churches in the African American community has produced a marked difference in risk communication on diseases and led to reduced mistrust of the healthcare system because such establishments are considered trustworthy and can increase community action.

The chapters in part 3, "Environmental Health," address the impact of COVID-19 on the environment. Michele Morrone, in chapter 6, considers the extent to which the virus highlighted the critical role played by environmental health practitioners, who at times became first responders, especially on cruise ships. The enhanced breadth and depth of their roles has significant implications on the current and future workforce. In chapter 7, Kujang Laki and colleagues explore the environmental effects of the disposal of medical waste such as personal protective equipment (PPE). They discuss the impact of PPE disposal mechanisms on marine life, the use of plastics and sterilization, and provide recommendations to curtail PPE littering.

Part 4, "Global Health Success with Other Pandemics," compares COVID-19 with other pandemics. Chapters in this section provide comparative data and perspectives from different countries, offering a multifaceted approach that can enhance future responses to another COVID-19 outbreak. Sonya Panjwani and colleagues, in chapter 8, examine past pandemics to identify what worked, and what didn't, to inform COVID-19 prevention and treatment efforts. They utilize the World Health Organization's Integrated, People-Centered Health Services Framework to examine opportunities for improving health systems in their response to current pandemic and future pandemics. In chapter 9, Katie Schenk and Jerry Okal ponder the lessons learned from other global infectious diseases, such as the HIV/AIDS pandemic, and how COVID-19 response strategies can utilize existing toolkits for responding to emerging infections.

The two chapters in part 5, "Policy and Politics," provide assessments of the conflict between individual autonomy and public health mandates.

The intersection of governmental policies and individual politics can impact the timeliness of effective response and development of sustainable interventions. In chapter 10, Adaeze Aroh and colleagues discuss the challenges associated with individual autonomy versus mandating the wearing of face masks, which are scientifically supported as efficacious in reducing transmission of COVID-19. Their objectives are geared toward enhancing the understanding of government mechanisms that address health policy problems and the intersection of health, politics, and policy. In chapter 11, Emma Biegacki and colleagues highlight the multilevel policy and practice efforts instituted to address the opioid crisis in the wake of the COVID-19 pandemic. Due in part to the reallocation of resources to address the pandemic, opioid overdose cases have skyrocketed. The authors provide insights that support the need to be creative and resourceful in order to improve health outcomes of people who use psychoactive drugs.

Finally, part 6, "Public Health Practice," addresses the extent to which COVID-19 exposed numerous challenges and gaps within the public health and medical systems. Lessons learned for the future of public health practice (e.g., in regard to better community partnerships, workforce capacity, and timely resources) are key to avoiding repeating mistakes. In chapter 12, Carolyne Nganga-Good and Adanna Agbo explore the extent to which COVID-19 uncovered weaknesses in healthcare facilities and systems globally. They identify specific areas for improvement—such as data and information systems, workforce, and infrastructure—that are critical in preparing the healthcare system for any future pandemics. In chapter 13, Pablo Dintrans and colleagues compare public health leadership globally across three countries: Chile, France, and the United States. They advocate for a concerted effort in determining the roles that public health leaders and competencies should play in mitigating further COVID-19 transmission. Their work is informed by a crisis leadership framework that identifies five critical tasks that are instrumental in addressing a health crisis: sense-making, decision-making, meaning-making, crisis termination, and learning.

COVID-19 upended medical and public health systems globally. Its impact has resulted in devastating outcomes among individuals, communities, governments, educational systems, corporations and other organizational environments, and much more. In response, this book is intended to promote equity through the application of public health theory and practice, to lay a framework that reflects on lived experiences, and to challenge all of us to participate in public health advocacy.

REFERENCES

Altiparmakis, Argyrios, Abel Bojar, Sylvain Brouard, Martial Foucault, Hanspeter Kriesi, and Richard Nadeau. 2021. "Pandemic Politics: Policy Evaluations of Government Responses to COVID-19." *West European Politics* 44, no. 5–6: 1159–79. https://doi.org/10.1080/01402382.2021.1930754.

Antwi-Boasiako, Joseph, Charles Othniel A. Abbey, Patrick Ogbey, and Rita Amponsah Ofori. 2021. "Policy Responses to Fight COVID-19: The Case of Ghana." *Brazilian Journal of Public Administration* 55, no. 1 (January–February): 122–39. https://dx.doi.org/10.1590/0034-761220200507.

Bashir, Muhammad Farhan, Benjiang Ma, and Luqman Shahzad. 2020. "A Brief Review of Socio-economic and Environmental Impact of Covid-19." *Air Quality, Atmosphere and Health* 13:1403–9. https://doi.org/10.1007/s11869-020-00894-8.

Bel, Germà, Óscar Gasulla, and Ferran A. Mazaira-Font. 2021. "The Effect of Health and Economic Costs on Governments' Policy Responses to COVID-19 Crisis under Incomplete Information." *Public Administration Review* 81, no. 6 (November–December): 1131–46. https://doi.org/10.1111/puar.13394.

Benavides, Lucía. 2020. "Spain Briefly Passes Italy in COVID-19 Cases but Officials See Growth Rate Slowing." *National Public Radio (NPR),* April 3, 2020. https://www.npr.org/sections/coronavirus-live-updates/2020/04/03/826699690/spain-briefly-passes-italy-in-covid-19-cases-but-officials-see-growth-rate-slowi.

Béland, Daniel, Shannon Dinan, Philip Rocco, and Alex Waddan. 2021. "Social Policy Responses to COVID-19 in Canada and the United States: Explaining Policy Variations between Two Liberal Welfare State Regimes." *Social Policy & Administration: An International Journal of Policy and Research* 55, no. 2 (March): 280–94. https://doi.org/10.1111/spol.12656.

Casaglia, Anna. 2021. "Borders and Mobility Injustice in the Context of the Covid-19 Pandemic." *Journal of Borderlands Studies* 36, no. 4: 695–703. https://doi.org/10.1080/08865655.2021.1918571.

Centers for Disease Control and Prevention. 2021a. "How to Protect Yourself and Others." Updated July 26, 2021. https://stacks.cdc.gov/view/cdc/108306.

———. 2021b. "Scientific Brief: SARS-CoV-2 Transmission." *Centers for Disease Control and Prevention,* May 7, 2021. https://www.cdc.gov/coronavirus/2019-ncov/science/science-briefs/sars-cov-2-transmission.html.

COVID-19 Vaccine Tracker. 2021. "8 Vaccines Approved for Use by WHO." December 13, 2021. https://covid19.trackvaccines.org/agency/who/.

Cucinotta, Domenico, and Maurizio Vanelli. 2020. "WHO Declares COVID-19 a Pandemic." *Acta Biomed* 91, no. 1: 157–60. https://pubmed.ncbi.nlm.nih.gov/32191675/.

Executive Office of the President Council of Economic Advisers. 2022. *Economic Report of the President.* PR JRB.9. Washington, DC: U.S. Government Publishing Office. https://www.govinfo.gov/app/details/ERP-2022.

Gadarian, Shana Kushner, Sara Wallace Goodman, and Thomas B. Pepinsky. 2021. "Partisanship, Health Behavior, and Policy Attitudes in the Early Stages of the

COVID-19 Pandemic." *PLOS ONE* 16, no. 4: e0249596. https://doi.org/10.1371/journal.pone.0249596.

Horwitz, Leora I., Simon A. Jones, Robert J. Cerfolio, Fritz Francois, Joseph Greco, Bret Rudy, and Christopher M. Petrilli. 2021. "Trends in COVID-19 Risk-Adjusted Mortality Rates." *Journal of Hospital Medicine* 16, no. 2 (February): 90–92. https://doi.org/10.12788/jhm.3552.

Jordan, Rachel E., Peymane Adab, and Kar Keung Cheng. 2020. "Covid-19: Risk Factors for Severe Disease and Death." *BMJ* 368:m1198. https://doi.org/10.1136/bmj.m1198.

Katella, Kathy. 2021. "Omicron, Delta, Alpha, and More: What to Know about the Coronavirus Variants." *Yale Medicine: News.* December 10. https://www.yalemedicine.org/news/covid-19-variants-of-concern-omicron.

Kaye, Alan D., Chikezie N. Okeagu, Alex D. Pham, Rayce A. Silva, Joshua J. Hurley, Brett L. Arron, Noeen Sarfraz, et al. 2021. "Economic Impact of COVID-19 Pandemic on Healthcare Facilities and Systems: International Perspectives." *Best Practice & Research Clinical Anaesthesiology* 35, no. 3 (October): 293–306. https://doi.org/10.1016/j.bpa.2020.11.009.

Lei, Yuxiao. 2021. "Hyper Focusing Local Geospatial Data to Improve COVID-19 Vaccine Equity and Distribution." *Journal of Urban Health* 98, no. 4 (August): 453–58. https://doi.org/10.1007/s11524-021-00552-z.

Liang, Li-Lin, Hsu-Sung Kuo, Hsiu J. Ho, and Chun-Ying Wu. 2021. "COVID-19 Vaccinations Are Associated with Reduced Fatality Rates: Evidence from Cross-Country Quasi-Experiments." *Journal of Global Health* 11. https://doi.org/10.7189/jogh.11.05019.

Loembé, Marguerite Massinga, and John N. Nkengasong. 2021. "COVID-19 Vaccine Access in Africa: Global Distribution, Vaccine Platforms, and Challenges Ahead." *Immunity* 54, no. 7 (July): 1353–62. https://doi.org/10.1016/j.immuni.2021.06.017.

Lucero-Prisno III, Don Eliseo, Isaac Olushola Ogunkola, Uchenna Frank Imo, and Yusuff Adebayo Adebisi. 2021. "Who Will Pay for the COVID-19 Vaccines for Africa?" *American Journal of Tropical Medicine and Hygiene* 104, no. 3 (March): 794–96. https://doi.org/10.4269/ajtmh.20-1506.

Nordling, Linda. 2020. "The Pandemic Appears to Have Spared Africa So Far. Scientists Are Struggling to Explain Why." *Science,* August 11, 2020. https://doi.org/10.1126/science.abe2825.

Phan, Thien Luan, and Congo Tak-Shing Ching. 2020. "A Reusable Mask for Coronavirus Disease 2019 (COVID-19)." *Archives of Medical Research* 51, no. 5 (July): 455–57. https://doi.org/10.1016/j.arcmed.2020.04.001.

Singh, Bawa, and Vijay Kumar Chattu. 2021. "Prioritizing 'Equity' in COVID-19 Vaccine Distribution through Global Health Diplomacy." *Health Promotion Perspectives* 11, no. 3 (August): 281–87. https://doi.org/10.34172/hpp.2021.36.

Tai, Don Bambino Geno, Aditya Shah, Chyke A. Doubeni, Irene G. Sia, and Mark L. Wieland. 2021. "The Disproportionate Impact of COVID-19 on Racial and Ethnic Minorities in the United States." *Clinical Infectious Diseases* 72, no. 4 (February): 703–6. https://doi.org/10.1093/cid/ciaa815.

Thompson, Mark G., Jefferey L. Burgess, Allison L. Naleway, Harmony L. Tyner, Sarang K. Yoon, Jennifer Meece, Lauren E. W. Olsho, et al. 2021. "Interim Estimates of Vaccine Effectiveness of BNT162b2 and mRNA-1273 COVID-19 Vaccines in Preventing SARS-CoV-2 Infection among Health Care Personnel, First Responders, and Other Essential and Frontline Workers—Eight U.S. Locations, December 2020–March 2021." *Morbidity and Mortality Weekly Report (MMWR)* 70, no. 13: 495–500. https://doi.org/10.15585/mmwr.mm7013e3.

US Food and Drug Administration. 2020. "Emergency Use Authorization for Vaccines Explained." November 20, 2020. Accessed December 14, 2021. https://www.fda.gov/vaccines-blood-biologics/vaccines/emergency-use-authorization-vaccines-explained.

Ward, Joseph L., Rachel Harwood, Clare Smith, Simon Kenny, Matthew Clark, Peter J. Davis, Elizabeth S. Draper, et al. 2022. "Risk Factors for PICU Admission and Death among Children and Young People Hospitalized with COVID-19 and PIMS-TS in England during the First Pandemic Year." *Nature Medicine* 28:193–200. https://doi.org/10.1038/s41591-021-01627-9.

World Health Organization. 2021a. "Less than 10% of African Countries to Hit Key COVID-19 Vaccination Goal." *WHO Africa,* October 18, 2021. https://www.afro.who.int/news/less-10-african-countries-hit-key-covid-19-vaccination-goal.

———. 2021b. "WHO-Convened Global Study of Origins of SARS-CoV-2: China Part." *Joint WHO-China Study: 14 January–10 February 2021.* March 30, 2021. Accessed December 13, 2021. https://www.who.int/publications/i/item/who-convened-global-study-of-origins-of-sars-cov-2-china-part.

———. n.d. *WHO Coronavirus (COVID-19) Dashboard.* Accessed March 14, 2023. https://covid19.who.int.

Worobey, Michael. 2021. "Dissecting the Early COVID-19 Cases in Wuhan." *Science,* November 18, 2021. Accessed December 14, 2021. https://www.science.org/doi/10.1126/science.abm4454.

Yu, Weijun, and Jessica Keralis. 2020. "Controlling COVID-19: The Folly of International Travel Restrictions." *Health and Human Rights Journal,* April 6, 2020. https://www.hhrjournal.org/2020/04/controlling-covid-19-the-folly-of-international-travel-restrictions/.

Part 1

COMMUNITY ENGAGEMENT

1

Building Community Collaborations in Challenging Times

TIMNIT BERHANE GHEBRETINSAE, DEVIN MADDEN,
TASMIM HOQUE, AND NITA VANGEEPURAM

In March 2020, the World Health Organization declared the coronavirus disease 2019 (COVID-19) a pandemic (WHO 2020). In the same month, the first COVID-19 case was confirmed in New York City, which quickly became the first epicenter of the pandemic in the United States (CDC-CRT 2020). As more cases began to emerge across the country, other public health and social threats started surfacing. Vulnerable and historically marginalized communities were disproportionately affected with higher morbidity and mortality rates (NCIRD 2021). National data reported on November 22, 2021, showed that American Native, African American, and Latinx populations experienced 2.5–3.3 times more hospitalizations and 1.9–2.2 times higher death rates due to COVID-19 in the United States than Whites (NCIRD 2021). These trends were also reflected in NYC, where Asian, Pacific Islander, African American, and Latinx populations had disproportionately higher hospitalization and death rates (NYCDH n.d.-b). Underlying conditions, socioeconomic status, access to care, and the day-to-day lived experiences of these vulnerable populations exposed them to higher rates of health risk factors and worse health outcomes (NCIRD 2021; NCIRD 2020). Similarly, the pandemic severely impacted the chronically ill and disabled, rural populations, LGBTQ+ individuals, those with lower incomes, people experiencing homelessness, and immigrants (Kantamneni 2020; Mueller et al. 2021; Clark et al. 2020; Zimmerman et al. 2009). Each of these populations is disproportionately represented in the essential, frontline, and critical infrastructure industries that were the vital engine keeping the United States running during the pandemic (Kantamneni 2020). This representation likely contributed to the higher COVID-19 case rates experienced in these populations, given that they are more likely to use public transportation, may not have health insurance, are less likely to receive paid leave from work, are less likely to have savings to sustain them, and often are not able to safely isolate in crowded housing situations (Do and Frank 2020).

As the country eventually found itself in a new stage of the pandemic, one where a vaccine was readily available to those ages five and up, similarly lower vaccination rates were observed within these same disproportionately hurt communities for various reasons.[1] Data from the NYC Department of Health and Mental Hygiene depicted racial/ethnic disparities in the percentage of fully vaccinated individuals older than five across the zip codes and boroughs. Based on November 2021 vaccination rates for NYC, it was reported that Black residents, followed by Latinx and White community members, had the lowest rates citywide; however, these rates were seen to be evolving at the time of reporting (NYCDH n.d.-a). Additionally, three of the five boroughs of New York (Brooklyn, the Bronx, and Queens) had a disproportionate percentage of unvaccinated adults (NYCDH n.d.-a). These same neighborhoods experience higher rates of limited English proficiency (LEP) and poverty, are medically underserved, and are majority Black, Latinx, or Asian communities (NYCDYCD 2022). Even in zip codes with higher vaccination rates, subgroups—including residents of public housing, individuals with LEP, LGBTQ+ community members, people who are food insecure, and those involved in the criminal justice system—experience lower vaccination rates and greater incidence of challenges due to social determinants of health (Do and Frank 2020).

It is important to highlight that we still do not fully understand the long-lasting effects of the pandemic and we will probably continue to see an increase in physical, emotional, and mental health challenges at a national and global level as the repercussions of the pandemic are felt. Now more than ever, it is important to engage vulnerable populations in public health research, messaging, and practice. They are the experts on the ground who are best able to speak to their needs and experiences, and can better advocate on the local issues they have pinpointed as important given their intimate understanding of these issues (O'Brien and Whitaker 2011). Engaging with community members directly also allows the community-based organizations that serve these local communities to tailor their services based on direct input (O'Brien and Whitaker 2011). However, the approaches and methods that have been traditionally employed in public health research involve new challenges presented by the nature of the pandemic. This calls for a swift adaptation of public health research in this time of crisis.

In this chapter, we will cover the basics and principles of community-based participatory research (CBPR), the essential and emerging role of virtual community engagement, and how to leverage virtual engagement for CBPR. Along the way, we will share real-life examples of how we, researchers and public health professionals working at the Icahn School of Medicine's Institute for Health Equity Research (IHER), found ourselves adapting to the virtual world and leveraging tools that were new to us to build fruitful collaborations with our community partners, from the beginning of the pandemic in March 2020 to the end of 2021, when this chapter was written.

COMMUNITY-BASED PARTICIPATORY RESEARCH

Despite the challenges imposed by the pandemic, the field of public health needs to utilize research approaches that engage the communities that have been the most impacted to understand their immediate and long-term needs. CBPR offers such an approach by bringing community and academic members together to equitably collaborate and contribute in all stages of research, recognizing that each group has expertise on topics that are of interest or relevant to the community (Horowitz, Robinson, and Seifer 2009). CBPR is grounded in some guiding principles that community-academic partners can jointly adapt based on the objectives of their research.

One core principle is that *community* is used to define a group brought together by a unit of identity; this can be any unit, ranging from a group of people in a certain geographical location to people with shared issues or values, or individuals facing the same health conditions or other challenges (Horowitz, Robinson, and Seifer 2009). While how a community is defined depends on the matter at hand, it is important to have a shared understanding of this definition for the scope of each project and to engage with members who self-identify as part of that community (Horowitz, Robinson, and Seifer 2009; Israel et al. 2005).

Another principle that follows on this emphasizes that community and academic members of the collaborative partnership contribute equally to the work in all phases and stages of the research process. Members from both sides constructively engage in shared decision-making, starting from recognizing the health issue to be addressed through to the final stages of disseminating results and developing strategies for improving community health outcomes based on study findings (Horowitz, Robinson, and Seifer 2009; Israel et al. 2005). Community members and academic researchers cultivate a bidirectional relationship in which they recognize each other's skills and learn from each other, fostering a co-learning process (Horowitz, Robinson, and Seifer 2009; Holkup et al. 2004). As such, strengths, skills, and resources of local community organizations and members are recognized and embraced as assets to address recognized health issues (Holkup et al. 2004). This community-academic partnership is based on mutual trust, shared decision-making, and shared ownership of research, and the gained knowledge benefits all partners involved (Horowitz, Robinson, and Seifer 2009; Holkup et al. 2004). Trust building is an essential part of this process and is strengthened through continued alliance over time; partners commit to a long-term research collaboration by employing a cyclical and iterative partnership collaboration (Israel et al. 2005).

Other important principles to highlight include that the process emphasizes multiple determinants of health from ecological perspectives, that there should be a healthy balance between the knowledge generated and the tangible action carried out in communities for the mutual benefit of all parties (Horowitz, Robinson, and Seifer 2009), and that the dissemination of knowledge gained is shared with all and by all community partners (Israel et al. 2005).

Given these principles, and the need to establish and nurture trust in the relationships these community-academic partnerships create, CBPR is traditionally a process that requires extensive in-person interaction with community members and stakeholders (Zimmerman et al. 2009). However, with the restrictions created by social distancing and stay-at-home orders, these face-to-face interactions were not possible in our case, and it was essential to find innovative ways of engaging with community partners virtually.

THE EMERGING ROLE OF VIRTUAL ENGAGEMENT

Researchers were not the only ones forced to discover how to innovate, transform relationships, and maintain productivity during the pandemic. Despite restrictions on holding in-person meetings, various organizations, communities, and even governmental entities continued to work collaboratively, engaging in meaningful conversations and decision-making in the virtual space. Though engagement has become a hybrid of in-person and remote interactions over the years, the transition to completely virtual engagement suddenly became a reality as we were pushed into work-from-home mode

(Parker, Horowitz, and Minkin 2020). For any organization that relies on collaboration, particularly with external stakeholders, this also meant reconsidering traditional methods of engagement.

Virtual engagement can refer to any interactive effort done remotely and can include online meetings, interviews, town halls, emails, and more. For it to be successful in building relationships and accomplishing goals, we have to consider how we leverage the tools available to us and reflect on both the facilitators of and barriers to meaningful online engagement.

AVAILABLE RESOURCES:
DIGITAL TOOLS AND PLATFORMS AT OUR FINGERTIPS

Virtual Meeting Platforms

Video conferencing platforms: Small- and large-scale meetings and webinars continue to be an essential way to engage community partners and organizations in conversations. The most popular platforms include Zoom, Microsoft Teams, GoToMeeting, Skype, and Cisco Webex, among others (Walsh, n.d.). Zoom became so popular in the early days of the pandemic that some went so far as to call it the "poster child of 2020," and it should be no surprise that it was the number one downloaded app that same year (Graham 2020).

Although many of us have likely become very familiar with at least one of these platforms for one-on-one or group meetings, town halls, webinars, and even social gatherings (Roy 2020), there are nuances to consider when deciding which to use, and it can feel like an overwhelming choice at times. While specific platforms are used by different organizations and employers, when collaborating outside your organization, it is important to consider features and costs, as well as the ease of learning certain platforms and what your external collaborators are most accustomed to using (Fedorowicz, Arena, and Burrowes 2020; COHE, n.d.). Fortunately, there are many technology websites and blogs that have outlined the multitude of available platforms to help users make informed choices (Boyarsky 2020; Walsh, n.d.). In addition, a quick search of Google can generate reviews of the latest trends and thoughts from tech-savvy individuals and may highlight new platforms and/or features to be considered. For example, while most users know that PowerPoint presentations can be shared on Zoom, not all know that these presentations can be used as the background while presenters appear live on the screen in front of a slide deck (Biegun 2021).

Our experience: During the period of activity described here, we relied heavily on these platforms and worked to find ways to innovate within them in order to engage and remain in communication with our community partners. When New York City became a COVID-19 epicenter (CDCCRT 2020), we brought together a large network of partners from across the city and beyond to develop (a) an online survey that would examine the needs and challenges of New Yorkers during the pandemic and (b) a resource repository to help address these needs. A lot of moving pieces and a rapidly changing public health crisis meant our team needed to adapt quickly to the fact that bringing our partners together for in-person meetings to share ideas and strategies was no longer a possibility. In subsequent sections, we will show how we leveraged different technologies to develop the survey and other initiatives born out of that work. Critical to our success from the start, however, was finding an appropriate virtual meeting platform that would make it easier to avoid technological fumbles in front of a live audience.

We generally hosted small workgroup meetings of about five to fifteen people via Zoom to engage in conversations with partners. We successfully conducted Zoom meetings to collaboratively plan our survey design, analysis, and outreach efforts. Once the survey was deployed, we also hosted larger groups of over a hundred people for virtual town halls to keep our local communities informed of the pandemic's evolution, provide space for them to share their concerns, and connect them to experts in various fields who could answer questions. That Zoom allows people without internet access to join via phone dial-in was an added benefit for us when we were considering accessibility for our participants. Additionally, the ability to screen share is a feature that helped make collaborative meetings and town halls engaging, as presenters and others could share agendas, notes, slides, graphs, and other visuals. However, it is important to note that when individuals call into meetings, this feature is not accessible for them.

Although Zoom was a very effective platform for us to engage with our CBPR partners, we realized that we needed new strategies to address the ever-growing Zoom fatigue that everyone was encountering (Ramachandran 2021). We continued to leverage commonly used strategies such as icebreakers and check-ins while exploring innovative methods and organizing formats we could adapt to online spaces to keep our communities engaged. To inspire creative brainstorming when we needed it most, we looked to one organizing tool in particular: Open Space Technology (Herman, n.d.). Traditionally hosted in person, Open Space meetings begin by inviting people to generate an exhaustive list of ideas or concerns that participants can then explore in an open dialogue in groups they self-select to join, based on their interests. Dialogues follow four key principles for the democratization of idea-sharing while fostering community building: (1) Whoever comes is the right person; (2) Whatever happens is the only thing that could have; (3) Whenever it starts is the right time; and (4) When it's over, it's over (Zentis 2017). Fortunately, others have been pioneers in bringing Open Space Technology to Zoom (Maljković 2020), and we were able to lean on their lessons learned to create events and make space for conversations that were engaging, inspiring, and generative.

Social Media Platforms

Social media: Social media platforms can be leveraged for various purposes to meet people where they are, which, for an average of two hours and twenty-four minutes a day, *is* on social media (Georgiev 2019). Several blog posts highlight the importance of social media to organizations and projects. Whether the goal is to share content relevant to the topic at hand, begin conversations with constituents, or drive traffic to an upcoming event, social media allows people and organizations to spotlight what they are doing and disseminate information. It can also be a great way to informally engage with communities in a way that establishes rapport and builds trust (Fedorowicz, Arena, and Burrowes 2020; LHS, n.d.). But not all users view all social media equally, and it is important to be able to distinguish among the ever-growing list of available social media tools to get maximum return on the often lofty investment that building a social media presence requires.

The most popular social networks globally in 2021 were Facebook, YouTube, WhatsApp, Instagram, WeChat, and TikTok (Statista 2023). Similarly, in the United States, YouTube, Facebook, Instagram, Snapchat, Twitter, and TikTok were among the most popular social network platforms (Pew Research Center 2021a). While young adults were and still are the ones with the highest usage percentages, recent years have seen a gradual increase in usage among older adults. Research from the Pew Research Center on social media trends and use in 2021 highlights the differences across demographics among users of various platforms. Figure 1.1 illustrates some of these distinctions and is a helpful reference point for organizations considering which channels will best meet their needs (Pew Research Center 2021a).

Our experience: From the trends noted above, it is clear that social media is an effective tool for reaching young people, but understanding the reach of each platform is helpful because people of all ages are using some type of social media (Fedorowicz, Arena, and Burrowes 2020). One example of how we have been able to leverage social media in our CBPR projects involves the vaccination equity research we are leading in NYC. The

Use of online platforms, apps varies – sometimes widely – by demographic group

% of U.S. adults in each demographic group who say they ever use …

0%   20   40   60   80   100

	YouTube	Facebook	Instagram	Pinterest	LinkedIn	Snapchat	Twitter	WhatsApp	TikTok	Reddit	Nextdoor
Total	81	69	40	31	28	25	23	23	21	18	13
Men	82	61	36	16	31	22	25	26	17	23	10
Women	80	77	44	46	26	28	22	21	24	12	16
White	79	67	35	34	29	23	22	16	18	17	15
Black	84	74	49	35	27	26	29	23	30	17	10
Hispanic	85	72	52	18	19	31	23	46	31	14	8
Ages 18-29	95	70	71	32	30	65	42	24	48	36	5
30-49	91	77	48	34	36	24	27	30	22	22	17
50-64	83	73	29	38	33	12	18	23	14	10	16
65+	49	50	13	18	11	2	7	10	4	3	8
<$30K	75	70	35	21	12	25	12	23	22	10	6
$30K-$49,999	83	76	45	33	21	27	29	20	29	17	11
$50K-$74,999	79	61	39	29	21	29	22	19	20	20	12
$75K+	90	70	47	40	50	28	34	29	20	26	20
HS or less	70	64	30	22	10	21	14	20	21	9	4
Some college	86	71	44	36	28	32	26	16	24	20	12
College+	89	73	49	37	51	23	33	33	19	26	24
Urban	84	70	45	30	30	28	27	28	24	18	17
Suburban	81	70	41	32	33	25	23	23	20	21	14
Rural	74	67	25	34	15	18	18	9	16	10	2

Note: White and Black adults include those who report being only one race and are not Hispanic. Hispanics are of any race. Not all numerical differences between groups shown are statistically significant (e.g., there are no statistically significant differences between the shares of White, Black or Hispanic Americans who say the use Facebook). Respondents who did not give an answer are not shown.
Source: Survey of U.S. adults conducted Jan. 25-Feb. 8, 2021.
"Social Media Use in 2021"

PEW RESEARCH CENTER

FIGURE 1.1. Use of online platforms and apps by demographic group (Pew Research Center, 2021).

Institute for Health Equity Research has been working in partnership with other research organizations (including the hospital NYU Langone Health and clinics forming part of the Institute for Family Health) and local community members and organizations to improve equity in the uptake of the COVID-19 vaccines and inclusion in clinical trials related to COVID-19, as part of the National Institutes of Health's Community Engagement Alliance (CEAL) efforts (NIH, n.d.). To inform this work, our community partners frequently examine New York City Department of Health vaccine data. The data have consistently demonstrated the importance of reaching young people, who are getting vaccinated at disproportionately lower rates than other age groups across the city (NYCDH n.d.-a). Given the soaring popularity of TikTok among Generation Z individuals, our community partners have suggested that social media efforts targeting this group center on TikTok. On the other hand, Facebook continues to be the better option for older individuals such as baby boomers (Pew Research Center 2021a). As in our example, data about health disparities and platforms most commonly used by different socio-demographic groups should shape outreach strategies for public health and CBPR initiatives.

In addition, when choosing which platform to leverage, it is also important to consider the functionality of the platform and how its features align with your goals. For example, certain social media platforms are a good option for sharing and promoting events. Our team has had success creating event pages on both Facebook and LinkedIn because each of these platforms has a dedicated space for events that makes it easy for individuals and organizations to upload flyers, provide event details, and link people to registration information (Fedorowicz, Arena, and Burrowes 2020). We have used these networks to promote town halls on the COVID-19 vaccine, the community-generated research brainstorming sessions mentioned above using Open Space, and panel discussions with virtual engagement and digital media experts, to name a few.

Social media platforms are also important to consider when trying to do targeted outreach or recruitment to identify research participants, share health promotion materials, and much more. While organizations and individuals can reach people in a variety of unpaid ways such as using popular hashtags, tagging relevant accounts, and getting their followers to share their content (Tay 2018), it is sometimes helpful to pay for advertisements through these channels (Gurd 2022). This is particularly true when targeting community members with particular interests or in a defined geographic area. For example, when recruiting participants for our community-based COVID survey, we used a small portion of our budget to promote the survey through Facebook to New Yorkers living in zip codes with high COVID-19 case rates who we were unable to reach through other mechanisms.

Additionally, several social media platforms have begun making it easy to reach audiences through "live" events. If people already follow a particular social media account, they may stumble upon these events when using the platform as part of their daily routine, but it is also possible to advertise them in advance (Facebook, n.d.). For example, through our collaborative work with some local partners, we found that one agency we worked with, in particular, had found some success leveraging Facebook Live to communicate important information to their primarily immigrant, Spanish-speaking community. We partnered with them to informally engage their followers in important conversations about COVID-19 and address misinformation about the available vaccines since Facebook was already a trusted portal for that community.

Survey and Polling Platforms

The tools: Social media polls are popping up all over Instagram, Facebook, and Twitter, to name a few (Gould 2019), providing some proof that polling is not only informative for the pollster but also engaging for the person responding to the poll. Many of the virtual meeting platforms mentioned above also allow organizers to poll participants in real time (Fedorowicz, Arena, and Burrowes 2020), and several additional tools have been developed to help gamify meeting experiences while also giving meeting or event facilitators some valuable information. Poll Everywhere (PollEverywhere, n.d.; UVaCollab, n.d.), Kahoot (Kahoot, n.d.), and Slido (Slido, n.d.) are three such tools that provide more variety than some of the polling features embedded into meeting platforms. With these interactive tools, audience members can be asked to anonymously rank options, answer multiple-choice questions, respond to open-ended prompts, and more. In addition, results can be shared in real time via a word cloud or with other compelling visual tools.

While polls are fun, accessible, and informative, there will be times when more information is needed than a catchy "this" or "that" vote in a 24-hour Instagram story, for example, can provide. In these instances, there are several survey platforms to choose from that can help gather feedback, comments, information about communities' needs and ideas on timely and relevant topics. Some of the commonly used online survey tools are Survey Monkey, Google Forms, and Qualtrics (Fedorowicz, Arena, and Burrowes 2020; COHE, n.d.), but there are many others to choose from, depending on a project's specific needs. While some of these survey tools are free, others offer free as well as fee-based, higher-tiered services with additional features, and some have an outright cost. If the surveys include any personal identifiers or information deemed secure or private, it may be best to use platforms that guarantee protection of this information, although such features often have a cost.

Our experience: Building rapport among a group of remote participants who have not themselves ever met can be a slow process. When we, in collaboration with a task force of community engagement partners, launched a CBPR online workshop series for local stakeholders, we set the stage for engagement early on with Poll Everywhere. With the prompt, "What comes to mind when you hear the word research?" front and center, participants shared their honest thoughts. We saw affirming, open words like "curiosity" and "engagement," but we also saw negatively charged words like "power" and "biased questions." Having this anonymous reflection allowed us to open the course in a way that acknowledged all of the feelings that the many words contained. While it helped the facilitators understand where people were coming from, it also appeared to help the participants feel like they could share openly in the virtual space we created.

To build and deploy our community-based COVID survey, we leveraged many different survey platforms at different times for different reasons. For example, when collaborating across the team, we would often solicit feedback through Google Forms surveys. When it came to the actual survey tool itself, we attempted programming the survey on other platforms before we landed with REDCap, a secure, HIPAA-compliant data collection platform that was developed by researchers at Vanderbilt University to allow researchers to program, manage and track their projects without needing to heavily rely on tech experts (PRC, n.d.). Using REDCap offered many benefits to our fast-paced team as we worked efficiently to deploy a survey that could be accessible to many and get us the information we felt was valuable. For one, the platform enabled us to program the survey in multiple languages under one user link that could be distributed to potential participants across the city; upon clicking the link, participants would be prompted to select their language before finding themselves in the survey, making it easier to manage outreach processes and keep track of incoming data. Additionally, REDCap features an opportunity for researchers to review all data on the back end through visual stats and charts, and even create special reports based on variables of interest. This was incredibly helpful to our research team as we considered our sample and identified any emerging trends.

Collaboration Platforms: Crowdsourcing, Brainstorming, and Getting Work Done

The tools: Coordinating work across so many partners and collaborators can feel daunting. Of course, there is email, which is still, in our minds at least, the gold standard for quickly communicating with colleagues and peers. However, there are a range of other tools that can help us have more interactive and iterative workflows. Adding some of these to your virtual-engagement processes might even increase the fun factor. In this section, we'll discuss a few of these resources. While we have utilized some of these tools, we are not (as with all those mentioned in this chapter) endorsing any particular tool, and also want to acknowledge that this list is incomplete.

Some platforms, such as Google Jamboard, are useful for taking shared digital notes during an online event or meeting, substituting for the large, blank, sticky Post-It notes that used to colorfully, and messily, capture our thoughts at in-person meetings. The benefit to this platform is that your board of thoughts gets saved on the cloud, making it easy to revisit the conversation and move it forward. As a bonus, Jamboard allows multiple people to add to the whiteboard at a time, removing the need for one lone notetaker who tries to capture and synthesize everyone's thoughts. Plus, there is no limit to how many Jamboards any one user can create, and they are free (Google, n.d.).

Padlet is another tool that may be of value for collaborative projects. While it can serve a similar function to Jamboard, Padlet provides a lot of opportunities for customizing the look, feel, and layout of projects. Their motto is, "It's a beautiful day. Make something beautiful," so if compelling aesthetics are of interest, Padlet may be an appropriate option. Documents of multiple file types may be uploaded to Padlet projects, making it easy to share content and solicit feedback from others. Padlet has both free and premium options (Padlet, n.d.).

Slack is another tool that has shown its staying power despite the many changes to technology over the years, and new tech tools being launched every day. On Slack, collaborators can create separate "channels" for various workflows, conversations, or topics, tag and message users they're working with, and upload files, among other things. Slack offers free and pro options (Slack, n.d.).

Ultimately, choosing between the many available collaboration platforms involves a careful consideration of which tools will work best for your specific community, so it is important to ask your communities and collaborators about the best ways to engage with them virtually. In the ever-changing landscape of virtual tools, it is likely that partners may suggest resources not included in this overview that may offer new and innovative features.

Our experience: Our IHER team and the community partners we work with decided to try Jamboard at the Open Space forum we hosted. We were previously unfamiliar with the platform, but at a community partner's suggestion, decided to utilize it to capture notes in breakout rooms in a way that could be visible to all attendees, regardless of the breakout room they were in. While it took some time to acclimate participants to the Jamboard experience, and some felt more comfortable with it than others, it provided us with a clear record of the concepts that emerged from each discussion and a record to easily share back with the audience.

To encourage collaboration after the Open Space event and as a way for people to see the research ideas they'd generated come to life, we created separate Padlet projects for each topic of discussion and shared links with all participants to join the projects of interest to them. Within each Padlet, we created a welcome post, inviting and orienting users to the space and providing a contact to reach out to with questions. We also included a link to the original Jamboard, providing visitors with a way to review the notes and remind themselves of key points from the discussion. In addition to a post inviting people to introduce themselves and share their interests in collaboration, we posted five questions that could serve as a jumping-off point for utilizing the space: (a) Why is this an important research topic or question? (b) Which stakeholders need to be involved in building out the research questions? (c) What are our goals? (d) How do we think the community would respond to this topic or idea? (e) How do we get community buy-in for this research and make sure they're involved every step of the way? While the Padlets ultimately were not leveraged to the degree we hoped for, we had discovered a new tool to keep in our arsenal for future collaborative endeavors.

BENEFITS OF VIRTUAL ENGAGEMENT AT A GLANCE

Virtual community engagement allows for wider participation of community members, across communities. People who were normally unable to participate in community events and meetings for various reasons are now able to join from the comfort of their homes without having to worry about spending money on transportation, commute time, or taking a day off from work (LHS, n.d.). Similarly, it is possible to reach a more diverse group by engaging hard-to-reach individuals who may, for instance, live in remote areas as well as groups of people traditionally underrepresented (Hussey 2021). While concerns about a "digital divide" have been frequently cited and should not be discounted as a reality for many individuals in this country, the 2018 American Community Survey suggests that 85% of Americans had a broadband internet subscription and 92% had a smart device to connect with (USCB 2021). Wider reach means more voices can be heard and considered; this may lead to better decision-making on issues and policies directly or indirectly impacting the communities we serve.

Virtual engagement is also a way of meeting various groups and individuals where they are since many people already engage with social media in some way. In the United States, the number of people with social media accounts has gradually increased: based on the 2021 data, about 82% of people have a social networking account, with approximately 70% of individuals actively using these sites monthly (Statista 2022).

Virtual engagement also allows for conversation to continue taking place over time, helping build positive relationships between organizations and

community members (Hussey 2021). This may ultimately lead to better retention rates of participants in studies or long-lasting partnerships on initiatives. Online platforms also provide a safe place for individuals to engage
in discussions and conversations in ways that feel comfortable for them. For
example, in a video conference, participants can choose to leverage the chat
function, react with emojis, speak through the microphone, and keep their
camera on or off.

Additionally, more attention is being paid—including by researchers at
the University of Colorado—and there is increasing discussion about how
we can make some of the tech platforms we use frequently, like Zoom, more
accessible to people with certain disabilities (CUDAO 2020). Some of the
platforms we referenced, like Slack, are already building in features and tips
for improving accessibility and inclusion (Slack, n.d.).

CHALLENGES TO VIRTUAL ENGAGEMENT AT A GLANCE

While virtual engagement has made events more accessible for some, it may
limit the inclusion of other people who could otherwise participate at in-
person events. Some groups (for example individuals experiencing homelessness, seniors, people with disabilities, and those living in rural areas) may
not have access to smart gadgets, broadband, or accessible platforms that
allow them to participate in all virtual events (LHS, n.d.). This means that
representation and opinions from these groups may be missing from the discussion. Specific barriers and challenges experienced by these populations
or subgroups may not surface if they are not adequately represented (LHS,
n.d.).

With the recent and in many cases almost total shift to remote work,
many people are already spending too much time on computers and in virtual back-to-back meetings. With more and more online events, we may see
increased fatigue and burden. It is necessary to be mindful that, just as with
in-person engagement, participants are humans who have time limits and a
healthy tendency toward participation fatigue (Fedorowicz, Arena, and Burrowes 2020; Epstein 2020).

While many applications and software for virtual engagement are available free of charge to participants, others require an investment, especially
if they offer additional safety and/or privacy features (Fedorowicz, Arena,
and Burrowes 2020). Despite cost challenges, it is always recommended to
go with the safest options to protect the privacy of community partners. For
example, when considering online surveys, it is best to avoid anything that

might raise suspicion of spam among users. This can be done by using a trusted survey platform, clearly presenting the name of the institution or survey team, attaching a logo, and including a description of the purpose of the survey.

While there are so many applications and tools to work with, it is also important to consider the compatibility of these platforms with all types of phones and other smart gadgets. When selecting tools or applications for wide use across partners, it is imperative to choose ones that can be easily accessible by all community members and stakeholders (COHE, n.d.). Last but not least, given that some of the platforms may be new to your collaborators, peers, and colleagues, and that individuals may have different levels of familiarity and comfort using such tools, it may take time and space to familiarize your partners with the tools and platforms you're using (Fedorowicz, Arena, and Burrowes 2020). Don't take it for granted that everyone has the same level of ease with technology.

As we've stated several times, there are a multitude of resources and tools available for virtual community engagement. It can sometimes be challenging to find the right tool that works best for your needs. In this chapter, we shared what we have researched, used, and found useful in our virtual community engagement efforts during the COVID-19 pandemic and highlighted some of the benefits and challenges associated with virtual engagement in general. Below are some additional considerations for ensuring equity and inclusion in your virtual collaborative work.

- To enhance your online marketing efforts, consider engaging members of your network and their networks as part of your outreach strategy. This is crucial because community organizations closely collaborate with various subgroups within communities, enabling outreach to a diverse population often underrepresented in virtual spheres.

- Acknowledge the fact that some community members may be non-English speaking or may have LEP and make sure that the utilized platforms can be accessed either in other applicable languages or provide translations or interpretation services (COHE, n.d.; Home for All 2020).

- Find ways to accommodate all persons with disabilities. Various streaming and meeting tools may have closed-caption features. When preparing graphs and other visual presentations, be mindful of the colors used and always include clear captions. When applicable, also provide virtual sign language interpreters (Brown 2020; Goldstein and Care 2012).

- Be understanding of members with low literacy and digital exposure and provide a safe environment that fosters learning and highlights the positive attributes of all participants (COHE, n.d.; Home for All 2020).

SUMMARY OF LESSONS LEARNED FROM VIRTUAL ENGAGEMENT AND VIRTUAL RESEARCH INITIATIVES

Transparency and trust building: These are priceless values when working on CBPR projects, and even more so when we are faced with an inability to build and foster relationships in a shared physical environment, as many of us are accustomed to doing. To earn partners' trust, it is important to be as transparent as possible about the intentions and goals of the work at hand, research or otherwise, and be as inclusive of partners as possible in all stages. It is also important to be continuously available to support partners' needs. Furthermore, in discussions and when making decisions, consider all options that people present and be open to group voting or other consensus decision-making models. We utilized tools such as Poll Everywhere, Microsoft Teams, Jamboard, Zoom chat features, and shared documents to make discussions and decision-making as easy and inclusive as possible for all members during and after virtual meetings.

Establishing and sustaining relationships: Working in times of crisis and uncertainty also creates unique personal challenges and insecurities. Therefore, when engaging with partners, it is essential to recognize the context and provide a safe space for people to share. To foster relationships, it is important to make time to get to know partners in smaller groups and individually. Similarly, to sustain strong relationships between workgroup members, it is important to provide a space where partners can engage with each other on a regular basis. Furthermore, it is imperative to acknowledge that virtual work has some striking differences compared to in-person meetings and team-building efforts. Finally, power dynamics can play a great role in fostering or discouraging relationship building. In virtual meetings, in particular, it can be easy for the organizer to unintentionally dominate the platform, so it is important to be deliberate in sharing ownership of the virtual space with others by doing things such as allowing screen-sharing privileges with other participants and providing sufficient talking time for everyone.

Work ethics, integrity, and data safety: Besides following the basics of all research safety protocols, it is essential to assure the safety of participants in the digital sphere, too, in ways that are particular to online research and collaborations. When collecting any sort of personal information, it is imperative to utilize HIPAA-compliant tools. Similarly, it is important to utilize safe and password-protected tools and software when recording, storing, and deleting data. Each organization's institutional review board or similar body may have specific guidelines and requirements for online privacy and data safety precautions.

Virtual Engagement in CBPR: What Has Been Shared by Researchers

One of the core tenets of community-based participatory research is that it's flexible and adaptive, making the transition to a virtual space an entirely feasible endeavor. In fact, as the severity of COVID-19 made physical gatherings a health risk for individuals, and researchers and community members alike found themselves at home more, the focus of many CBPR studies also began shifting to virtual platforms and leveraging several of the tools detailed above. Although this sudden change came with its challenges, continuing CBPR virtually has been crucial in building and sustaining relationships between community and academic partners who share common goals, including but not limited to understanding the impact of the pandemic from the viewpoint of the most vulnerable communities.

Depending on the goals and scope of the CBPR project, both qualitative and quantitative methods can be well supported by virtual platforms, and researchers who have shifted online during the pandemic have had success with both. In Thayer et al.'s (2021) qualitative research on best practices for virtually engaged community research, their findings indicate that using video conferencing mimics many of the benefits of in-person interactions that have otherwise been lost during the COVID-19 pandemic. These benefits include observing facial expressions, making eye contact, and analyzing body language, all of which help establish accountability and familiarity within a group. However, while there are opportunities for building comfort and trust through interactions on camera, video conferencing can also create a sense of distance—but one that can have some unexpected benefits, as well. For example, Valdez and Gubrium (2020) have speculated that the sense of distance created by Zoom, which they used for interviews on participants' sexual and reproductive health experiences, was a potential facilitator in making them feel safer talking about sensitive topics than they might in person.

Along with encouraging accountability and comfort, video conferencing for qualitative research also helps promote inclusivity by overcoming geographical limitations and expanding research platforms to communities that have limited opportunities to engage in person. Furthermore, individuals from distant locations who could only engage remotely during in-person meetings pre-COVID-19 felt they were more included in the discussion, now that everyone was engaging virtually (Marsh et al. 2021). Additionally, using video conferencing allowed this team, normally doing only in-person outreach, to recruit nationwide for research projects and thus increased research participation. These findings are also reflected in other studies, such as research carried out at the University of Alabama at Birmingham that highlights how virtual focus groups allowed participants who were traditionally excluded due to travel challenges to take part and contribute to the discussions (Dos Santos Marques et al. 2021). Perceptions and experiences of researchers and participants using Zoom in the health research context further reflect the above findings, with individuals across the board rating the platform as highly satisfactory and even better when compared to alternative traditional approaches (Archibald et al. 2019).

Survey platforms for both quantitative and qualitative data collection were common before the pandemic but have been critical to CBPR efforts during the pandemic. Since social distancing made it difficult to distribute physical surveys in person, several community research studies transitioned completely to online survey distribution. Similar to the benefit of video conferencing, online surveys may also facilitate inclusivity by improving our capacity to share them widely across networks, including social media networks. For instance, research partners at the Michigan Institute for Clinical and Health Research (MICHR) employed an online survey to identify how they could best meet the community's emergent needs and learn more about which channels would be best for communication with the community. Results from this survey allowed them to tailor their communication strategies, address some immediate community needs, and develop educational materials that could close the identified cultural, generational, and linguistic gaps (Marsh et al. 2021). As the MICHR team pivoted their community engagement infrastructure to a largely virtual platform, they saw an increase in participation in more rural areas and communities of color around the state (Marsh et al. 2021). Also, similar to how video conferencing created a more comfortable space for research participants to discuss sensitive topics (e.g., sexual practices or drug use), online surveys on similarly sensitive topics may also be preferred over surveys administered in person (Hlatshwako et al. 2021). The benefits of online surveys can be seen in their quicker pace, too, as the time and cost investment in creating and administering online surveys is a fraction of that for similar surveys conducted in person (Hlatshwako et al. 2021).

Virtual CBPR done throughout the COVID-19 pandemic has shown that technology has made it possible to create meaningful community-engaged and community-driven research and that doing so also offers some benefits by removing the need for participants to travel, expanding reach to more communities, and creating comfortable spaces for sensitive conversations that may induce anxiety during face-to-face interactions. Of course, the virtual CBPR resources and tools cited in this chapter only highlight a small number of the technologies available to community and academic partners engaging in this work. We hope that as more public health practitioners and community health advocates learn about the different tools available to them, we will see future publications that detail their processes of engaging communities online and highlight the benefits of doing this work virtually, even if only in part. We also feel that, while the potential for virtual CBPR is only now starting to be recognized, our work and other studies to date highlight the crucial role virtual CBPR tools have played throughout the pandemic to continue critical research, dialogue, and collaboration.

RECOMMENDATIONS FOR FUTURE PRACTICE

- While we've now reached a time when we can use a hybrid approach to public health work that allows collaborators to be together in person and online, it's important to recognize that technology and leveraging it to build collaborative partnerships will likely continue to be an important part of this work. Therefore, finding a system, or systems, that feel comfortable, engaging, and accessible while fostering a sense of belonging among individual contributors is paramount. Considering innovative ways of integrating technology to enhance public health research and programs should be a goal all public health professionals pursue.

- Explore and experiment with others to learn which new tools can be adapted, but be cognizant of the fact that people might have different levels of comfort. While some people may love to try new tools, others might still be trying to learn the old ones. Create spaces that engage all participants, but acknowledge that there will likely be a few missteps along the way.

- Nurture relationships even when you can't hold physical meetings that allow you to break bread together or share a hug or handshake. Many of us and our community partners who have been engaged in various projects over the years can fondly remember the times when the community-academic research groups we worked with would go on team-building retreats to bond and get bold with our thinking. Since holding such events may be hard now or in the future, it is more important than ever to identify innovative ways to virtually build new partnerships and strengthen existing ones. Healthy and sustainable relationships are the cornerstones of CBPR, and we must continue to find ways to bond with each other. At some of the recurrent meetings our community partners join, for example, individuals take turns telling jokes. Sometimes, the jokes fall flat, but that in itself enables the team to laugh together and create memories, even through our boxes on the screen.

- If the plan is to engage on social media, be strategic. Consider the time and effort it takes to garner a following and meet any set goals for the project. Sometimes, it's better to turn to existing social media accounts. Most organizations have a Facebook, Instagram, or Twitter profile at this point, and have spent a lot of time and resources to build loyal followings, engage their communities, and become trusted sources for information. Would it be more generative to distribute project-specific content through such existing pages than to create a new project profile and start from scratch? The answer depends on a lot of factors that are worth taking the time to think through and weigh.

- Zoom and survey platforms are clearly invaluable to the work researchers and others in public health do, but they're not the only tools we need to leverage in this work, particularly when it comes to its relationship-building component. Use new technologies, and use old technologies in new ways. Experiment with what works and doesn't work for building strong communicative and collaborative relationships with stakeholders. Then, write about it and share your findings. Let others in the field know about the ins and outs of the behind-the-scenes processes of leveraging technology to make a positive impact in the lives of many.

DISCUSSION QUESTIONS

- What do you see as the benefits and limitations of relying on technology to bring a CBPR project, or other community-engaged projects, to life?

- Do you know of other tools that would contribute to community building in the virtual setting? What are they? How would you efficiently and effectively leverage these tools?

- Do you think technology lends itself to more equitable research practices, or do you think it has the potential to hurt our work toward equity? Why?

NOTE

1. This chapter was written in late 2021, when the COVID-19 vaccine was available only for children over five years old. The vaccine has been made available to anyone over six months old since then. However, the racial/ethnic disparities in vaccination rates remain very similar to what is reported here.

REFERENCES

Archibald, Mandy M., Rachel C. Ambagtsheer, Mavourneen G. Casey, and Michael Lawless. 2019. "Using Zoom Video Conferencing for Qualitative Data Collection: Perceptions and Experiences of Researchers and Participants." *International Journal of Qualitative Methods* 18. https://doi.org/10.1177/1609406919874596.

Biegun, Daniel. 2021. "10 Powerful Things You Didn't Know You Could Do on Zoom." Visionaryteaching.com, March 8, 2021. https://visionaryteaching.com/10-powerful-things-you-didnt-know-you-could-do-on-zoom/.

Boyarsky, Katherine. 2020. "The 10 Best Free Video Conferencing Platforms." OwlLabs.com, March 2, 2020. https://resources.owllabs.com/blog/video-conferencing-tools.

Brown, Lydia X. Z. 2020. "How to Center Disability in the Tech Response to COVID-19." Brookings Institution website, July 20, 2020. https://www.brookings.edu/techstream/how-to-center-disability-in-the-tech-response-to-covid-19/.

CDCCRT (CDC COVID-19 Response Team). 2020. "Geographic Differences in COVID-19 Cases, Deaths, and Incidence—United States, February 12–April 7, 2020." *Morbidity and Mortality Weekly Report (MMWR)* 69, no. 15: 465–71. http://dx.doi.org/10.15585/mmwr.mm6915e4.

Clark, Eva, Karla Fredricks, Laila Woc-Colburn, Maria Elena Bottazzi, and Jill Weatherhead. 2020. "Disproportionate Impact of the COVID-19 Pandemic on Immigrant Communities in the United States." July 13. *PLOS Neglected Tropical Diseases* 14, no. 7: e0008484. https://doi.org/10.1371/journal.pntd.0008484.

COHE (Colorado Office of Health Equity). n.d. *Inclusive Virtual Community Engagement during COVID-19.* Denver: Colorado Office of Health Equity, Department of Public Health and Environment. https://covid19.colorado.gov /sites/covid19/files/Inclusive%2C%20Virtual%20Community%20Engagement %20During%20COVID-19.pdf.

CUDAO (Colorado University Digital Accessibility Office). 2020. "Zoom Accessibility Best Practices." Colorado University Digital Accessibility Office website, March 25, 2020. https://www.colorado.edu/accessible-technology/resources /zoom-accessibility-best-practices.

Do, D. Phuong, and Reanne Frank. 2020. "Unequal Burdens: Assessing the Determinants of Elevated COVID-19 Case and Death Rates in New York City's Racial/Ethnic Minority Neighbourhoods." *Journal of Epidemiology and Community Health* 75, no. 4: 321–26. https://doi.org/10.1136/jech-2020-215280.

Dos Santos Marques, Isabel C., Lauren M. Theiss, Cynthia Y. Johnson, Elise McLin, Beth A. Ruf, Selwyn M. Vickers, Mona N. Fouad, Isabel C. Scarinci, and Daniel I. Chu. 2021. "Implementation of Virtual Focus Groups for Qualitative Data Collection in a Global Pandemic." *American Journal of Surgery* 221, no. 5 (May): 918–22. https://doi.org/10.1016/j.amjsurg.2020.10.009.

Epstein, Helen-Ann Brown. 2020. "Virtual Meeting Fatigue." *Journal of Hospital Librarianship* 20, no. 4: 356–60. https://doi.org/10.1080/15323269.2020.1819758.

Facebook. n.d. "Best Practices for Major Broadcasts on Facebook Live." Meta Business Help Center. Accessed September 10, 2021. https://www.facebook.com /business/help/626637251511853.

Fedorowicz, Martha, with Olivia Arena and Kimberly Burrowes. 2020. *Community Engagement during the COVID-19 Pandemic and Beyond: A Guide for Community-Based Organizations.* Washington, DC: Urban Institute. https:// www.urban.org/sites/default/files/publication/102820/community-engagement -during-the-covid-19-pandemic-and-beyond.pdf.

Georgiev, Deyan. 2019. "How Much Time Do People Spend on Social Media in 2021?" Techjury.net, March 8, 2019. Accessed September 13, 2021. https:// techjury.net/blog/time-spent-on-social-media/.

Goldstein, Daniel, and Gregory Care. 2012. "Disability Rights and Access to the Digital World: An Advocate's Analysis of an Emerging Field." *Federal Lawyer,* December 2012, 54–59. https://lawreview.law.miami.edu/wp-content/uploads/2013 /02/Goldstein-Care-Disability-Rights-and-Access-to-the-Digital-World.pdf.

Google. n.d. "Google Jamboard: Interactive Business Whiteboard." Google Workspace. Accessed September 10, 2021. https://workspace.google.com/products /jamboard/.

Gould, Ryan. 2019. "5 of the Best Social Media Poll Apps." SuperMonitoring.com, April 29, 2019. https://www.supermonitoring.com/blog/best-social-media-poll -apps/.

Graham, Jefferson. 2020. "Top Tech of the Year: Zoom as 'Poster Child for 2020.'" *USA Today*, December 29, 2020. https://www.usatoday.com/story/tech/2020/12/29/zoom-top-2020-technology-coronavirus/4048606001/.

Gurd, James. 2022. "Understanding the Role of Organic vs Paid Social Media Strategy." SmartInsights.com, April 20, 2022. https://www.smartinsights.com/social-media-marketing/social-media-strategy/understanding-role-organic-paid-social-media/.

Herman, Michael. n.d. "What Is Open Space Technology?" OpenSpaceWorld.org. Accessed September 10, 2021. https://openspaceworld.org/wp2/what-is/.

Hlatshwako, Takhona G., Sonam J. Shah, Priya Kosana, Emmanuel Adebayo, Jacqueline Hendriks, Elin C. Larsson, Devon J. Hensel, Jennifer Toller Erausquin, Michael Marks, Kristen Michielsen, Hanna Saltis, Joel M. Francis, Edwin Wouters, and Joseph D. Tucker. 2021. "Online Health Survey Research during COVID-19," *Lancet Digital Health* 3, no. 2 (February): e76–77. https://doi.org/10.1016/s2589-7500(21)00002-9.

Holkup, Patricia A., Toni Tripp-Reimer, Emily Matt Salois, and Clarann Weinert. 2004. "Community-Based Participatory Research: An Approach to Intervention Research with a Native American Community." *ANS: Advances in Nursing Science* 27, no. 3 (July): 162–75. https://doi.org/10.1097/00012272-200407000-00002.

Home for All. 2020. *Technology Tools for Virtual Community Engagement—August 2020 Supplements.* San Mateo, CA: Home for All SMC. https://homeforallsmc.org/wp-content/uploads/2020/09/Technology-Tools-for-Virtual-Community-Engagement.pdf.

Horowitz, Carol R., Mimsie Robinson, and Sarena Seifer. 2009. "Community-Based Participatory Research from the Margin to the Mainstream: Are Researchers Prepared?" *Circulation* 119, no. 19: 2633–42. https://doi.org/10.1161/circulationaha.107.729863.

Hussey, Sally. 2021. "Benefits of Online Community Engagement." Granicus.com. https://www.bangthetable.com/benefits-of-online-community-engagement/.

Israel, Barbara A., Eugenia Eng, Amy J. Schulz, and Edith A. Parker, eds. 2005. *Methods for Community-Based Participatory Research for Health.* London: Jossey-Bass.

Kahoot. n.d. "Kahoot!" Kahoot.com. Accessed September 10, 2021. https://kahoot.com.

Kantamneni, Neeta. 2020. "The Impact of the COVID-19 Pandemic on Marginalized Populations in the United States: A Research Agenda." *Journal of Vocational Behavior* 119:103439. https://doi.org/10.1016/j.jvb.2020.103439.

LHS (Local Housing Solutions). n.d. "Conducting Virtual Community Engagement." Localhousingsolutions.org. Accessed September 13, 2021. https://localhousingsolutions.org/plan/conducting-virtual-community-engagement/.

Maljković, Nenad. 2020. "Fearless Experimentation: Doing Open Space Event Online." *Medium.com*, March 24, 2020. https://medium.com/virtual-teams-for-systemic-change/fearless-experimentation-5a8695bbd10e.

Marsh, Erica E., Michael D. Kappelman, Rhonda G. Kost, Gia Mudd-Martin, Jackilen Shannon, Louisa A. Stark, and Olveen Carrasquillo. 2021. "Community

Engagement during COVID: A Field Report from Seven CTSAs." *Journal of Clinical and Translational Science* 5, no. 1: e104. https://doi.org/10.1017/cts.2021 .785.

Miller, Ron, and Alex Wilhelm. 2020. "Salesforce Buys Slack in a $27.7B Megadeal." *TechCrunch,* December 1, 2020. http://techcrunch.com/2020/12/01/salesforce -buys-slack/.

Mueller, J. Tom, Kathryn McConnell, Paul Berne Burow, Katie Pofahl, Alexis A. Merdjanoff, and Justin Farrell. 2021. "Impacts of the COVID-19 Pandemic on Rural America." *Proceedings of the National Academy of Sciences of the United States of America (PNAS)* 118, no. 1: 2019378118. https://doi.org/10.1073/pnas .2019378118.

NCIRD (National Center for Immunization and Respiratory Diseases). 2020. "Health Equity Considerations and Racial and Ethnic Minority Groups." Centers for Disease Control and Prevention, July 24, 2020. https://stacks.cdc.gov/view/cdc/91049.

———. 2021. "Risk for COVID-19 Infection, Hospitalization, and Death by Race/ Ethnicity." Centers for Disease Control and Prevention, April 23, 2021. https:// stacks.cdc.gov/view/cdc/105453.

NIH (National Institutes of Health). n.d. "NIH Community Engagement Alliance (CEAL)." National Institutes of Health. Accessed September 10, 2021. https:// covid19community.nih.gov.

NYCDH (New York City Department of Health). n.d.-a. "COVID-19: Data on Vaccines—NYC Health." New York City Department of Health. Accessed September 10, 2021. https://www1.nyc.gov/site/doh/covid/covid-19-data-vaccines .page.

———. n.d.-b. "COVID-19: Data Totals—NYC Health." New York City Department of Health. Accessed September 10, 2021. https://www1.nyc.gov/site/doh/covid /covid-19-data-totals.page.

NYCDYCD (New York City Department of Youth and Community Development). 2022. "Demographic Statistics by Zip Code." New York City Department of Youth and Community Development. Last updated May 9, 2022. https://data .cityofnewyork.us/City-Government/Demographic-Statistics-By-Zip-Code /kku6-nxdu.

O'Brien, Matthew J., and Robert C. Whitaker. 2011. "The Role of Community-Based Participatory Research to Inform Local Health Policy: A Case Study." *Journal of General Internal Medicine* 26:1498–501. https://doi.org/10.1007 /s11606-011-1878-3.

Padlet. n.d. "Padlet Features." Padlet.com. Accessed September 10, 2021. https:// padlet.com/features.

Parker, Kim, Juliana Menasce Horowitz, and Rachel Minkin. 2020. "How the Coronavirus Has—and Hasn't—Changed the Way Americans Work." Pew Research Center, December 9, 2020. https://www.pewresearch.org/social-trends /2020/12/09/how-the-coronavirus-outbreak-has-and-hasnt-changed-the-way -americans-work/.

Pew Research Center. 2021a. "Social Media Fact Sheet." Pew Research Center, April 7, 2021. https://www.pewresearch.org/internet/fact-sheet/social-media/.

———. 2021b. "Use of Online Platforms, Apps Varies—Sometimes Widely—by Demographic Group." Pew Research Center, April 5, 2021. https://www .pewresearch.org/internet/2021/04/07/social-media-use-in-2021/pi_2021-04 -07_social-media_0-03/.

Pierce, David. 2020. "How Slack Lost the Pandemic." Protocol.com, December 1, 2020. https://www.protocol.com/newsletters/sourcecode/how-slack-lost-the-pandemic.

PollEverywhere. n.d. Accessed September 10, 2021. https://www.polleverywhere.com.

PRC (Project REDCap). n.d. "About [REDCap]." Projectredcap.org. Accessed September 10, 2021. https://projectredcap.org/about/.

Ramachandran, Vignesh. 2021. "Stanford Researchers Identify Four Causes for 'Zoom Fatigue' and Their Simple Fixes." *Stanford News,* February 23, 2021. https://news.stanford.edu/2021/02/23/four-causes-zoom-fatigue-solutions/.

Roy, Jessica. 2020. "How to Have Zoom Parties That Are Actually Fun." *Los Angeles Times,* April 20, 2020. https://www.latimes.com/lifestyle/story/2020-04-20 /zoom-party-tips-etiquette-virtual-hangout-ideas-fun-game-night.

Slack. n.d. Accessed September 10, 2021. https://slack.com.

Slido. n.d. Accessed September 10, 2021. https://www.sli.do.

Statista. 2022. "Average Daily Time Spent on Social Networks by Users in the United States from 2018 to 2022." Statista.com. Last modified June 2, 2022. https://www .statista.com/statistics/1018324/us-users-daily-social-media-minutes/.

———. 2023. "Most Popular Social Networks Worldwide as of January 2023, Ranked by Number of Monthly Active Users." Statista.com. Last modified February 14, 2023. https://www.statista.com/statistics/272014/global-social-networks-ranked -by-number-of-users/.

Tay, Daniel. 2018. "10 Ways to Generate More Engagement with Your Social Media Posts." Socialmediatoday.com, July 24, 2018. https://www.socialmediatoday.com /news/10-ways-to-generate-more-engagement-with-your-social-media-posts /528351/.

Thayer, Erin K., Molly Pam, Morhaf Al Achkar, Laura Mentch, Georgia Brown, Traci M. Kazmerski, and Emily Godfrey. 2021. "Best Practices for Virtual Engagement of Patient-Centered Outcomes Research Teams during and after the COVID-19 Pandemic: Qualitative Study." *Journal of Participatory Medicine* 13, no. 1: e24966. https://doi.org/10.2196/24966.

USCB (US Census Bureau). 2021. "Computer and Internet Use in the United States: 2018." US Census Bureau, April 21, 2021. https://www.census.gov/newsroom /press-releases/2021/computer-internet-use.html.

UVaCollab. n.d. "What Is the Poll Everywhere Tool?" UVaCollab, University of Virginia. Accessed September 10, 2021. https://uvacollab.screenstepslive.com/s /help/m/integrations/l/1285840-what-is-the-poll-everywhere-tool.

Valdez, Elizabeth Salerno, and Aline Gubrium. 2020. "Shifting to Virtual CBPR Protocols in the Time of Corona Virus/COVID-19." *International Journal of Qualitative Methods* 19:1609406920977731. https://doi.org/10.1177/1609406920977315.

Walsh, Mike. n.d. "The 7 Best Videoconferencing Software Platforms for 2021." DGI Communications. Accessed September 10, 2021. https://www .dgicommunications.com/video-conferencing-software/.

WHO (World Health Organization). 2020. "WHO Director-General's Opening Remarks at the Media Briefing on COVID-19—11 March 2020." World Health Organization, March 11, 2020. https://www.who.int/director-general/speeches /detail/who-director-general-s-opening-remarks-at-the-media-briefing-on -covid-19---11-march-2020.

Zentis, Nancy. 2017. "OD Facilitation Tools—Open Space Technology." Institute of Organization Development, March 8, 2017. https://instituteod.com/od -facilitation-tools-open-space-technology/.

Zimmerman, Sheryl, Jane Tilley, Lauren Cohen, and Karen Love. 2009. *A Manual for Community-Based Participatory Research: Using Research to Improve Practice and Inform Policy in Assisted Living.* Chapel Hill, NC: Center for Excellence in Assisted Living, University of North Carolina. https://theceal.org/resources /a-manual-for-community-based-participatory-research-using-research-to -improve-practice-and-inform-policy-in-assisted-living/.

2

Battle of the Sexes

The Gendered Impact of the COVID-19 Pandemic

KOBI V. AJAYI, ELIZABETH WACHIRA, OBASANJO AFOLABI BOLARINWA,
AND SONYA PANJWANI

Male and female differences are unique, complex, and multifaceted. These differences are biological—that is, sex differences—physical, or socially engineered (Alexander et al. 2020; WHO 2007). However, a person's sex often may not be the same as their gender or gender identity. This is because, whereas sex refers to the biological difference, including differences in reproductive organs and chromosomes between males and females, gender is determined by other factors, including societal, cultural, and legal aspects. Gender identity, on the other hand, is subjective and reflects a person's acceptance of being male, female, or nonbinary. While biological sex may influence gender identity, a person's gender identity does not necessarily equate to biological sex (WHO 2007).

Because a person's sex is not always consistent with their gender or gender identity, accurately understanding or assessing infectious disease patterns across sex or gender may be challenging (WHO 2007). Still, there are distinct differences observable between males and females in this context, including variations in medication reaction, disease outcome, and vulnerability, making it crucial to examine the effect of sex and gender through the lens of the COVID-19 pandemic.

This chapter presents a discourse on gender dimensions of and perspectives on public health emergencies, infectious disease outbreaks, and response, focusing on the 2019 coronavirus (COVID-19) pandemic and using historical underpinnings and underlying theories to explain gender disparities in public health response to disease outbreaks. Insights from previous pandemics are used to assess the success or lack thereof of global health initiatives in incorporating a gender lens into the COVID-19 pandemic response. Understanding gender diversity can aid knowledge in the epidemiology, patterns, diagnosis, outcomes, treatments, and prevention of infectious disease across genders to foster equitable and targeted public health programs and policies.

While acknowledging that a person's gender does not always align with their sex, the argument presented here is based on the traditional biological definition of males and females and will use the terms sex and gender interchangeably.

SEX AND GENDER DIFFERENCES IN COVID-19 MORBIDITY AND MORTALITY

Since not long after its emergence in Wuhan, China, in December 2019, demographic reports on COVID-19 and the pandemic have indicated differential patterns of morbidity and mortality between males and females. In the first half of 2020, data from Europe showed males experiencing significantly higher mortality, with male-female relative risk ranging from 1.11 in Portugal to 1.54 in France (Ahrenfeldt et al. 2021). Other studies conducted in China, the United States, and Africa reported similar findings (Demombynes 2020). Consequently, risky health behaviors prevalent in males, poor testing for the SARS-CoV-2 virus, and limited vaccine uptake may be associated with higher rates of COVID-19 mortality (Promislow 2020; Ahrenfeldt et al. 2021). Although the authors argue for gender-sensitive approaches in the COVID-19 response, we do not undermine or disregard the impact of the pandemic on males. However, we bring to light the unintended consequences of exclusionary approaches to infectious disease prevention and control measures on certain populations.

Although males are more likely to report COVID-19 consequences, females experience disproportionate burdens of the pandemic, largely because of socially constructed gender norms (Connor et al. 2020; Wenham, Smith, and Morgan 2020). Traditionally, females bear a significant responsibility for caregiving and familial roles (Smith 2019). Since the start of the pandemic, "stay-at-home" orders elevated caregiving burdens informally designated to females, with heightened social, economic, and political consequences (Lightfoot and Moone 2020). These included a substantial increase in caregiving burdens, unpaid healthcare work in the home, loss of employment, gender-based violence, poor access to reproductive health services, and low-paying jobs or earnings. Females were also less likely to be included in COVID-19 vaccine clinical trials, making it more challenging to understand the vaccine's primary or side effects on females or the fetus (Van Spall 2021).

Moreover, response to some vaccines differs between sexes due to hormonal and chromosomal differences (WHO 2007). Additionally, among pregnant women, those who contracted the virus had higher chances of negative birth outcomes, were more frequently admitted to the intensive care unit, in need of a ventilator, and in severe cases, died from the disease as opposed to their nonpregnant counterparts (Zambrano et al. 2020). Other gender dimensions include women's roles as frontline health and social workers, as employees of health government structures, research, and surveillance organizations, and in leadership positions in health systems (Smith 2019).

While the reporting on gender-sensitive responses since the pandemic is a great improvement from previous epidemics, such as Ebola and the Zika virus, the negative impact of the pandemic on females suggests missed opportunities to integrate gender dimensions in COVID-19 preparedness and responses. According to the Global Health 50/50 COVID-19 Sex-Disaggregated Data Tracker, only 50% of countries reported sex-disaggregated COVID-19 data for cases and/or death in mid-June 2021 (Global Health 50/50 2021). In response to the shortage of sex-disaggregated data on COVID-19, international and national organizations have recommended strategic frameworks to include gender analysis in COVID-19 research, policy, surveillance, decision-making, and implementation (United Nations 2020; WHO 2020).

The underlying reasons for the lack of a gender-related approach to COVID-19 surveillance and reporting are unclear. However, the current COVID-19 prevention approach does not address the specific and diverse needs of minority populations and females, exacerbating existing vulnerabilities.

SEX AND GENDER DIFFERENCES IN THE INFECTIOUS DISEASE PROCESS

Sex and gender differences influence infectious disease processes. Understanding these variations will help us answer two important questions: (a) Who will be ill? and (b) What are the course and outcomes of illness? Examples of sex and gender differences that influence these matters are included in table 2.1.

TABLE 2.1. EXAMPLES OF SEX AND GENDER DIFFERENCES THAT INFLUENCE
WHO BECOMES ILL AND THE COURSE AND OUTCOME OF ILLNESS

Sex differences	Examples of sex differences that influence who becomes ill and the course and outcome of illness
Who becomes ill depends on susceptibility and exposure to an infectious disease agent. Differences between males and females can be measured by calculating separate incidence rates and can be tracked during an outbreak by plotting separate epidemic curves for males and females.	Differences in immune responses between males and females. Anatomical differences—particularly important for sexually transmitted infections.
Gender differences	Examples of gender differences that affect who becomes ill and the course and outcome of illness
The course and outcome of an illness are influenced by factors such as the nature and severity of symptoms, mortality rate, and disease sequelae. These depend both on biological responses to exposure and on treatment. Differences between males and females can be measured by calculating separate case-fatality and disability rates for males and females and by constructing different symptom profiles.	Differing access to immunization. Differing exposure because of gender roles. Differing nutritional status. Differing access to and use of preventive and curative healthcare, including differences in how males and females get treatment outside the home.

Table reproduced from WHO 2007, with permission of the World Health Organization.

SEX AND GENDER DIFFERENCES IN INFECTIOUS DISEASE PATTERNS USING THE LIFE COURSE APPROACH

In addition to differences in transmission, infectious disease patterns change over the life cycle among males and females. The life cycle includes infancy, childhood, adulthood, pregnancy, and old age. Table 2.2 shows the typical differences between males and females in the infectious disease process.

TABLE 2.2. TYPICAL DIFFERENCES BETWEEN MALES AND FEMALES
IN THE INFECTIOUS DISEASE PROCESS THROUGH THE "WHO BECOMES
AND COURSE AND OUTCOMES OF ILLNESS" FRAMEWORK

| Life cycle | Who becomes ill | | Course and outcome | |
	Susceptibility and immunity	Exposure	Treatment	Morbidity and mortality
Infants	Males have naturally weaker immune systems.	Exposure is similar for male and female infants.	In some countries, boys are more often and/or more quickly taken for treatment outside the home.	There is greater male mortality from infectious diseases.

Children	Levels of immunization for boys and girls are similar in most parts of the world. There are lower rates of immunization of females in south-central Asia.	In some societies, there are mobility differences (boys spend more time outside the home), which may account for differences in incidence and mortality for some diseases.	In some countries, boys are more often and/or more quickly taken for treatment outside the home.	There are disease-specific differences in severity and outcome. For example, mortality from measles and whooping cough is greater in females. Morbidity and disability may have different consequences for girls and boys.
Adults	For most infectious diseases, differences in incidence rates between males and females are more likely due to differences in exposure than to differences in immunity.	Men and women have different occupational exposures. Women have greater exposure in homes; men have greater exposure outside. Women are exposed in caretaker roles within the family and in caregiving occupations.	In some societies, women have poorer access to healthcare outside the home; access to outside care is controlled by males or other family members. Research on treatment often uses males—so there is less evidence for results for females.	There are disease-specific differences in severity and outcome. Morbidity and disability may have different consequences for males and females.
Pregnant and lactating women	Important changes in the immune system occur during pregnancy. Large knowledge gaps exist about the specific changes.	Exposures to some diseases may change during pregnancy. Pregnant women have more exposure to healthcare settings, so they may be at greater risk for some nosocomial infections.	Some treatments and control measures harm pregnant women, fetuses, and breastfeeding babies. Pregnant women are excluded from research on treatment. Some treatments are not given to pregnant women because of insufficient evidence of their safety.	Some diseases are particularly virulent during pregnancy. Some diseases adversely affect the fetus or breastfeeding baby.
Elderly	Both males and females have poorer immune systems in old age.	Lack of evidence.	Diagnosis is more difficult in the elderly for both males and females due to atypical presentations.	There are more women than men in this age group. Males die younger. Very little information is available on sex and gender differences and infectious diseases in this age group.

Table reproduced from WHO 2007, with permission of the World Health Organization.

THEORETICAL DIMENSIONS OF SEX AND GENDER

In conceptualizing sex, gender, health, and their relation to the COVID-19 pandemic, it is important to explore the theoretical underpinnings that predict or inform observed gender differences. Gender has been deemed a unique social determinant of health but is also related to sex differences that formulate widening health disparities (Springer, Stellman, and Jordan-Young 2012; Rich-Edwards et al. 2018; Connor et al. 2020). These disparities are compounded further in females with intersecting identities such as non-White race, low socioeconomic status, lower education, immigrant status, older age, disability, and rural location (Connor et al. 2020).

In the following section, we explore three theories, as outlined in table 2.3, that conceptualize the role of gender in health and how it results in male-female health differences. We note that this is not an exhaustive list but that these are important and relevant theories that can provide meaningful insights.

TABLE 2.3. GENDER-BASED THEORETICAL DIMENSIONS

Theory	Description	Relation to COVID-19 pandemic
Relational gender theory	This theory focuses on how social structures that create gender positionalities are shaped, addressed, and modified by social practices. Intrinsic patterns that result in gender inequalities must be surfaced to challenge existing structures and encourage movement toward equity in gender and health issues (Connell 2012).	Offers a holistic approach to differentiating between male and female COVID-19 transmission rates, accounting for divisions of labor and social roles. Could assist in challenging social practices and forming health policies that will help modify gender inequalities.
Theory of gender and power	The theory of gender and power analyzes social structures and explores gender dynamics and power differences between males and females. It posits that negative health outcomes occur due to the socialization of women and their being subordinate to men (Connell 2014).	Addresses the role of cultural expectations and power dynamics within the COVID-19 response at the family level. It recognizes that social structures sometimes place additional stress on women to serve as caregivers and discount their labor roles as stay-at-home orders disrupt day-to-day life for families.
Multi-facet gender and health model	This theory recognizes the complex relationships that exist and lead to sex differences in health, such as the prevalence of illness, illness behavior, treatment outcomes, and implications of disease. Understanding the interconnectedness of these various factors is critical to influencing health outcomes for both males and females (Bekker 2003).	Takes into account the differences between male and female self-presentation of complaints (i.e., women's tendency to dismiss illness to fulfill their role as caregivers). Public health COVID-19 campaigns should stress the importance of equality in diagnostics to reduce sex differences in illness behaviors.

SEX-GENDER RESPONSES IN PREVIOUS
INFECTIOUS DISEASE OUTBREAKS

The WHO's primary role is to direct international efforts and lead partners in global health responses. Therefore, how nations and local authorities respond to various outbreaks directly reflects what international organizations like the WHO deem important. The WHO coordinates and provides guidance when outbreaks are considered public health emergencies of international concern (PHEICs). Partners or countries representing the United Nations system are many. They include countries with different income levels and healthcare systems to consider in studying outbreak responses. A review of recent PHEICs can provide insight into how the WHO and its member nations respond to outbreaks. Although many outbreaks have occurred to date, we focus on two recent and major public health emergencies in countries with varying systems of healthcare to reflect on the gendered responses that were taken. These include the 2014–16 Ebola outbreak in West Africa and the 2015–16 Zika virus outbreak in the Americas.

Ebola Outbreak 2014–16

We start this exploration with the 2014–16 Ebola outbreak. The first case of Ebola was reported in Guinea in December 2013; after five additional cases, a medical alert was issued on January 24, 2014. Ebola virus disease (EVD) is caused by the *Zaire ebolavirus,* and on March 23, 2014, with 49 confirmed cases and 29 deaths, the WHO declared an outbreak of EVD (CDC 2019). This outbreak quickly spread to neighboring countries, including Guinea, Liberia, and Sierra Leone, which were widely affected, prompting the WHO to declare this a PHEIC on August 8, 2014 (CDC 2019). Weak surveillance systems and poor public health infrastructure, coupled with poor governance and corruption contributed to the outbreak's difficulties (CDC 2019; O'Brien and Tolosa 2016). A total of 28,616 cases of EVD and 11,310 deaths were reported in these three countries, with an additional 36 cases and 15 deaths outside these countries (CDC 2019).

The WHO's response to the EVD outbreak in these three countries focused on treatment, containment, and prevention. The few resources and healthcare centers, including hospitals and clinics, were converted largely or exclusively to Ebola treatment centers (Smith 2019; Strong and Schwartz, 2016). In the first months, before the WHO declared an outbreak, clinics and programs not diverted were initially closed down due to staff safety concerns, highlighting the implications of a delayed international response (Smith 2019; O'Brien and Tolosa 2016; Carter, Dietrich, and Minor 2017). Aside from shifting existing resources to emergency responses, containment efforts included using military control and passing laws that criminalized individuals or families taking care of their loved ones or burying them without reporting to local authorities. Militarized control included enforcing quarantines and imposing heavy fines and imprisonment on those who did not follow these statutes or welcomed strangers into their homes. The unintended consequence of this policing and criminalizing of the sick was individuals choosing to hide the sick, perform secret burials, and stigmatize both those who followed and those who disobeyed these laws (Carter, Dietrich, and Minor 2017; Minor 2017; Coltart et al. 2017). Despite these efforts, gendered responses to the outbreak were largely missing and there was a failure to consider how diseases affect and are experienced by men and women, respectively.

In these countries and globally, gendered roles identify women as primary caretakers in informal and formal health sectors. Containment efforts that criminalized these roles put women in a difficult situation as they had to choose between obeying laws or being good mothers, as society expected (Béland et al. 2021; Smith 2019). Their risk was increased due to these roles, but the diverting of services and resources led to limited access to maternal care. Messaging focused on disease prevention, particularly through handwashing, highlighted women's role as caretakers, and called on them to prevent transmission by not taking care of loved ones. To put this in context, when healthcare systems are overwhelmed in developing countries, there is an overreliance on women's informal and gendered care roles (Strong and Schwartz 2016; Fawole et al. 2016; Harman 2016). This increases their risk, and with no provision of protective equipment in both formal and informal settings, they suffer the brunt during these PHEICs. Despite their roles, they are not considered in the process of developing solutions, which is reflected in the decision-making and messaging used to contain and prevent disease spread (Smith 2019).

Zika Outbreak 2015–16

The second outbreak of interest is the 2015–16 Zika outbreak in the Americas. The first report to the WHO was from Brazil in March 2015, of an illness characterized by a skin rash that was found to be caused by Zika in May 2015. Zika is an arboviral disease spread by the *Aedes aegypti* mosquito. The common signs of infection include skin rash and minor flu-like symptoms with no lasting consequences (Wenham, Smith, and Morgan 2020). By January 2016, growing evidence of the impact Zika had on pregnant women and on babies contracting Congenital Zika Syndrome (CZS) prompted further attention to its implications. CZS results in babies being born with a neonatal malformation where their heads are smaller than expected, and they experience other developmental conditions. The link found between CZS and Zika prompted the WHO to declare Zika virus–related microcephaly a PHEIC on February 1, 2016. From 2015 to 2016, Zika transmission was confirmed in forty-eight countries and territories in the Americas, with 707,133 virus cases (Ikejezie et al. 2017).

Unlike the Ebola outbreak setting, the Americas include countries like Brazil with strong health systems evident in their quick vector control. Primary response efforts focused on fumigation and the destruction of mosquitoes and their breeding grounds, with the military deployed to assist in these efforts (Wenham, Smith, and Morgan 2020; Forero-Martínez et al. 2020). However, it is important to note that the Zika virus can be sexually transmitted, yet response efforts focused on access to sexual and reproductive health services were lacking (Forero-Martínez et al. 2020). Instead, education efforts included encouraging people to prevent mosquito bites by wearing long sleeves and using insecticide, while advising women of reproductive age to avoid getting pregnant. Further complicating these recommendations is the reality that, despite having strong healthcare systems, countries like Brazil still have major systematic gaps in women's health promotion or provision, lacking routine access to sexual and reproductive health services (Wenham, Smith, and Morgan 2020).

The focus on behavior modification messaging targeting women of reproductive age implies a woman's individual choice and responsibility to self-manage her increased risk during outbreaks—and that men do not have similar responsibilities. In addition, these efforts did not consider how a woman's social status can render her powerless to negotiate condom use and other behaviors that could prevent pregnancy and sexual transmission of Zika (Coutinho et al. 2021).

As in West Africa, messaging focused on avoiding pregnancy reinforces the unequal power relations between women and governments. One example of this is the disregard of power relations in condom negotiation among women from poor backgrounds or the right to refuse to care for sick loved ones. This targeted messaging yet again relied on motherhood concepts that create different expectations for women and men (Coutinho et al. 2021). This puts the burden of prevention on women, further reinforcing stereotypes and inequalities where women are only seen as caregivers or mothers when it comes to healthcare access and rights. Furthermore, these Zika prevention messages indicate a missed opportunity for gender inclusion in informing prevention efforts where men should be included and nonpregnant older women still are at risk of illness (Coutinho et al. 2021).

GENDERED RESPONSE TO THE COVID-19 PANDEMIC

In this section, we highlight the disproportionate impact of the COVID-19 pandemic on females by discussing aspects of daily lives where the consequences of the pandemic are more pronounced.

Caregiving Roles

Globally, unprecedented caregiving and familial responsibilities were germane issues brought to the fore by the pandemic. Since the pandemic, women have shouldered a disproportionate share of caregiving roles. Interestingly, both formal and informal caregiving roles experienced significant increases as stay-at-home orders saw the closures of daycare centers, schools, and workplaces. This has increased females' vulnerability to the negative effects of pandemic situations (Wenham 2020). Restricted movement and infection control measures during the pandemic led to many homes being turned into remote/virtual work environments, thus tasking mothers with combining their job roles and familial duties, while acting as educators for school-aged children (Béland et al. 2021).

Gender-Based Violence

Pandemics aside, gender-based violence of varying degrees (e.g., physical, emotional, and/or sexual abuse) is a global public health problem. Violence against women affects up to 35% of women worldwide at some point in their lifetimes (World Bank 2019). In extreme cases, gender-based violence can lead to the loss of a woman's life. Globally, an estimated 38% of murders of women are committed by an intimate partner (World Bank 2019). Sadly, gender-based violence is one of the key social vices exacerbated by pandemics. Abuse skyrocketed as women with abusive partners could not escape them or seek help from social services. This has been particularly true for women with poor financial and employment status (Béland et al. 2021). Furthermore, as the work modality in many industries switched from physical to virtual during the lockdown, gender-based violence also took a virtual form through hate speech and online harassment (European Commission 2021).

Mental Health and Psychological Burden

Amidst COVID-19, rapidly implemented infection control measures regarding obstetric care, intended to mitigate against cross-contamination of the virus, combined with limited social support during labor and delivery, have been found to be related to maternal distress (Ajayi et al. 2021). However, women tend to be exposed to multiple stressors (e.g., increased caregiving burden, fear of the COVID-19 virus, job losses, and gender-based violence, among others) that adversely affect their psychological well-being.

Access to Family Planning and Other Sexual and Reproductive Health Services

Access to family planning and sexual and reproductive health services has been one of the core goals of the United Nations Population Fund (UNFPA) since the 1994 International Conference on Population and Development (Mousky 2002; UNFPA 2020). However, despite several interventions and behavioral changes, reproductive-aged women's need for family planning and sexual and reproductive health services remains unmet (Gómez-Suárez et al. 2019; Gahungu, Vahdaninia, and Regmi 2021). Besides stigmatization in accessing these services, which adolescent girls and young women frequently feel, many women have unmet needs due to partners' opposition, resulting in covert use (Gómez-Suárez et al. 2019; Prata et al. 2017). Meanwhile, with the sudden emergence of the COVID-19 pandemic, the shuttering of clinics, restrictions on movement, and even border closures affected access to and use of these services (Dasgupta, Kantorová, and Ueffing 2020; Temmerman 2021).

Women's sexual and reproductive health decision-making, including choices on family planning, should be without interference. It's expected that when women fully control their sexual and reproductive health, their overall health is optimized (Sen 2014). COVID-19 lockdown altered the scope of this right by restricting women's access to family planning and sexual and repro-ductive services (Bolarinwa et al. 2021).

Economic and Financial Dimensions

The recession triggered by the pandemic, coupled with the strict mitigation measures enforced in female-dominated labor sectors, increased the risk of job insecurity (Wenham 2020). The chances of losing previous gains regard-ing gender equity are high. Statistics reveal that while employment prospects rose by 1.4% for men, they increased by only 0.8% for women in the second and third quarters of 2020 (Alon et al. 2020; European Commission 2021; Wenham 2020). In other instances, women deliberately opted out of work because it became too challenging to navigate their conflicting roles as moth-ers, wives, employees, or employers.

LESSONS LEARNED AND RECOMMENDATIONS FOR FUTURE PRACTICE

COVID-19 was in many respects unprecedented. One thing it has revealed is that our legal and societal actions to bridge the existing inequalities between males and females are more or less a mirage. There is a need for concerted and intentional global efforts to address the imbalances laid bare by the COVID-19 pandemic. The time is now for global health leaders, policy-makers, and government institutions to develop and implement gender-responsive frameworks for infection control measures. To inform equitable public health efforts, we propose including a theoretically informed gendered analysis, increased representation of women, and assurance of continued access to key support services amidst pandemics and beyond.

Theoretical Gendered Analysis

The role of gender and power must be explored to understand better the differential impact women experience during outbreaks. This gendered analysis must be employed from the onset rather than waiting for data that confirm women are disproportionately affected or underrepresented. Inquiry into how gender and power shape women's realities before, during, and after outbreaks must be considered. Therefore, this conceptualization of gender, health, and its relation to the COVID-19 pandemic must explore the theoretical underpinnings that predict or inform observed gender differences.

Increased Representation

Historically, national and global response efforts have excluded women from the table. Meanwhile, aside from the equity issues involved, as a simple matter of public health, socially prescribed care roles place women in key positions to notice trends at the local level that can signal the start of outbreaks and thus ultimately improve global health security. Therefore, it is necessary to increase women's representation to help ensure early response to the rise of epidemics and pandemics.

This representation could very effectively include formally recognized "gender advisers" who are knowledgeable about and actively engage with local women's groups and those traditionally excluded due to organizational differences. Gender-aware data collection should inform policy and response efforts. Such measures can ensure access to services and support for all, particularly those most vulnerable, and avoid exacerbating existing gender inequalities or creating gender injustices.

Continued Services and Support

A pattern evident in all pandemic responses is that resources and services are shifted to focus on immediate biomedical needs, as opposed to structural issues. This shift leads to decreased access to and affordability of services, and further compounds existing vulnerabilities that women experience, leading to increased risk of illness and unmet health needs. It is important to note that women are at the front lines in both formal and informal employment sectors, especially during outbreaks. Therefore, they require support services, including providing information and resources. Benefits should extend beyond sexual and reproductive health to include economic, mental health, and domestic violence services to ensure women's emotional well-being and physical and psychological safety during these stressful times.

Application to COVID-19 and Other Pandemics

Although in many instances considerations of gender have been integrated into the response to COVID-19, by and large, deliberate inclusion of gender frameworks or reporting has been suboptimal, signifying missed opportunities. It is crucial that collaborative public health efforts include key stakeholders to articulate gender perspective in policies, programs, and documentation. This approach can be expected to mitigate the negative consequences of COVID-19 and other pandemics on females. In addition, attention must be paid to the psychosocial implications of the pandemics. Increased burdens from caregiving roles, loss of employment, and poor social support magnify women's vulnerabilities during public health emergencies. Though recognized, these factors are often not considered in global health planning and outbreak response. Therefore, a gendered analysis must be incorporated into preparedness and response efforts to improve effectiveness while promoting gender and health equity goals.

DISCUSSION QUESTIONS

- Considering the male exclusionary approach to infectious disease prevention, who should be tasked with ensuring infectious disease prevention adopts a gendered framework? Why?

- Looking at the COVID-19 pandemic response so far, how has gender shaped global efforts to mitigate the spread of the virus?

- Identify and discuss at least one organization, policy, or program that has successfully integrated gender in its framework during a public health emergency.

- What is missing in the global health approach to gender-responsive strategies in infectious disease control efforts?

REFERENCES

Ahrenfeldt, Linda Juel, Martina Otavova, Kaare Christensen, and Rune Lindahl-Jacobsen. 2021. "Sex and Age Differences in COVID-19 Mortality in Europe." *Wiener klinische Wochenschrift* 133, no. 7–8 (April): 393–98. https://doi.org/10.1007/s00508-020-01793-9.

Ajayi, Kobi V., Idethia S. Harvey, Sonya Panjwani, Inyang Uwak, Whitney Garney, and Robin L. Page. 2021. "Narrative Analysis of Childbearing Experiences during the COVID-19 Pandemic." *MCN: The American Journal of Maternal/Child Nursing* 46, no. 5 (September/October): 284–92. https://doi.org/10.1097/nmc.0000000000000742.

Alexander, Linda Lewis, Judith H. LaRosa, Helaine Bader, and Susan Garfield. *New Dimensions in Women's Health.* 8th ed. Burlington, MA: Jones & Bartlett Learning, 2020.

Alon, Titan, Matthias Doepke, Jane Olmstead-Rumsey, and Michèle Tertilt. 2020. *The Impact of COVID-19 on Gender Equality.* NBER Working Paper no. W26947. Cambridge, MA: National Bureau of Economic Research.

Bekker, Marrie H. J. 2003. "Investigating Gender within Health Research Is More Than Sex Disaggregation of Data: A Multi-facet Gender and Health Model." *Psychology, Health & Medicine* 8, no. 2: 231–43. https://doi.org/10.1080/1354850031000087618.

Béland, Louis-Philippe, Abel Brodeur, Joanne Haddad, and Derek Mikola. 2021. "Determinants of Family Stress and Domestic Violence: Lessons from the COVID-19 Outbreak." *Canadian Public Policy* 47, no. 3 (September): 439–59. https://muse.jhu.edu/pub/50/article/807571.

Bolarinwa, Obasanjo Afolabi, Bright Opoku Ahinkorah, Abdul-Aziz Seidu, Edward Kwabena Ameyaw, Balsam Qubais Saeed, John Elvis Hagan Jr., and Ugochinyere Ijeoma Nwagbara. 2021. "Mapping Evidence of Impacts of COVID-19 Outbreak on Sexual and Reproductive Health: A Scoping Review." *Healthcare* 9, no. 4 (April): 436. https://doi.org/10.3390/healthcare9040436.

Carter, Simone E., Luisa Maria Dietrich, and Olive Melissa Minor. 2017. "Mainstreaming Gender in WASH: Lessons Learned from Oxfam's Experience of Ebola." *Gender & Development* 25, no. 2 (2017): 205–20. https://doi.org/10.1080/13552074.2017.1339473.

CDC (Centers for Disease Control and Prevention). 2019. "2014–2016 Ebola Outbreak in West Africa." Centers for Disease Control and Prevention. Last updated March 8, 2019. https://www.cdc.gov/vhf/ebola/history/2014-2016-outbreak/index.html.

Coltart, Cordelia E. M., Benjamin Lindsey, Isaac Ghinai, Anne M. Johnson, and David L. Heymann. 2017. "The Ebola Outbreak, 2013–2016: Old Lessons for New Epidemics." *Philosophical Transactions of the Royal Society B: Biological Sciences* 372, no. 1721: 20160297. https://doi.org/10.1098/rstb.2016.0297.

Connell, Raewyn. 2012. "Gender, Health and Theory: Conceptualizing the Issue, in Local and World Perspective." *Social Science & Medicine* 74, no. 11 (June): 1675–83. https://doi.org/10.1016/j.socscimed.2011.06.006.

———. 2014. *Gender and Power: Society, the Person and Sexual Politics.* New York: John Wiley & Sons.

Connor, Jade, Sarina Madhavan, Mugdha Mokashi, Hanna Amanuel, Natasha R. Johnson, Lydia E. Pace, and Deborah Bartz. 2020. "Health Risks and Outcomes That Disproportionately Affect Women during the Covid-19 Pandemic: A Review." *Social Science & Medicine* 266:113364. https://doi.org/10.1016/j.socscimed.2020.113364.

Coutinho, Raquel Zanatta, Aida Villanueva Montalvo, Abigail Weitzman, and Letícia Junqueira Marteleto. 2021. "Zika Virus Public Health Crisis and the Perpetuation of Gender Inequality in Brazil." *Reproductive Health* 18:1–21. https://doi.org/10.1186/s12978-021-01067-1.

Dasgupta, Aisha, Vladimíra Kantorová, and Philipp Ueffing. 2020. "The Impact of the COVID-19 Crisis on Meeting Needs for Family Planning: A Global Scenario by Contraceptive Methods Used." *Gates Open Research* 4:102. https://doi.org/10.12688/gatesopenres.13148.2.

Demombynes, Gabriel. 2020. "COVID-19 Age-Mortality Curves Are Flatter in Developing Countries." World Bank Policy Research Working Paper no. 9313 (July). https://doi.org/10.1596/1813-9450-9313.

European Commission [Directorate-General for Justice and Consumers]. 2021. *2021 Report on Gender Equality in the EU.* Luxembourg: Publications Office of the European Union. https://data.europa.eu/doi/10.2838/57887.

Fawole, Olufunmilayo I., Olufunmi F. Bamiselu, Peter A. Adewuyi, and Patrick M. Nguku. 2016. "Gender Dimensions to the Ebola Outbreak in Nigeria." *Annals of African Medicine* 15, no. 1 (January–March): 7–13. https://doi.org/10.4103/1596-3519.172554.

Forero-Martínez, Luz J., Rocío Murad, Mariana Calderón-Jaramillo, and Juan C. Rivillas-García. 2020. "Zika and Women's Sexual and Reproductive Health: Critical First Steps to Understand the Role of Gender in the Colombian Epidemic." *International Journal of Gynecology & Obstetrics* 148, no. S2 (January): S15–19. https://doi.org/10.1002/ijgo.13043.

Gahungu, Jumaine, Mariam Vahdaninia, and Pramod R. Regmi. 2021. "The Unmet Needs for Modern Family Planning Methods among Postpartum Women in Sub-Saharan Africa: A Systematic Review of the Literature." *Reproductive Health* 18:1–15. https://doi.org/10.1186/s12978-021-01089-9.

Global Health 50/50. 2021. "The Sex, Gender and COVID-19 Project: Dataset." Global Health 50/50. Last updated August 24, 2021. https://globalhealth5050.org/the-sex-gender-and-covid-19-project/dataset/.

Gómez-Suárez, Marcela, Maeve B. Mello, Mónica Alonso Gonzalez, Massimo Ghidinelli, and Freddy Pérez. 2019. "Access to Sexual and Reproductive Health Services for Women Living with HIV in Latin America and the Caribbean: Systematic Review of the Literature." *Journal of the International AIDS Society* 22, no. 4 (April): e25273. https://doi.org/10.1002/jia2.25273.

Harman, Sophie. 2016. "Ebola, Gender and Conspicuously Invisible Women in Global Health Governance." *Third World Quarterly* 37, no. 3: 524–41. https://doi.org/10.1080/01436597.2015.1108827.

Ikejezie, Juniorcaius, Craig N. Shapiro, Jisoo Kim, Monica Chiu, Maria Almiron, Ciro Ugarte, Marcos A. Espinal, and Sylvain Aldighieri. 2017. "Zika Virus Transmission—Region of the Americas, May 15, 2015–December 15, 2016."

Morbidity and Mortality Weekly Report (MMWR) 66, no. 12: 329–34. https://doi
.org/10.15585/mmwr.mm6612a4.

Lightfoot, Elizabeth, and Rajean P. Moone. 2020. "Caregiving in Times of Uncertainty: Helping Adult Children of Aging Parents Find Support during the COVID-19 Outbreak." *Journal of Gerontological Social Work* 63, no. 6–7 (August–October): 542–52. https://doi.org/10.1080/01634372.2020.1769793.

Minor, Olive Melissa. 2017. "Ebola and Accusation: Gender and Stigma in Sierra Leone's Ebola Response." *Anthropology in Action* 24, no. 2: 25–35. https://doi
.org/10.3167/aia.2017.240204.

Mousky, Stafford. 2002. "UNFPA's Role in the Population Field." In *An Agenda for People: The UNFPA through Three Decades,* edited by Nafis Sadik, 211–47. New York: New York University Press.

O'Brien, Melanie, and Maria Ximena Tolosa. 2016. "The Effect of the 2014 West Africa Ebola Virus Disease Epidemic on Multi-level Violence against Women." *International Journal of Human Rights in Healthcare* 9, no. 3: 151–60. http://dx
.doi.org/10.1108/IJHRH-09-2015-0027.

Prata, Ndola, Suzanne Bell, Ashley Fraser, Adelaide Carvalho, Isilda Neves, and Benjamin Nieto-Andrade. 2017. "Partner Support for Family Planning and Modern Contraceptive Use in Luanda, Angola." *African Journal of Reproductive Health* 21, no. 2 (June): 35–48. https://doi.org/10.29063/ajrh2017/v21i2.5.

Promislow, Daniel E. L. 2020. "A Geroscience Perspective on COVID-19 Mortality." *Journals of Gerontology: Series A* 75, no. 9 (September): e30–e33. https://doi
.org/10.1093/gerona/glaa094.

Rich-Edwards, Janet W., Ursula B. Kaiser, Grace L. Chen, JoAnn E. Manson, and Jill M. Goldstein. 2018. "Sex and Gender Differences Research Design for Basic, Clinical, and Population Studies: Essentials for Investigators." *Endocrine Reviews* 39, no. 4 (August): 424–39. https://doi.org/10.1210/er.2017-00246.

Sen, Gita. 2014. "Sexual and Reproductive Health and Rights in the Post-2015 Development Agenda." *Global Public Health* 9, no. 6: 599–606. https://doi.org/10
.1080/17441692.2014.917197.

Smith, Julia. 2019. "Overcoming the 'Tyranny of the Urgent': Integrating Gender into Disease Outbreak Preparedness and Response." *Gender & Development* 27, no. 2: 355–69. https://doi.org/10.1080/13552074.2019.1615288.

Springer, Kristen W., Jeanne Mager Stellman, and Rebecca M. Jordan-Young. 2012. "Beyond a Catalogue of Differences: A Theoretical Frame and Good Practice Guidelines for Researching Sex/Gender in Human Health." *Social Science & Medicine* 74, no. 11 (June): 1817–24. https://doi.org/10.1016/j.socscimed.2011.05
.033.

Strong, Adrienne, and David A. Schwartz. 2016. "Sociocultural Aspects of Risk to Pregnant Women during the 2013–2015 Multinational Ebola Virus Outbreak in West Africa." *Health Care for Women International* 37, no. 8 (August): 922–42. https://doi.org/10.1080/07399332.2016.1167896.

Temmerman, Marleen. 2021. "Family Planning in COVID-19 Times: Access for All." *Lancet Global Health* 9, no. 6 (June): e728–29. https://doi.org/10.1016
/S2214-109X(21)00231-X.

UNFPA (United Nations Population Fund). 2020. *Impact of the COVID-19 Pandemic on Family Planning and Ending Gender-Based Violence, Female Genital Mutilation and Child Marriage.* Interim Technical Note, April 27, 2020. New York: UNFPA. https://www.unfpa.org/resources/impact-covid-19-pandemic-family-planning-and-ending-gender-based-violence-female-genital.

United Nations. 2020. United Nations General Assembly, Resolution 75/157, Women and Girls and the Response to the Coronavirus Disease (COVID-19). December 23, 2020. https://undocs.org/en/A/RES/75/157.

Van Spall, Harriette Gillian Christine. 2021. "Exclusion of Pregnant and Lactating Women from COVID-19 Vaccine Trials: A Missed Opportunity." *European Heart Journal* 42, no. 28: 2724–26. https://doi.org/10.1093/eurheartj/ehab103.

Wenham, Clare. 2020. *The Gendered Impact of the COVID-19 Crisis and Post-crisis Period.* Study PE 658.227 (September). European Parliament, Directorate-General for Internal Policies, Policy Department for Citizens' Rights and Constitutional Affairs. https://www.europarl.europa.eu/RegData/etudes/STUD/2020/658227/IPOL_STU(2020)658227_EN.pdf.

Wenham, Clare, Julia Smith, and Rosemary Morgan. 2020. "COVID-19: The Gendered Impacts of the Outbreak." *Lancet* 395, no. 10227: 846–48. https://doi.org/10.1016/S0140-6736(20)30526-2.

WHO (World Health Organization). 2007. *Addressing Sex and Gender in Epidemic-Prone Infectious Diseases.* Geneva, Switzerland: World Health Organization. https://apps.who.int/iris/handle/10665/43644.

———. 2020. *Gender and COVID-19.* Advocacy Brief, May 14, 2020. Geneva, Switzerland: World Health Organization. https://www.who.int/publications/i/item/WHO-2019-nCoV-Advocacy_brief-Gender-2020.1.

World Bank. 2019. "Gender-Based Violence (Violence against Women and Girls)." World Bank, September 25, 2019. https://www.worldbank.org/en/topic/socialsustainability/brief/violence-against-women-and-girls.

Zambrano, Laura D., Sascha Ellington, Penelope Strid, Romeo R. Galang, Titilope Oduyebo, Van T. Tong, Kate R. Woodworth, et al. 2020. "Update: Characteristics of Symptomatic Women of Reproductive Age with Laboratory-Confirmed SARS-Cov-2 Infection by Pregnancy Status—United States, January 22–October 3, 2020." *Morbidity and Mortality Weekly Report (MMWR)* 69, no. 44: 1641–47. http://dx.doi.org/10.15585/mmwr.mm6944e3.

3

Leveraging Social Networks for COVID-19

The Other Socially Transmitted Infection

JAIH B. CRADDOCK, MARQUITTA DORSEY,
RACHEL LUDEKE, AND VASHTI ADAMS

In 2020, COVID-19 became the leading cause of death in the United States, with an average of more than three thousand people dying of COVID-19 per day. As of August 16, 2021, there were more than 36.7 million COVID-19 cases and 619,000 COVID-19–related deaths in the United States alone (CDC 2021a). Even though three COVID-19 vaccines (Pfizer, Moderna, and Johnson & Johnson) were developed in record time and made available to the US public for free starting in December 2020, as of August 16, 2021, only 50.8% of the US population aged 12 or older was fully vaccinated for COVID-19 (CDC 2021c).

Because COVID-19 is a socially transmitted infection, in which our social interactions directly and indirectly increase the spread, social network–based methods (e.g., contact tracing and social distancing) have been used to identify and isolate individuals and communities at risk of COVID-19. Although social network–based methods of contact tracing and social isolation have had a significant impact on decreasing the spread of COVID-19 in some communities (CDC 2021d), social network methods can also be leveraged to better understand social determinants of COVID-19 health disparities; inform scientists and policy-makers of the gaps in vaccine and testing dissemination; increase vaccine access in underserved communities; and disseminate COVID-19–based interventions that can decrease vaccine hesitancy and increase COVID-19 prevention behaviors (e.g., mask wearing, social distancing, and COVID-19 testing and vaccinations). Yet even with widespread COVID-19 testing and vaccine dissemination, systemic inequities among racial and ethnic minorities have led to substantial differences in COVID-19 testing, diagnosis, treatment, vaccinations, and death rates (Bibbins-Domingo 2020). This chapter examines how social network methods (a) have been leveraged to examine and address social determinants of health and health disparities in various communities and settings, (b) are currently being used to address COVID-19 risk and health outcomes, and (c) can be leveraged to better address COVID-19 and other health inequities related to socially transmitted infections in communities of color.

AN OVERVIEW OF SOCIAL NETWORK METHODS IN PUBLIC HEALTH

The study of human networks via social networks serves as a methodological tool and research paradigm to explore the intricacies of relationships. Social networks are networks of social interactions and personal relationships salient in influencing communication (Valente 2010). At its core, social network analysis focuses primarily on the social relationships that are achieved or attributed among individuals, families, communities, countries, and other objects (Bandyopadhyay, Rao, and Sinha 2011; Kadushin 2012). Social network analyses encompass (a) whole-network approaches whereby researchers attempt to understand the interconnections of each actor or person in a network and their interconnections and (b) personal-network analysis wherein the focus is on an individual and their interconnections with others in their social networks (see figures 3.1a and 3.1b). Networks can manifest as conceptual or theoretical models, real-world structures or systems, simulations of given phenomena in society, or strictly mathematical models used to show relationships between variables (see figure 3.2). Because this chapter uses a social network lens, there is an assumption that all communities are made up of various types of social networks. Thus, when the terms *community* or *communities* are used in this chapter, the authors are inherently referring to one or more types of social networks.

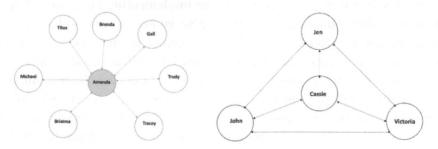

FIGURE(S) 3.1A (LEFT) AND 3.1B (RIGHT). Examples of social network types: (a) personal network (egocentric); (b) whole network (sociometric).

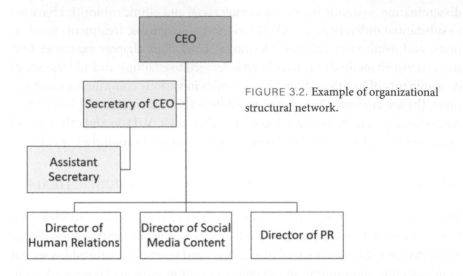

FIGURE 3.2. Example of organizational structural network.

The field of public health has long acknowledged the significance of relational characteristics in understanding disease, social issues, and population health (Luke and Harris 2007). With the explosion in the use of social network analysis in public health, researchers have the ability to examine all aspects of human interaction when it comes to the influence of peers and family members in health situations. But although the field of public health has long adopted an ecological approach, researchers in the field have only recently adopted a more nuanced approach to the analysis of social networks. According to Luke and Harris (2007), their review of the use of social network analysis in public health revealed that researchers generally use the method to explore three categories: transmission networks, support networks, and organizational networks.

In transmission networks, researchers tend to study the flow of disease or information in a given social network. This line of inquiry influences the majority of network-based interventions for implementing behavioral change strategies, which could include exploring social norms, peer influence, and social influence (Valente 2010). For instance, social network analysis has been used by researchers to understand how HIV/AIDS spreads in high-risk networks and how engaging with social networks can decrease transmission in high-risk populations by increasing prevention through network mobilization (Heckathorn et al. 1999; Rothenberg et al. 1998). A more recent study explored HIV transmission to understand how the advent of social media has played a role in adoption of safe-sex practices among groups with greater risk of transmission (Pagkas-Bather et al. 2020). Other studies have explored the intersection of race and ethnicity and transmission in urban areas (Pivnick et al. 1994; Ragonnet-Cronin et al. 2021). In Ragonnet-Cronin and colleagues' study (2021), they found that HIV transmission networks in New York, Los Angeles County, and Cook County, Illinois, were more assortative by race and ethnicity than age or transmission risk, particularly for Black individuals. In addition to examining transmission of disease or infections, for instance in mapping the effect of social distancing on reducing COVID-19 viral transmission (Bailey et al. 2020; Gutin et al. 2021), analysis of transmission networks can also focus on the spread of information throughout a social network, as in examining where public-trusted information regarding adherence to social distancing comes from and how it is shared (Fridman et al. 2020).

Network analysis has also been used by public health researchers to study support networks and forms of social support and social capital among individuals and community groups (Albrecht and Goldsmith 2003). In this way, researchers can explore health behaviors affected by social support systems and resource allocation in communities. Significant aspects of social support have shown correlations with having an established support network of friends and families that can help to modify health behavior. Perhaps the most famous longitudinal examination of health behaviors and social support is the long-running Framingham Heart Study, which began data collection in 1948 and is ongoing (Andersson et al. 2019). The original cohort consisted of 5,209 people in Framingham, Massachusetts, and the offspring cohort is composed of most of the children of those who participated in the original study, their spouses, and their children (Mahmood et al. 2013). The study has used a sociometric or whole-network approach to understand the development of coronary artery disease and factors related to developing the disease in randomly selected populations (Tsao and Vasan 2015). It remains a hallmark study in the epidemiology field because it changed the way that researchers conduct cohort study data collection. It has been cited in more than two thousand peer-reviewed articles (Oppenheimer 2010) spanning many subjects beyond the study's original purpose, including research on the epidemiology of cardiovascular disease (Mahmood et al. 2013; Manson and Bassuk 2017), risk of developing congestive heart failure (Kenchaiah and Vasan 2015; Lloyd-Jones 2001; Mahmood and Wang 2013), obesity (Elias et al. 2003; Hubert et al. 1983; Xu et al. 2018), diabetes (Hempler, Joensen, and Willaing 2016), and even the dynamic transmission of happiness within networks of social support (James and Christakis 2008). The use of social network analysis to understand social support continues to be a major way in which researchers in public health interact not only with the individual but also their environment to create meaningful and holistic frameworks for interventions that consider the effect of social influence and support.

Organizational networks in public health have been examined using a systems approach to design and evaluate public health programs, primarily to explore communication networks among employees, agency stakeholders, and others in a public health setting (Valente 2010). Researchers in the field of public health have utilized a systems approach in designing and evaluating health interventions (Luke and Harris 2007). The systems approach considers different components of an intervention or program, including how these moving pieces interact, and requires thinking beyond a singular field of inquiry to create a mechanism for change (Leischow and Milstein 2006; Midgley 2006). Organizational social network analysis recently gained steam in the field of public health but is still evolving as a way to explore health systems research (Blanchet and James 2012). Organizational social network analysis has been used to study communication links among health department staff members to support agency decision-making for public health managers (Merrill et al. 2007), inform agency intervention in reducing youth violence (Bess, Speer, and Perkins 2011), and explore how researchers can best exchange evidence-based practices in the development of health policy (Shearer, Dion, and Lavis 2014). Thus, social network analysis provides a mechanism for public health researchers to explore, understand, and describe different types of structural and relational issues that can affect the overall health and well-being of individuals, families, groups, and communities (Luke and Harris 2007), including when it comes to understanding the transmission and spread of COVID-19 and implementing community-based COVID-19 prevention efforts.

SEXUALLY TRANSMITTED INFECTIONS: LEVERAGING WHAT WE KNOW ABOUT SOCIAL NETWORK IMPACT ON BEHAVIORAL CHANGE

During the last thirty years, researchers have worked to understand and implement methods to help stop the spread of HIV and other sexually transmitted infections. Because there are many similarities between how HIV and COVID-19 spread in social networks (see table 3.1), these lessons can be and have been leveraged in the efforts to stop the spread of COVID-19 (Logie 2020; McMahon et al. 2020; Quinn 2020).

TABLE 3.1. COMMONALITIES BETWEEN THE SPREAD
AND PREVENTION OF HIV AND COVID-19

Factors	HIV	COVID-19
Social networks	Current and previous exposure to HIV by sexual or needle-sharing network members can increase an individual's risk of, exposure to, and acquisition of HIV.	Current and previous exposure to COVID-19 by social network members can increase an individual's risk of, exposure to, and acquisition of COVID-19.
Testing: awareness of current status	Testing and knowing one's status is the first step to preventing the spread of HIV. Informing the individuals who you have been in contact with about potential exposure and the need for testing is important in the efforts to slow the spread.	Testing and knowing one's status is the first step to preventing the spread of COVID-19. Informing the individuals who you have been in contact with about potential exposure and the need for testing is important in the efforts to slow the spread.
Window between exposure, testing, and results	The time between exposure and testing detection is a large window that can vary from 10 to 90 days postexposure, depending on the test. A negative test result can indicate that a person either did not have HIV at the time of testing or testing took place too early for detection.	The time between exposure and COVID-19-related symptoms can range from 2 to 14 days. COVID-19 testing is point-in-time, meaning that the test results only indicate your COVID-19 status at the time of testing and cannot tell you if you contracted COVID-19 between testing and receiving your results. A negative test result only means that you did not have COVID-19 at the time of testing.

Source: CDC (2021b; 2021e).

Leveraging health communication with social network members has been shown to be an important factor in HIV prevention (Craddock 2020; Craddock et al. 2020), and these lessons can be leveraged to increase COVID-19 prevention in the United States (Gunther-Grey, Wolitski, and Reitmeijer, n.d.). HIV interventions that focus on behavioral change in social networks have been shown to be effective in reducing the spread and new acquisitions of HIV (Rice et al. 2018). Behavior change theories, such as Bandura's (1999) social cognitive theory and Rogers's (2010) diffusion of innovation theory, highlight the importance of social interactions in driving behavior change. Both theories emphasize how interpersonal communication between social network members can be important in influencing behaviors, knowledge, and beliefs, which in turn shape individual-level HIV or COVID-19 behaviors.

A core component of social cognitive theory is that people can learn from observing the behaviors of others (Bandura 1999). Vicarious learning is one form of observational learning in which individuals acquire new behaviors after observing a person of similar or higher status engage in a behavior and receive a "reinforcing consequence" (Bandura 1965; Huitt and Monetti 2008). This vicarious learning typically takes place in a network or interaction setting. Applying this concept to socially or sexually transmitted infection prevention behaviors, an individual may decide to wear a mask (new behavior) after witnessing a social network member not wearing a mask (observation) while attending a social gathering of vaccinated and nonvaccinated individuals (behavior) and later learning that the social network member who did not wear a mask has contracted COVID-19 (reinforcing consequence). Vicarious learning can also take place via videos or live feeds on various platforms including social media such as TikTok, YouTube, Instagram, Facebook, and X (formerly known as Twitter). Thus, these platforms can be leveraged for COVID-19 prevention efforts.

Diffusion of innovation theory similarly underscores the importance of social interactions in driving behavior change, but it is primarily useful for understanding how new behaviors spread throughout communities. This theory suggests that members of a community can be categorized into five groups, each of which adopts new behaviors at different rates: innovators, early adopters, early majority, late majority, and laggards (Rogers 2010). Except among the risk-taking innovators, who are the first to adopt new behaviors, the diffusion of new behaviors is influenced by subjective evaluations from members of a social network. Although individuals can be introduced to a new behavior through communication channels, including mass and social media (e.g., TV, magazines, TikTok, YouTube, Instagram), Rogers (2010) suggests that interpersonal communication is the most effective (talking or directly interacting with social network members). Other structural network factors, such as homophily, size, and density, can also influence the rate and success of diffusion. For instance, if everyone in a small (size), tight-knit (density) social network has the same averse beliefs (a function of homophily) about being vaccinated for COVID-19, the likelihood that the diffusion of new information about the safety of the COVID-19 vaccine would spread and change behaviors is low due to shared beliefs and modeling of behaviors (see figure 3.3a). Compare this to a larger (size), less connected (density) social network where individuals have differing beliefs (heterogeneity) about the COVID-19 vaccine. In this network, the likelihood that the diffusion of new information about the safety of the COVID-19 vaccine would change behaviors is probably higher because the variation in beliefs, behaviors, and strength of ties (weak or strong connections) creates space for modeling of new behaviors and beliefs (figure 3.3b).

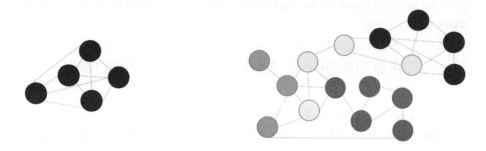

FIGURE 3.3A (LEFT) AND 3.3B (RIGHT). Social networks of various densities: (a) high density and high homophily in beliefs indicated by shade of nodes; (b) moderate density and heterogeneity in beliefs indicated by shade of nodes.

COVID-19 VACCINATION HESITANCY AND UNCERTAINTY

COVID-19 vaccination hesitancy and uncertainty have led to disparities in vaccination rates in the US population. Including after the vaccine became available for individuals twelve years and older (CDC 2021c), there have continued to be varyingly low rates of vaccination uptake, particularly among Black individuals. Among marginalized and minority populations in general, similarities have been found between HIV and COVID-19 hesitancy and uncertainty in the realm of prevention, regarding the use of preexposure prophylaxis, postexposure prophylaxis, and antiviral medications.

Studies examining vaccine uptake by race have found that Black adults younger than forty-five are most reluctant to get vaccinated, with 41% of adults aged eighteen to forty-four stating that they did not plan to get a COVID-19 vaccine and about 21% stating that they were unsure (NFID 2021). Similarly, Black Americans make up 14% of the US population but 42% of new diagnoses of HIV, with rates twice as high among Black men compared to Latino men (second highest rate) and Black women with the highest rate among women at 58% (Kaiser Family Foundation 2020). Yet when it comes to HIV prevention, a study of preexposure prophylaxis use among men who have sex with men found that only 26% of Black men used the preventive measure (Kanny et al. 2019). These numbers are even lower in the larger Black population. Given that Black individuals represent about 8.5% of individuals fully vaccinated for COVID-19 (CDC 2021c) and the continued low utilization of pharmaceutical HIV prevention methods (e.g., preexposure prophylaxis, postexposure prophylaxis, antiviral measures), we have to consider factors (e.g., systemic racism and intersections of oppression in large networks [CDC 2021d]) beyond those at the individual level that can lead to these syndemic disparities.

THE SYNDEMIC NATURE OF THE COVID-19 PANDEMIC

Defined as a population-level clustering of social and health problems, a syndemic involves two or more diseases or health conditions clustered in a specific population with certain contextual and social factors that result in adverse disease interactions (Singer et al. 2017). Essentially, syndemic theory suggests that co-occurring epidemics interact with individuals and populations concurrently while enhancing various consequences regarding health or health disparities (Singer 1994). For example, Black young adults who live with and navigate racial oppression in US society contend with greater risks of contracting sexually transmitted infections and COVID-19, largely due to the historical lineage of racism and discrimination.

In 2020, the COVID-19 pandemic along with heightened awareness of police brutality against Black and Brown individuals presented unprecedented health disparities. Across the nation, as protests against systemic racism and police brutality filled the streets of major cities, Black and Brown (Latinx and Indigenous) communities engaged in social action activities that encouraged close contact and community when COVID-19 rates were at their peak. The syndemic nature of the COVID-19 pandemic in the US, particularly its comorbidity with the pandemic of racism and persistent HIV pandemic, continue to inherently marginalize the health and well-being of Black and Brown social networks, particularly as it relates to social determinants of health such as race, access to health resources, and timely delivery of preventive knowledge.

Consider the 2020 COVID-19 testing rollout. Health disparities in COVID-19 cases and deaths may be linked to a slow governmental response and rollout of COVID-19 testing (Blake 2021; Kates et al. 2020) and historical exploitation of Black and Brown Americans' health for scientific gains. Black and Brown individuals are enduring disproportionate health disparities experienced simultaneously, in large part due to the historical underpinnings of discrimination and systemic racism. These factors could all have links to the HIV and sexually transmitted infection epidemic, the epidemic of racism, and the COVID-19 pandemic. Instead of seeing two or more epidemics as simply occurring at the same time and contributing to one health outcome, more attention to how each epidemic compounds experiences with other epidemics and how health outcomes may contribute to these health crises is warranted. This can be done using social network analysis methods.

SOCIAL NETWORK METHODS FOR STUDYING SYNDEMICS: HOW SOCIAL NETWORKS CAN BE LEVERAGED TO BETTER ADDRESS COVID-19 INEQUITIES IN COMMUNITIES OF COLOR

Some scholars have examined syndemic theory in the context of sexually transmitted infections and HIV transmission among young adults (Hill et al. 2019; Lyons, Johnson, and Garofalo 2013). Through twenty-one interviews with an ethnically diverse sample of men aged eighteen to twenty-four who have sex with men, Lyons and colleagues (Lyons, Johnson, and Garofalo 2013) reported the colliding impact of polysubstance use, weak familial support, high-risk lifestyles, and education. As a result of grounded theory analysis, these scholars identified causal links between HIV infection and other meso and macro factors such as lack of role models, preventive education, and goal planning, which are all important to emerging adulthood development.

According to syndemic theory, if Black and Brown individuals experience higher risk of COVID-19 transmission and HIV, social factors and conditions are plausible factors to explain behaviors, rather than individual-level factors such as genetics and intergenerational transmission of practices and behaviors (Bibbins-Domingo 2020). Types of syndemic interaction may be important considerations among Black and Brown populations. Transmission of sexually and socially transmitted diseases intersect when resources, information, and access at macro levels of society are limited (e.g., low dissemination of prevention knowledge [Singer et al. 2017]). Some scholars have suggested that behaviors are contingent on the culture's norms, whereby behaviors reflect the advantages or limitations present in the culture (e.g., ideas, beliefs, knowledge, resources) of the social network (Airhihenbuwa, Ford, and Iwelunmor 2014). Because syndemic behaviors are representative of current resources or the lack thereof, considering multicomponent interventions where factors linked to each epidemic are addressed is essential.

Several scholars have explored various interventions that target or moderate the impact of syndemics on health outcomes. Disruptions to effective interventions may lie at the structural level, at which prevention efforts cannot excel. Da Silva and colleagues (2020) posited that social networks can be a method for buffering the impact of syndemic conditions on HIV contraction. Utilizing a representative cohort of 618 young Black transgender men and men who have sex with men, they found that engaging in social networks with more family members and friends buffered the syndemic impact (i.e., community violence, poverty, history of justice system involvement, illicit substance use, and depression) on HIV contraction. In other words, greater social support gained through friends and family may contribute to engaging in healthy sexual behaviors while experiencing structural barriers and ultimately prevent HIV contraction (da Silva et al. 2020). Social networks and culturally relevant considerations may be the best approach for prevention and intervention efforts when considering the syndemic impact of COVID-19, systemic racism, and increasing sexual health disparities related to HIV and sexually transmitted infection contraction (Airhihenbuwa et al. 2014; da Silva et al. 2020).

HOW SOCIAL NETWORK METHODS ARE CURRENTLY USED TO ADDRESS COVID-19 RISK

Although social network–based methods of contact tracing and social isolation have had a significant impact on decreasing the spread of COVID-19, social network methods can also be leveraged to better understand social determinants of COVID-19 health disparities; inform scientists and policymakers of the gaps in vaccine and testing dissemination; increase vaccine access in underserved communities; and disseminate COVID-19–based interventions that can decrease vaccine hesitancy and increase COVID-19 prevention behaviors (e.g., mask wearing, social distancing, and COVID-19 testing and vaccinations).

A great example of how social networks have been leveraged to track breakthrough COVID-19 cases (fully vaccinated people who test positive for COVID-19) is the data collected by Michael Donnelly, a data scientist from New York (Simmons-Duffin 2021). Donnelly tracked COVID-19 breakthrough case leads in his personal network after several friends and their network members reported testing positive for COVID-19 after being vaccinated. Donnelly then shared these data with the Centers for Disease Control and Prevention in real time. Some have argued that Donnelly's data prompted the federal agency to change its guidance for how those who have been vaccinated should keep themselves safe (Simmons-Duffin 2021). Donnelly stated that the norms of his social network, which he identifies as a gay community, include sharing their risk and medical history, stemming from experiences with the HIV/AIDS epidemic (Simmons-Duffin 2021). This example highlights the impact of the HIV/AIDS epidemic for specific communities and networks during the COVID-19 pandemic. In this case, the behaviors of this social network, whose norm is for members to communicate openly about their health status and share with whom they have interacted, have translated in a beneficial way to a different pandemic, COVID-19. This same translation of previous behaviors and experiences (e.g., of racism, discrimination, stigma, or medical mistrust) surrounding the HIV epidemic in Black communities is disadvantageous to the health outcomes of Black individuals during COVID-19.

As part of recent social network–based efforts to increase vaccinations among communities of color that have been historically underserved, many US cities are leveraging social media influencers as popular opinion leaders or change agents to disseminate accurate and positive messaging about the COVID-19 vaccine to their large social networks of followers (Anderson 2021). As previous research has indicated, popular opinion leader models are effective in disseminating new behaviors and interventions in specific networks (Quinn 2020), and using this model on social media platforms is a great way to reach large networks of individuals in a short amount of time to increase COVID-19 prevention behaviors. In addition to leveraging social media–based influencers to increase COVID-19 vaccination in social networks, social network methods can be used to disseminate COVID-19–based behavioral interventions that can decrease vaccination hesitancy and increase other COVID-19 prevention behaviors (e.g., mask wearing, social distancing, and COVID-19 testing) in underserved communities.

Similar to using social media influencers to share up-to-date and accurate COVID-19 information, community-based (e.g., churches, schools, community centers, families) popular opinion leaders or change agents who are dispersed across the community-based network can be trained to educate and share COVID-19 information with friends and family members in their network (Bondi et al. 2018). Other COVID-19 interventions include Colorado's #PowertheComeback (CDPHE 2021), which focuses on leveraging employee networks of businesses to increase vaccinations in Colorado, or the Vaccination Ambassadors Program offered in partnership between the Chicago Department of Public Health and Malcolm X College (City of Chicago 2021), which provides training opportunities for individuals to became certified and trusted messengers regarding the COVID-19 vaccine. These vaccination ambassadors go into their communities to educate community members about COVID-19 and provide accurate resources and information (City of Chicago 2021). Maryland has taken a different social network approach with its "Don't Invite COVID" campaign (MDH 2021), which asks Marylanders to check with their network members about their COVID-19 symptoms and status before socializing. These campaigns are prime examples of how cities and states use network-based methods to increase COVID-19 education and vaccinations among various communities.

In addition to leveraging social networks to disseminate information in social networks and communities, social network methods can be used to trace the dissemination of COVID-19 information in social networks by collecting social network data. These data, which may be gathered using questions such as "Who have you communicated with about COVID-19 via text, phone, in person, or on social media?" could help to determine how and through what means COVID-19 information is spreading through various social networks (Bondi et al. 2018). Based on this information, we can track what social networks have higher rates of testing and vaccination for COVID-19 and use this information to better tailor interventions for similar communities. At the macro level, social network–based COVID-19 data, like those collected by Michael Donnelly (Simmons-Duffin 2021), can be leveraged to inform city, state, and federal health agencies and policy-makers.

LESSONS LEARNED

Research in the realm of HIV prevention and intervention has taught us a great amount about what has and has not worked when it comes to decreasing the spread of a sexually and socially transmitted infection, like COVID-19, within social networks of individuals. We have learned that we must not only consider individual-level risk factors that may contribute to the spread of infection, but must also consider social network characteristics (e.g., size, density, behaviors, and beliefs) and environmental factors. Additionally, HIV research has illustrated the impact that historical trauma and medical mistrust has on new intervention implementation, dissemination, and adoption within communities of color. These lessons have highlighted the need for age-appropriate and culturally tailored interventions that address the concerns of target populations and meet them where they are in their communities (e.g., social media, community organizations, clinics) and in stages of behavioral change. HIV research has also highlighted the ability to leverage technology to reach large populations and to educate and address misinformation and misconceptions. These lessons can be applied to the prevention and intervention efforts for COVID-19.

CONCLUSION

To address this urgent COVID-19 pandemic, public health experts do not have to reinvent the wheel when it comes to prevention and tracking efforts. Because COVID-19 is a socially transmitted infection, social network methods can and should be used to understand and examine the spread of COVID-19 in social networks (communities), disseminate information and interventions in various communities, examine the syndemic nature of health disparities related to COVID-19, and shape policy development at the city, state, and federal levels. Leveraging lessons learned and prevention methods from other socially and sexually transmitted infections, such as HIV, can help with quicker implementation of COVID-19 prevention efforts in social networks across the US and throughout the world.

RECOMMENDATIONS FOR FUTURE PRACTICE

- Think beyond the individual level when it comes to prevention and intervention efforts. Think about how social networks can be leveraged to improve both individual- and community-level health outcomes.

- Consider potential syndemics (two or more diseases or health conditions clustered in a specific population with certain contextual and social factors, resulting in adverse disease interactions) when addressing public health concerns, particularly in Black and Brown communities.

- Do not be afraid to borrow, adapt, and combine ideas, methods, and interventions (as long as the originals are cited) to meet the needs of different populations and different diseases, infections, and viruses.

DISCUSSION QUESTION

- Think about an intervention effort shown to be effective in the prevention, intervention, or treatment of a disease, virus, or infection. How would you transform or adapt this intervention or prevention effort to address a different public health challenge (e.g., disease, virus, or infection)? Provide a detailed example.

REFERENCES

Airhihenbuwa, Collins O., Chandra L. Ford, and Juliet I. Iwelunmor. 2014. "Why Culture Matters in Health Interventions: Lessons from HIV/AIDS Stigma and NCDs." *Health Education and Behavior* 41, no. 1 (February): 78–84. https://doi .org/10.1177/1090198113487199.

Albrecht, Terrance L., and Daena J. Goldsmith. 2003. "Social Support, Social Networks, and Health." In *Handbook of Health Communication,* edited by Teresa L. Thompson et al., 263–84. Mahwah, NJ: Lawrence Erlbaum.

Anderson, James. 2021. "Can Social Media Influencers Change Vaccine Skeptics' Minds?" *Los Angeles Times,* August 10, 2021. https://www.latimes.com /world-nation/story/2021-08-10/can-social-media-influencers-change-vaccine -skeptics-minds.

Andersson, Charlotte, Andrew D. Johnson, Emelia J. Benjamin, Daniel Levy, and Ramachandran S. Vasan. 2019. "70-Year Legacy of the Framingham Heart Study." *Nature Reviews Cardiology* 16:687–98. https://doi.org/10.1038/s41569-019-0202-5.

Bailey, Michael, Drew M. Johnston, Martin Koenen, Theresa Kuchler, Dominic Russel, and Johannes Strobel. 2020. *Social Networks Shape Beliefs and Behavior: Evidence from Social Distancing during the COVID-19 Pandemic.* Cambridge, MA: National Bureau of Economic Research.

Bandura, Albert. 1965. "Vicarious Processes: A Case of No-Trial Learning." *Advances in Experimental Social Psychology* 2:1–55. https://doi.org/10.1016/S0065 -2601(08)60102-1.

———. 1999. "Social Cognitive Theory of Personality." In *Handbook of Personality: Theory and Research,* 2nd ed., edited by Lawrence A. Pervin and Oliver P. John, 154–96. New York: Guilford Press.

Bandyopadhyay, Suraj, A. R. Rao, and Bikas K. Sinha. 2011. *Models for Social Networks with Statistical Applications.* Thousand Oaks, CA: Sage.

Bess, Kimberly D., Paul W. Speer, and Douglas D. Perkins. 2011. "Ecological Contexts in the Development of Coalitions for Youth Violence Prevention: An Organizational Network Analysis." *Health Education & Behavior* 39, no. 5: 526–37. https://doi.org/10.1177/1090198111419656.

Bibbins-Domingo, Kirsten. 2020. "This Time Must Be Different: Disparities during the COVID-19 Pandemic." *Annals of Internal Medicine* 173, no. 3: 233–34. https://doi.org/10.7326/m20-2247.

Blake, Aaron. 2021. "How Politics Infected Trump's Coronavirus Response, in One Key Case." *Washington Post,* November 15, 2021. https://www.washingtonpost .com/politics/2021/11/15/politics-infected-trump-virus-response.

Blanchet, Karl, and Philip James. 2012. "How to Do (or Not to Do) . . . a Social Network Analysis in Health Systems Research." *Health Policy and Planning* 27, no. 5 (August): 438–46. https://doi.org/10.1093/heapol/czr055.

Bondi, Elizabeth, Jaih Craddock, Rebecca Funke, Chloe LeGendre, and Vivek Tiwari. 2018. "Maximizing the Spread of Sexual Health Information in a Multimodal Communication Network of Young Black Women." In *Artificial Intelligence and Social Work,* edited by Milind Tambe and Eric Rice, 93–118. Cambridge: Cambridge University Press.

CDC (Centers for Disease Control and Prevention). 2021a. "COVID Data Tracker: Cases, Deaths, and Testing." https://covid.cdc.gov/covid-data-tracker /#cases_casesper100klast7days.

———. 2021b. "COVID-19 Testing Overview." https://www.cdc.gov/coronavirus /2019-ncov/symptoms-testing/testing.html.

———. 2021c. "COVID-19 Vaccinations in the United States." https://covid.cdc.gov /covid-data-tracker/#vaccinations_vacc-total-admin-rate-total.

———. 2021d. "HIV and African American People: HIV Prevention." https://www .cdc.gov/hiv/group/racialethnic/africanamericans/index.html.

———. 2021e. "Types of HIV Testing." https://www.cdc.gov/hiv/basics/hiv-testing /test-types.html.

CDPHE (Colorado Department of Public Health and Environment). 2021. "Power the Comeback Resources." https://covid19.colorado.gov/bizpledgetoolkit.

City of Chicago. 2021. "Protect Chicago." https://www.chicago.gov/city/en/sites /covid-19/home/protect-chicago.html.

Craddock, Jaih B. 2020. "Sexual Health Communication among Young Black Women and Their Social Network Members." *Journal of the Society for Social Work and Research* 11, no. 4: 569–89. https://psycnet.apa.org/doi/10.1086/711701.

Craddock, Jaih B., Anamika Barman-Adhikari, Kattie Massey Combs, Anthony Fulginiti, and Eric Rice. 2020. "Individual and Social Network Correlates of Sexual Health Communication among Youth Experiencing Homelessness." *AIDS and Behavior* 24:222–32. https://doi.org/10.1007/s10461-019-02646-x.

da Silva, Daniel Teixeira, Alida Bouris, Dexter Voisin, Anna Hotton, Russell Brewer, and John Schneider. 2020. "Social Networks Moderate the Syndemic Effect of Psychosocial and Structural Factors on HIV Risk among Young Black Transgender Women and Men Who Have Sex with Men." *AIDS and Behavior* 24:192–205. https://doi.org/10.1007/s10461-019-02575-9.

Elias, M. F., P. K. Elias, L. M. Sullivan, P. A. Wolf, and R. B. D'Agostino. 2003. "Lower Cognitive Function in the Presence of Obesity and Hypertension: The Framingham Heart Study." *International Journal of Obesity* 27, no. 2 (February): 260–68. https://doi.org/10.1038/sj.ijo.802225.

Fowler, James H., and Nicholas A. Christakis. 2008. "Dynamic Spread of Happiness in a Large Social Network: Longitudinal Analysis over 20 Years in the Framingham Heart Study." *BMJ* 337:a2338. https://doi.org/10.1136/bmj.a2338.

Fridman, Ilona, Nicole Lucas, Debra Henke, and Christina K. Zigler. 2020. "Association between Public Knowledge about COVID-19, Trust in Information Sources, and Adherence to Social Distancing: Cross-Sectional Survey." *JMIR Public Health and Surveillance* 6, no. 3: 1–17. https://doi.org/10.2196/22060.

Gunther-Grey, J., M. A. Wolitski, and O. R. Reitmeijer. n.d. *Building Our Understanding: Key Concepts of Evaluation Applying Theory in the Evaluation of Communication Campaigns.* Atlanta, GA: Centers for Disease Control and Prevention, Healthy Communities Program. https://www.cdc.gov/nccdphp/dch /programs/healthycommunitiesprogram/tools/pdf/apply_theory.pdf.

Gutin, Gregory, Tomohiro Hirano, Sung-Ha Hwang, Philip R. Neary, and Alexis Akira Toda. 2021. "The Effect of Social Distancing on the Reach of an

Epidemic in Social Networks." *Journal of Economic Interaction and Coordina-tion* 16:629–47. https://doi.org/10.1007/s11403-021-00322-9.

Heckathorn, Douglas D., Robert S. Broadhead, Denise L. Anthony, and David L. Weakliem. 1999. "AIDS and Social Networks: HIV Prevention through Net-work Mobilization." *Sociological Focus* 32, no. 2: 159–79. https://doi.org/10.1080 /00380237.1999.10571133.

Hempler, Nana F., Lene E. Joensen, and Ingrid Willaing. 2016. "Relationship be-tween Social Network, Social Support and Health Behaviour in People with Type 1 and Type 2 Diabetes: Cross-Sectional Studies." *BMC Public Health* 16:1–7. https://bmcpublichealth.biomedcentral.com/articles/10.1186/s12889-016-2819-1.

Hill, Ashley V., Natacha M. De Genna, Maria J. Perez-Patron, Tamika D. Gilreath, Carmen Tekwe, and Brandie DePaoli Taylor. 2019. "Identifying Syndemics for Sexually Transmitted Infections among Young Adults in the United States: A Latent Class Analysis." *Journal of Adolescent Health* 64, no. 3 (March): 319–26. https://doi.org/10.1016/j.jadohealth.2018.09.006.

Hubert, Helen B., Manning Feinleib, Patricia M. McNamara, and William P. Cas-telli. 1983. "Obesity as an Independent Risk Factor for Cardiovascular Disease: A 26-Year Follow-Up of Participants in the Framingham Heart Study." *Circula-tion* 67, no. 5 (May): 968–77. https://doi.org/10.1161/01.cir.67.5.968.

Huitt, William G., and David M. Monetti. 2008. "Social Learning Perspective." In *International Encyclopedia of the Social Sciences,* 2nd ed., edited by William A. Darity, 602–3. Farmington Hills, MI: Macmillan.

Kadushin, Charles. 2012. *Understanding Social Networks: Theories, Concepts, and Findings.* New York: Oxford University Press.

Kaiser Family Foundation. 2020. "Black Americans and HIV/AIDS: The Basics." Kaiser Family Foundation, February 7, 2020. https://www.kff.org/hivaids/fact -sheet/black-americans-and-hivaids-the-basics/.

Kanny, Dafna, William L. Jeffries IV, Johanna Chapin-Bardales, Paul Denning, Susan Cha, Teresa Finlayson, Cyprian Wejnert, and National HIV Behavioral Surveillance Study Group. 2019. "Racial/Ethnic Disparities in HIV Preex-posure Prophylaxis among Men Who Have Sex with Men—23 Urban Areas, 2017." *Morbidity and Mortality Weekly Report (MMWR)* 68, no. 37 (Septem-ber 20): 801–6. https://stacks.cdc.gov/view/cdc/83360/cdc_83360_DS1.pdf.

Kates, Jennifer, Josh Michaud, Larry Levitt, Karen Pollitz, Tricia Neuman, Mi-chelle Long, Robin Rudowitz, MaryBeth Musumeci, Meredith Freed, and Juliette Cubanski. 2020. "Comparing Trump and Biden on COVID-19." Kai-ser Family Foundation, September 11, 2020. https://www.kff.org/coronavirus -covid-19/issue-brief/comparing-trump-and-biden-on-covid-19/.

Kenchaiah, Satish, and Ramachandran S. Vasan. 2015. "Heart Failure in Women—Insights from the Framingham Heart Study." *Cardiovascular Drugs and Therapy* 29, no. 4 (August): 377–90. https://doi.org/10.1007/s10557-015 -6599-0.

Leischow, Scott J., and Bobby Milstein. 2006. "Systems Thinking and Modeling for Public Health Practice." *American Journal of Public Health* 96, no. 3 (March): 403–5. https://doi.org/10.2105/AJPH.2005.082842.

Lloyd-Jones, Donald M. 2001. "The Risk of Congestive Heart Failure: Sobering Lessons from the Framingham Heart Study." *Current Cardiology Reports* 3:184–90. https://doi.org/10.1007/s11886-001-0021-1.

Logie, Carmen H. 2020. "Lessons Learned from HIV Can Inform Our Approach to COVID-19 Stigma." *Journal of the International AIDS Society* 23, no. 5 (May): e25504. https://doi.org/10.1002/jia2.25504.

Luke, Douglas A., and Jenine K. Harris. 2007. "Network Analysis in Public Health: History, Methods and Applications." *Annual Review of Public Health* 28:69–93. https://doi.org/10.1146/annurev.publhealth.28.021406.144132.

Lyons, Thomas, Amy K. Johnson, and Robert Garofalo. 2013. "'What Could Have Been Different': A Qualitative Study of Syndemic Theory and HIV Prevention among Young Men Who Have Sex with Men." *Journal of HIV/AIDS & Social Services* 12, no. 3–4: 368–83. https://doi.org/10.1080/15381501.2013.816211.

Mahmood, Syed S., Daniel Levy, Ramachandran S. Vasan, and Thomas J. Wang. 2013. "The Framingham Heart Study and the Epidemiology of Cardiovascular Disease: A Historical Perspective." *Lancet* 383, no. 9921: 999–1008. https://doi.org/10.1016/s0140-6736(13)61752-3.

Mahmood, Syed S., and Thomas J. Wang. 2013. "The Epidemiology of Congestive Heart Failure: Contributions from the Framingham Heart Study." *Global Heart* 8, no. 1: 77–82. https://doi.org/10.1016/j.gheart.2012.12.006.

Manson, JoAnn E., and Shari S. Bassuk. 2017. "The Framingham Offspring Study—A Pioneering Investigation into Familial Aggregation of Cardiovascular Risk." *American Journal of Epidemiology* 185, no. 11: 1103–8. https://doi.org/10.1093/aje/kwx068.

McMahon, James H., Jennifer F. Hoy, Adeeba Kamarulzaman, Linda-Gail Bekker, Chris Beyrer, and Sharon R. Lewin. 2020. "Leveraging the Advances in HIV for COVID-19." *Lancet* 396, no. 10256: 943–44. https://doi.org/10.1016/S0140-6736(20)32012-2.

MDH (Maryland Department of Health). 2021. "Don't Invite COVID." Maryland Department of Health, May 10, 2021. https://health.maryland.gov/newsroom/Pages/Maryland-Department-of-Health-Launches-%E2%80%98Don%E2%80%99t-Invite-COVID%E2%80%99-campaign-to-encourage-continued-COVID-testing,-contact-tracing.aspx.

Merrill, Jacqueline, Suzanne Bakken, Maxine Rockoff, Kristine Gebbie, and Kathleen M. Carley. 2007. "Description of a Method to Support Public Health Information Management: Organizational Network Analysis." *Journal of Biomedical Informatics* 40, no. 4 (August): 422–28. https://doi.org/10.1016/j.jbi.2006.09.004.

Midgley, Gerald. 2006. "Systemic Intervention for Public Health." *American Journal of Public Health* 96, no. 3 (March): 466–72. https://doi.org/10.2105/AJPH.2005.067660.

NFID (National Foundation for Infectious Disease). 2021. National Foundation for Infectious Disease. https://www.nfid.org.

Oppenheimer, Gerald M. 2010. "Framingham Heart Study: The First 20 Years." *Progress in Cardiovascular Diseases* 53, no. 1 (July–August): 55–61. https://doi.org/10.1016/j.pcad.2010.03.003.

Pagkas-Bather, Jade, Lindsay E. Young, Yen-Tyng Chen, and John A. Schneider. 2020. "Social Network Interventions for HIV Transmission Elimination." *Current HIV/AIDS Reports* 17, no. 5: 450–57. https://doi.org/10.1007/s11904-020 -00524-z.

Pivnick, Anitra, Audrey Jacobson, Kathleen Eric, Lynda Doll, and Ernest Drucker. 1994. "AIDS, HIV Infection, and Illicit Drug Use within Inner-City Families and Social Networks." *American Journal of Public Health* 84, no. 2 (February): 271–74. https://doi.org/10.2105/ajph.84.2.271.

Quinn, Katharine G. 2020. "Applying the Popular Opinion Leader Intervention for HIV to COVID-19." *AIDS and Behavior* 24, no. 12: 3291–94. https://doi.org/10 .1007/s10461-020-02954-7.

Ragonnet-Cronin, Manon, Nanette Benbow, Christina Hayford, Kathleen Poortinga, Fangchao Ma, Lisa A. Forgione, Zhijuan Sheng, Yunyin W. Hu, Lucia V. Torian, and Joel O. Wertheim. 2021. "Sorting by Race/Ethnicity across HIV Genetic Transmission Networks in Three Major Metropolitan Areas in the United States." *AIDS Research and Human Retroviruses* 37, no. 10: 784–92. https://doi.org/10.1089/aid.2020.0145.

Rice, Eric, Amanda Yoshioka-Maxwell, Robin Petering, Laura Onasch-Vera, Jaih Craddock, Milind Tambe, Amulya Yadav, Bryan Wilder, Darlene Woo, Hailey Winetrobe, and Nicole Wilson. 2018. "Piloting the Use of Artificial Intelligence to Enhance HIV Prevention Interventions for Youth Experiencing Homelessness." *Journal of the Society for Social Work and Research* 9, no. 4: 551–73. https:// doi.org/10.1086/701439.

Rogers, Everett M. 2010. *Diffusion of Innovations.* 4th ed. New York: Simon and Schuster.

Rothenberg, Richard B., John J. Potterat, Donald E. Woodhouse, Stephen Q. Muth, William W. Darrow, and Alden S. Klovdhal. 1998. "Social Network Dynamics and HIV Transmission." *AIDS* 12, no. 12: 1529–36. https://doi.org/10.1097 /00002030-199812000-00016.

Shearer, Jessica C., Michelle Dion, and John N. Lavis. 2014. "Exchanging and Using Research Evidence in Health Policy Networks: A Statistical Network Analysis." *Implementation Science* 9: article 126. https://doi.org/10.1186/s13012-014-0126-8.

Simmons-Duffin, Selena. 2021. "How a Gay Community Helped the CDC Spot a COVID Outbreak—And Learn More about Delta." National Public Radio, August 6, 2021. https://www.npr.org/sections/health-shots/2021/08/06/1025553638 /how-a-gay-community-helped-the-cdc-spot-a-covid-outbreak-and-learn-more -about-de.

Singer, Merrill. 1994. "AIDS and the Health Crisis of the U.S. Urban Poor: The Perspective of Critical Medical Anthropology." *Social Science & Medicine* 39, no. 7 (October): 931–48. https://doi.org/10.1016/0277-9536(94)90205-4.

Singer, Merrill, Nicola Bulled, Bayla Ostrach, and Emily Mendenhall. 2017. "Syndemics and the Biosocial Conception of Health." *Lancet* 389, no. 10072: 941–50. https://doi.org/10.1016/S0140-6736(17)30003-X.

Tsao, Connie W., and Ramachandran S. Vasan. 2015. "The Framingham Heart Study: Past, Present, and Future." *International Journal of Epidemiology* 44, no. 6 (December): 1763–66. https://doi.org/10.1093/ije/dyv336.

Valente, Thomas W. 2010. *Social Networks and Health: Models, Methods, and Applications*. New York: Oxford University Press.

Xu, Hanfei, Adrienne Cupples, Andrew Stokes, and Ching-Ti Liu. 2018. "Association of Obesity with Mortality over 24 Years of Weight History." *JAMA Network Open* 1, no. 7: e184587. https://doi.org/10.1001/jamanetworkopen.2018.4587.

Part 2

RISK COMMUNICATION

4

Social Media Content and Engagement Strategies during the COVID-19 Pandemic

A Risk Communication and Community Engagement Campaign
Targeting University Students in the United States

AGGREY WILLIS OTIENO, GHANEM AYED ELHERSH, AND LAEEQ KHAN

The significance of effective Risk Communication and Community Engagement (RCCE) strategies cannot be overstated as the world wrestles with the effects of the COVID-19 pandemic. Originating in Wuhan, China, in December 2019, the highly pathogenic coronavirus (CoV) following SARS-CoV-1 and MERS-CoV had led to over 660 million confirmed cases and 6 million deaths globally by the end of December 2022 (WHO 2022). These figures are still increasing every day as new COVID-19 variants emerge. A few weeks after its emergence, the causative agent was identified as a new coronavirus (2019-nCoV), and the disease was later named COVID-19 by the World Health Organization (Keni et al. 2020). The WHO officially declared the emergence of a new pandemic on March 11, 2020 (Huang et al. 2020). The first confirmed COVID-19 case in the United States was documented on January 19, 2020, in Snohomish County, Washington. It wasn't long before the US became the epicenter of COVID-19, as the number of reported cases surpassed those of any other country worldwide (Huang et al. 2020). At the time of this writing, over 103,436,829 infected individuals and more than 1 million deaths have been confirmed in the US (WHO, n.d.). Reported COVID-19 cases in the US account for 18% of global prevalence. This necessitated the adoption of major behavioral, clinical, and intervention policies aimed at mitigating the transmission and preventing the virus's persistence among humans globally (Huang et al. 2020).

As the number of deaths from COVID-19 continues to rise worldwide, it is becoming increasingly essential to understand RCCE tools and strategies used in mitigating the spread of the disease among at-risk populations (Dryhurst et al. 2020). From the reported COVID-19 cases, it was documented that the elderly, individuals with preexisting chronic health conditions, and those experiencing immune suppression were at higher risk of suffering from COVID-19–related morbidity and mortality (Thng et al. 2021). According to Thng and colleagues, individuals belonging to or having a particular gender, race, ethnicity, social position, education, class, physical and cognitive ability, sexual orientation, citizen status, and other stigmatized identities were more predisposed to experiencing adverse outcomes from COVID-19. This is because inequities rooted in fundamental social causes affect the ability of individuals and groups to implement recommended precautions such as handwashing, observing physical distancing, and accessing vaccines, with implications for increasing the risk and spread of COVID-19 transmission (Thng et al. 2021). Moreover, Thng and colleagues documented that the risk of exposure to COVID-19 is higher in crowded environments, such as jails and prisons, immigrant detention centers, refugee camps, homeless shelters, impoverished neighborhoods, naval ships, crowded workplaces, and learning institutions.

Early evidence indicated that younger populations were vulnerable to acquiring and transmitting COVID-19 but were less susceptible to adverse effects of COVID-19 in comparison to the adult population (Snape and Viner 2020; Morrow-Howell and Gonzales 2020). This perception was further buoyed by reports that younger individuals infected with COVID-19 mostly recovered from the disease (Morrow-Howell and Gonzales 2020). Students from higher learning institutions in the US mostly belonged to this age group. Due to the younger populations having low perceptions of being susceptible to COVID-19, there was low adherence to WHO regulations aimed at mitigating the spread of COVID-19 within this age group (Nivette et al. 2021). Therefore, the media was awash with reports of young individuals, primarily students, who held parties and other activities where social distancing was not observed. Since the institutions of higher learning acted as a bridge to households and communities, asymptomatic students had a higher possibility of experiencing viral shedding, which created a pool of viral circulation responsible for introducing the virus to the students' homes and beyond (Snape and Viner 2020).

University students, as a result, became transmitters of COVID-19 to other vulnerable populations, especially when they traveled back to their homes after the closure of learning institutions (CDC 2021). In addition, reports of COVID-19 outbreaks and hospitalization among children and teenagers indicated the importance of targeting the younger population with anti-COVID-19 messaging (Snape and Viner 2020). Moreover, targeting students from higher learning institutions is strategic, as they represent a unique subset of individuals at risk of COVID-19 that have more autonomy and pressing needs to live independently (CDC 2021). With over 77 million students attending various learning institutions in the US, out of which not less than 20 million are at the college level (US Census Bureau 2019), there is a manifold risk of increased COVID-19 infection. Therefore, educational institutions in the US became epicenters in combating the spread of COVID-19. Yet there is limited information on the online RCCE strategies used by institutions of higher learning and how they mitigated the spread of COVID-19. Even though anecdotal evidence indicates that RCCE is a critical pillar in adopting behavioral responses against the spread of epidemics, little is known about the aspects of the online RCCE techniques that elicited significant engagement from the online target audience in the context of the COVID-19 pandemic.

To alleviate the spread of COVID-19 among university students, a sizable midwestern university established a special COVID-19 operations task force that was active in disseminating information to the general public to raise awareness of COVID-19 in terms of general knowledge, community updates, risk factors, and preventive measures. Drawing from the health communication campaign implemented by this university, we used the lens of RCCE to examine how it implemented a health communication campaign targeting university students during the ongoing COVID-19 pandemic. Specifically, we aimed to analyze the content and online engagement with the Instagram posts made by the university as part of its health communication campaign against COVID-19.

EPIDEMIOLOGY AND EFFECTS OF COVID-19

According to the Centers for Disease Control, COVID-19 is transmitted from one person to another when an individual breathes in a droplet containing the virus when they contact infected persons. Besides breathing in contaminated air particles through the mouth, individuals can also acquire the virus through their eyes and noses, including in situations where they touch contaminated surfaces and then use unclean hands to touch their mouths, eyes, or noses (CDC 2022). The CDC (2022) further documents that those closer than six feet from the infected person are most likely to get infected. The COVID-19 incubation period is mainly between two to fourteen days, and the most common symptoms are cough, fever, loss of taste, and shortness of breath (CDC 2022).

As viruses are prone to mutation, the emergence of new COVID-19 variants has been documented in various parts of the world (CDC 2022). By 2021, the CDC (2022) had confirmed five notable variants of COVID-19 worldwide: (a) B.1.1.7 (Alpha), popularly known as the United Kingdom variant; (b) B.1.351 (Beta), first detected in South Africa; (c) P.1 (Gamma), which originated in Brazil; (d) B.1.617.2 (Delta), initially identified in India, and (e) the B.1.1.529 variant (Omicron), which emerged in Botswana and was confirmed as a new variant by scientists in South Africa. Omicron became a variant of concern to the WHO and various governments, including that of the US. Even though the Delta variant spread more easily and quickly, leading to more morbidity and mortality worldwide, Omicron was more lethal than all the other four variants. This is because Omicron's genomic sequencing had an "extremely high number" of mutations that drove further waves of disease by evading individuals' immune systems (Malabadi et al. 2021).

As the medical community in various parts of the world raced to develop COVID-19 treatments and vaccines, ongoing government and community efforts were devoted mainly to early detection, prevention, and containment of the spread of the virus (Kashte et al. 2021). The most common prevention strategies recommended by the WHO are regular handwashing or hand sanitization, wearing face masks, and social distancing (Thng et al. 2021). The spread of COVID-19 has also been curtailed by aggressive COVID-19 testing campaigns, which ensured that infected individuals were identified and quarantined in good time, even before they became symptomatic (Keni et al. 2020). Though vaccines are available for emergency use, there is no known effective treatment for COVID-19 (WHO 2020). The most widely adopted intervention is to provide symptomatic management and supportive therapy to the infected individuals (CDC 2022). So far, the US Food and Drug Administration (FDA) has approved Johnson & Johnson, Moderna, and Pfizer-BioNTech COVID-19 vaccines for emergency use in the US (Center for Biologics Evaluation and Research, 2023). Protective behavior such as (a) frequent washing of hands for at least twenty seconds, (b) covering of mouths while sneezing or coughing, (c) disinfecting surfaces, (d) wearing of face masks, (e) observing social distancing, and (f) isolating oneself if in contact with infected individuals was found to be effective in combating the spread of COVID-19 (Keni et al. 2020). Regular symptomatic testing and getting COVID-19 vaccinations are highly recommended (Keni et al. 2020). Meanwhile, due to individual and group perceptions of low risk—locally and globally—adoption of recommended protective behaviors was and remains very slow. As a result, COVID-19 continued unabated and still does. This year's variants are relatively benign, as of this writing, but nothing in regard to pandemic is sure.

Besides the high mortality rates and morbidities resulting from COVID-19, the pandemic also sparked socioeconomic crises and recession across the world. Measures against the spread of COVID-19—that is, to prevent the spread of the virus, particularly to vulnerable individuals—had widespread socioeconomic implications. Social distancing, self-isolation, and travel restrictions have led to a reduced workforce across multiple economic areas (Nicola et al. 2020). To take one critical sector in a globalized economy for example, COVID-19 led to an immediate crash in demand for hotels and restaurants due to lockdowns, enforcement of social distancing measures, and fear of travel. The COVID-19 outbreak also dampened the demand for oil due to a price war that led to grave implications for the global economy (Nicola et al. 2020).

The education sector, from preschool to university, has also been affected by COVID-19. Different countries have introduced various policies, ranging from partial to complete closure of educational institutions (Yeshaswini 2020). According to UNESCO, close to 900 million students worldwide were affected by the closure of educational institutions (UNESCO 2021). Institutions across the globe placed field-based research in areas not related to the pandemic on hold. In some countries, funding for research, both related and not related to COVID-19, was suspended in order to allow clinically trained staff deployed to teach in institutions of higher learning to return to the front line (Nicola et al. 2020). Several scientific conferences were canceled or postponed (Yeshaswini 2020).

The specific mortality, morbidities, and socioeconomic effects of COVID-19 underscore the importance of sustained RCCE campaigns. People must be empowered to effectively adopt preventive measures, no matter how obvious: being vaccinated, going for COVID-19 and other tests, wearing facemasks, regular handwashing, covering one's mouth while coughing or sneezing, maintaining social distance, or self-isolating (Prasad Singh, Sewda, and Shiv 2020).

CONCEPTUAL FRAMEWORK

The ongoing COVID-19 pandemic has shown us that adoption of RCCE principles for health-protective behaviors is critical to breaking the COVID-19 and other transmission chains. This study adopted the online RCCE conceptual framework, as summarized in figure 4.1. The following section further investigates the relationship between the utilization of digital platforms in risk communication and virtual community engagement in the fight against COVID-19.

During disease outbreaks, especially in emerging pandemics such as COVID-19, public health communication specialists grapple with the challenge of designing and disseminating information about impending risks presented by an emerging disease while at the same time dealing with anxieties and misinformation experienced by affected individuals and the public at large. This underscores the importance of executing carefully planned health communication campaigns. The COVID-19 pandemic presented a global public health crisis that called for changes in communication strategies and collective responsibility from all global citizens. Consequently, the World Health Organization (WHO) in early 2020 recommended the utilization of RCCE strategies to prevent the spread of COVID-19. RCCE is a framework utilized by public health professionals to develop and execute a system for communicating risks by an organization or agency mandated to curtail the spread of diseases (Costantino and Fiacchini 2020). In addition, RCCE involves coordinated communication that targets internal and external stakeholders intending to implement strategic public communication and community engagement that leads to the management of existing uncertainties, false perceptions, and misinformation among vulnerable populations (Costantino and Fiacchini 2020).

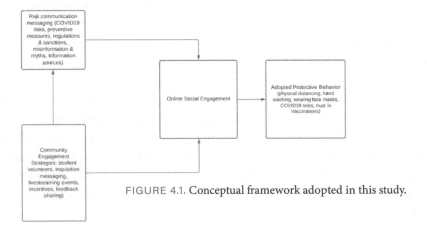

FIGURE 4.1. Conceptual framework adopted in this study.

As a global public health crisis, the COVID-19 pandemic has presented an environment where people are unprepared and do not possess adequate knowledge for dealing with uncertain circumstances (Timmis and Brüssow 2020). Several studies have documented the vital role played by RCCE in raising awareness about the existence of health threats such as the COVID-19 pandemic. Scholars such as Blanchard-Boehm (1998) argue that RCCE campaigns should be informative, flexible, and able to propagate the adoption of preventive and protective measures that mitigate both physical and psychological threats presented by diseases such as COVID-19. Prior research has explored how risk perception mediates the relationship between risk communication and adopting protective behavior against COVID-19, and how risk communication and risk perception have affected behavior change among students during the COVID-19 pandemic.

According to Fang et al. (2012), risk communication content conditioned by high degrees of trust can drive the target audience to comply with the recommended behavior change. Generally, risk communication enables individuals to perform the following actions: (a) consume warning messages; (b) figure out the related content; (c) trust the significance of the message; (d) evaluate the truth of provided explanations with other people; and (e) adopt actions or measures recommended in the disseminated risk communication messages to save lives and properties (Blanchard-Boehm 1998; Heydari et al. 2021). However, according to Blanchard-Boehm (1998), the level and type of risk communication depend on the complexity of the risk and level of potential risk, as well as risk perception held by the targeted populations.

Varghese et al. (2021) argue that risk communication is key to improving familiarity with and adherence to protective measures in normal times and during pandemics. They further contend that failure to communicate the right message effectively results in distrust, negative consequences to the economy, and loss of lives. In addition, for risk communication to be effective, it has been documented that risk messages have to be shared with the public in an open and timely manner, to reduce the knowledge gap and to convince the public to change their behavior during a pandemic (Varghese et al. 2021). In addition to disseminating recommendations that are easy for the public to understand and comply with, trust in the message's source is essential for effective risk communication (Fang et al. 2012). Available evidence indicates that risk communication leads to awareness of the nature, magnitude, and significance of existing risks to combat the transmission of diseases in the long term (Fang et al. 2012). Furthermore, through the communication of risks, individuals are not only aware but also able to adopt preventive and protective behavior changes necessary to alleviate the existing threat (Fang et al. 2012).

Strategic risk communication campaigns contribute to achieving the following deliverables: mitigating threats, information provision, enhancement of recovery, public relations, and generation of calls to action (Fang et al. 2012). Studies done by Fang et al. (2012) indicate that risk communication has helped reduce harm to the involved parties through different but credible communication channels. Moreover, during public health emergencies, such as the COVID-19 pandemic, a well-coordinated and efficient communications strategy helps stakeholders define risks, identify hazards, assess weaknesses, and promote community resilience, thereby increasing the capacity to cope with the global health challenge (Fang et al. 2012). However, there is a shortage of information about the content of risk communication messages disseminated by higher learning institutions to curb the spread of diseases such as COVID-19.

On the other hand, various studies have documented that the utilization of digital platforms in RCCE campaigns is vital in (a) reaching diverse audiences, (b) establishing interactive and ongoing community engagement, (c) facilitating public control and empowerment, and (e) increasing the likely impact or broadening the transmission of urgent public health communications (Abrams and Greenhawt 2020; Malik, Khan, and Quan-Haase 2021). This realization became essential as millions worldwide turned to digital platforms for work and social functions under pandemic conditions. With a rapidly growing segment of the global population living under government lockdown as part of COVID-19 mitigation, the demand for video conferencing apps such as Microsoft Teams, Google Hangouts, and Zoom surged worldwide (Nellis and Menn 2020). Meanwhile, a study conducted by Auxier (2021) documented that 72% of Americans had access to various media technologies such as Twitter, YouTube, and Facebook, while the use of Instagram, Snapchat, and TikTok was more prevalent among adults under thirty. Teenagers, such as those targeted in this study, are among the most active users of various media technologies (Prasad Singh, Sewda, and Shiv 2020).

Over the years, media technology and digital platforms such as Instagram have been handy tools for strategic health communication during a crisis like that presented by the COVID-19 pandemic (Bao et al. 2020). They provide an environment that enhances the sharing of global health information between public health specialists and their intended audiences (Strekalova 2017; Otieno et al. 2021). As much as various health communication scholars have documented the growing utilization of social media for health communication, little attention has been focused on adopting social media in advancing RCCE campaigns. Social media both carry distinct benefits and present unique health communication and education challenges. Analysis of social media content may enhance our understanding of the RCCE mechanisms, and feeds from digital platforms such as Instagram present evidence of how RCCE strategies can be adopted in mitigating the spread of diseases. According to the WHO (2020), community engagement strategies involve holding public health education events and providing support services to populations facing threats to their health and economic or social well-being. Various researchers have documented the importance of executing strategic community engagement over the years (Heydari et al. 2021). During avian influenza, SARS, and Ebola outbreaks, governments of the affected countries used community engagement strategies to coordinate and collaborate with other strategic stakeholders to mitigate potential health risks (Fang et al. 2012). Nevertheless, in the era of social distancing and lockdowns, where face-to-face community engagement is limited, little attention has been focused on understanding the online community engagement strategies used by health communication practitioners to mobilize and organize their target audience to adopt COVID-19 containment measures.

Media technologies, including social networking sites, have become essential in RCCE campaigns. As a result, engagement of the online audience with the content of social media campaigns is necessary for any RCCE intervention. The level of engagement of the target audience and their perception of the public health agency in charge of deploying RCCE can be observed through indicators like the number of likes, mentions, tags, replies, shares, and retweets in a dialogic communication (Ngai, Einwiller, and Singh 2020; Otieno et al. 2021). An online audience can be engaged on social media through comments and likes and co-creating additional messages while maintaining and reinforcing connections with other social media users on the same topic. A "like" indicates a target audience member's endorsement of what is being communicated, while sharing or retweeting a post requires more effort and is, therefore, a demonstration of higher engagement (Ngai, Einwiller, and Singh 2020). Previous studies have established that there are crucial drivers that health communication specialists need to consider for their health communication campaigns to elicit optimal online engagement by their target audience. Some of these include the usefulness of information to the target audience, culturally induced communication styles adopted by health communication practitioners, and the kind of images used on social media posts (Ngai, Einwiller, and Singh 2020).

Nevertheless, there is a scarcity of information about the factors that drive online engagement with social media content posted within the context of online RCCE interventions targeting university students during pandemics. We therefore utilized data from Instagram posts published by a large midwestern university in the US to answer the following three research questions:

- RQ1: What kind of online risk communication content from their university did students access during the COVID-19 pandemic?
- RQ2: Which online community engagement strategies did the university adopt in its efforts to curb COVID-19 transmission among students?
- RQ3: What kind of social media content elicited significant social engagement by the audience interacting with the online Risk Communication and Community Engagement campaign?

COLLECTION AND CONTENT ANALYSIS OF INSTAGRAM POSTS

To answer the above three research questions, in August 2021 we collected 456 Instagram posts from a large midwestern university's COVID-19 operations task force Instagram account. All the posts/images, associated captions, and metadata shared by the COVID-19 operations task force on Instagram from September 30, 2020, to August 12, 2021, were gathered and recorded in a spreadsheet. We developed a coding scheme to guide the systematic classification of Instagram posts. The coding scheme was tested by analyzing 50 Instagram posts that formed the base for coding scheme development, with agreement among the coders established through extensive discussions about various aspects of the coding. Cohen's Kappa reliability above 0.7 was realized by the coders in all the identified categories. Cohen's Kappa in this study was thus used as a measure of interrater reliability. This is because it's essential to test intercoder agreements in order to ensure that coding categories are clear and the final ratings are accurate and reliable (Rau and Yu-shan 2021).

Generally, content analysis was employed to scrutinize COVID-19 Instagram posts, and coding was performed on three main dimensions: image used, risk communication messaging, and community engagement strategies adopted. The images used were coded into image type, person portrayal, and gender depiction. The risk communication dimension was coded into five categories: risk and crisis information, addressing myths and misinformation, COVID-19 regulations and sanctions, recommended personal preventive measures, and utilization of authoritative health information sources in the Instagram posts. Community engagement was coded as live streaming of public health education events, provision of incentives, sharing contacts for feedback from the target audience, using inquisitive messaging, student involvement in the RCCE campaign, and updates about public health events.

Risk Communication Content

In assessing the content of these 452 Instagram posts, the coauthors of this study established five main categories of risk communication content. Most of the Instagram posts discussed risks associated with COVID-19 infections (70.4%), outlined preventive measures to be adopted by individuals (46.1%), and provided updates on new COVID-19 regulations and sanctions (25.9%). Only 4.9% of the Instagram posts addressed online misinformation and myths about COVID-19. Looking at the information provided, 58.2% of the Instagram posts included content from authoritative sources, such as state and university officials, with the mandate to curb the spread of COVID-19 within their respective spheres. In addition, many of the Instagram posts had infographic images (67.7%), and were animated (63.9%) with nonhuman beings (74.8%), as seen in table 4.1.

TABLE 4.1. CONTENT OF RISK COMMUNICATION MESSAGES POSTED ON INSTAGRAM

Categories	Reliabilities	Frequency and Percentage
		Type of images used
Image type	1.00	Photograph = 146 (32.2%)
		Infographic = 306 (67.7%)
Person portrayal	1.00	Frontline health worker – 18 (4%)
		Ordinary individual = 12 (2.7%)
		Student = 48 (10.6%)
		Government/state official = 8 (1.8%)
		University official = 6 (1.3%)
		Group images = 16 (3.5%)
		Animated images = 289 (63.9%)
		Images of nonhuman beings 55 (12.2%)
Gender	1.00	Male = 42 (9.3%)
		Female = 72 (15.9%)
		Nonhuman being = 338 (74.8%)
		Risk communication messaging
Risks and crisis information	0.922	No = 134 (29.6%)
		Yes = 318 (70.4%)
Addressing misinformation	1.00	No = 430 (95.1%)
		Yes = 22 (4.9%)
Provision of incentives	1.00	No = 398 (88.1%)
		Yes = 54 (11.9%)
Regulations and sanctions	1.00	No = 335 (74.1%)
		Yes = 117 (25.9%)
Personal preventive measures	1.00	No = 240 (53.1%)
		Yes = 212 (46.1%)
Authoritative information sources	0.917	No = 189 (41.8%)
		Yes = 263 (58.2%)

COMMUNITY ENGAGEMENT STRATEGIES

This study also aimed at determining the community engagement strategies deployed as part of the COVID-19 RCCE campaign. From the content analysis of Instagram posts, the most prominent community engagement strategies deployed to reach the students were: (a) the involvement of student volunteers such as campus ambassadors and public health liaisons in the health communication campaign (26.1%), (b) the use of inquisitive messaging techniques on Instagram posts (13.7%), (c) organizing of special offline events around campus such as COVID-19 vaccinations and asymptomatic testing (12.8%), (d) provision of incentives to students (such as providing some form of scholarships to vaccinated students) to encourage adoption of the recommended behavior (11.9%), (e) live streaming of health education events (9.3%), and (f) gathering and sharing feedback through calls, online surveys, and email communications (6.9%), as shown in table 4.2.

TABLE 4.2. ONLINE COMMUNITY ENGAGEMENT STRATEGIES DEPLOYED BY THE UNIVERSITY

Categories	Reliabilities	Frequency and percentage
Community engagement strategies		
Live streaming of events	1.00	No = 410 (90.7%) Yes = 42 (9.3%)
Sharing feedback	1.00	No = 421 (93.1%) Yes = 31 (6.9%)
Use of inquisitive messaging	0.852	No = 390 (86.3%) Yes = 62 (13.7%)
Involvement of student volunteers	1.00	No = 334 (73.9%) Yes = 118 (26.1%)
Events information	0.790	No = 394 (87.2%) Yes = 58 (12.8%)
Provision of incentives to students	1.00	No = 398 (88.1%) Yes = 54 (11.9%)

FACTORS THAT ELICITED SIGNIFICANT ENGAGEMENT BY THE ONLINE AUDIENCE

In addition, this study documented 7,080 likes on Instagram posts between September 30, 2020, and August 12, 2021. We transposed the total likes for each month from the beginning of the campaign, as shown in figure 4.2. The study showed a significant upward trend in attracting online engagement from those following the Instagram account. However, downward trends were witnessed in January and February 2021, before likes shot up again in March and April. The same upward trend was observed further in August 2021.

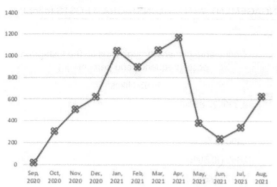

FIGURE 4.2. Time sequencing of online engagement.

There was, however, minimal two-way dialogic communication between the COVID-19 operations staff and their online audience, as there were very few comments generated by Instagram users who interacted with the posts made by the health communication campaign team. As a result, we determined the level of online engagement elicited by the RCCE campaign by only analyzing the number of likes made by the online audience vis-à-vis the type of images used, the content of the posts, and the kind of people portrayed on the Instagram posts, as summarized in table 4.3.

TABLE 4.3. TARGET AUDIENCE ENGAGEMENT WITH THE INSTAGRAM POSTS

Category	Online engagement through likes on the Instagram posts (frequency and percentage)
Image type	7,080 likes
Photograph	3,284 (46.38%)
Infographic	3,796 (58.62%)
Person portrayal	6,980 likes
Frontline health worker	407 (5.83%)
Ordinary individual	210 (3.01%)
Student	1,138 (16.30%)
Government/state official	155 (2.22%)
University official	204 (2.92%)
Group image (three or more people)	309 (4.43%)
Animated image	3,615 (51.79%)
Nonhuman being	942 (13.50%)
Gender depiction	7,080 likes
Male	1,016 (14.35%)
Female	1,571 (22.19%)
Nonhuman being	4,493 (63.46%)

TABLE 4.3. TARGET AUDIENCE ENGAGEMENT WITH THE INSTAGRAM POSTS (*cont.*)

Category	Online engagement through likes on the Instagram posts (frequency and percentage)
Risk communication messaging	15,650 likes*
Risks and crisis information	4,395 (28.08%)
Addressing myths and misinformation	323 (2.06%)
Provision of incentives for COVID-19	1,490 (9.52%)
Updates on new regulations	1,652 (10.56%)
Personal preventive measures to be adopted	4,312 (27.55%)
Authoritative information sources	3,478 (22.22%)
Community engagement strategies deployed	4,911 likes
Live streaming of events	494 (10.06%)
Sharing contacts for feedback	342 (6.96%)
Quizzes and soliciting feedback	854 (17.39%)
Involvement of student volunteers in the risk communication campaign	2,267 (46.16%)
Information about events/activities	954 (19.43%)

*The number of likes in this section is more than 7,080 because several Instagram posts had more than one category of risk communication messaging.

As shown in table 4.3, generally, social media posts with nonhuman beings (63.46%), specifically those with infographic images (58.62%), elicited significant engagement by the online audience. In addition, risk communication messages that had higher engagement were those that provided risks and crisis information (28.08%), recommended personal preventive measures to be adopted by the target audience (27.55%), and cited authoritative information sources (22.22%). On the other hand, community engagement strategies that attracted significant online engagement with the Instagram posts involved student volunteers in risk communication campaigns (46.16%), had information about anti-COVID-19 events/activities (19.43%), and featured quizzes or other solicitations of feedback from the online audience (17.39%).

DISCUSSION

This study aims to understand the deployment of Risk Communication and Community Engagement (RCCE) campaigns against the COVID-19 pandemic. Our research model is based on the understanding that innovative RCCE strategies are at the center of any effort influencing desired behavior change during global health pandemics. Due to the social distancing measures during the COVID-19 pandemic, at-risk populations relied heavily on digital platforms, mainly social media, to inform their level of risk perception and determine their degree of involvement with community engagement (Abrams and Greenhawt 2020). The availability of various digital platforms has provided health communication practitioners with the opportunity to deploy these platforms to conduct online RCCE interventions.

A considerable amount of the previous research in this field has been conducted following a disease outbreak to investigate the impact of risk communication on individuals' perceptions of risk. For example, a study on an outbreak in New York City of *Neisseria meningitidis* serogroup C infection among men who have sex with men employed RCCE strategies that led to multisectoral intervention and increased vaccine administration and curbed the outbreak (Kratz et al. 2015). RCCE was also used in Kenya to establish a tuberculosis clinical decision support system that enhanced aggressive case-finding and treatment of patients living with HIV/AIDS (Catalani et al. 2014). However, the present study was conducted in the real-time context of the COVID-19 outbreak.

This study advances our understanding of social media's online risk communication content during a pandemic. It unearths the online community engagement strategies one US university adopted in a public health crisis. The approaches documented here can be used by other academic institutions in other parts of the world still grappling with enforcing COVID-19 regulations, especially as the world struggles with new variants and waves of COVID-19 morbidity and mortality.

Through the findings of this study, it becomes further evident that digital platforms such as Instagram play a vital role in enhancing virtual community engagement in the mitigation of pandemics. Through the content analysis of Instagram posts, we established that the involvement of campus ambassadors and public health liaisons attracted higher engagement by the targeted audience. Inquisitive messages also generated significant attention. This is in line with the public engagement model for social media communication described by Khan et al. (2021), which highlighted three key factors that promote online public engagement: self-disclosure, positive attitude, and inquisitiveness. In addition, this study found that infographics and animated images grabbed greater attention on Instagram. This is in line with an investigation by Malik, Khan, and Quan-Haase (2021), which revealed that infographics could be an engaging way to convey health-related messages on social media.

Even though RCCE has primarily been utilized to study and execute offline interventions, this study contributes to the expanding literature that shows RCCE is a practical framework for analyzing risk communication and online community engagement during pandemics. Capabilities provided by social media technology thus offer opportunities for innovative health communication campaigns that can trigger offline activities like the ones documented in this study. There were, however, minimal online interactions in terms of likes and user-generated content under the Instagram comment section. The campaign, therefore, missed opportunities to enhance online engagement by taking advantage of the audience as secondary sources of information through the health communication campaign's Instagram account. Scholars such as Otieno et al. (2021), Khan et al. (2021), and Heydari et al. (2021) have documented the importance of enhanced online engagement. According to these scholars, dialogic engagement between health communication professionals and their online audience is a crucial metric in measuring the success of online health communication campaigns. As Khan et al. (2021) argued, posting a humorous message for followers creates impressions of reciprocity and recognition that help harness their willingness to stay engaged. Moreover, the number of retweets, likes, comments, and shares a social media post generates is an indicator of what the targeted population thinks about the posted health information and thus in turn functions as a cue to draw people's attention and increase perceptions of message credibility (Heydari et al. 2021; Otieno et al. 2021).

Nevertheless, some practical implications can be gleaned from this exploratory study regarding audience engagement behavior. First, this study's drop in online engagement indicates lower audience attention and involvement when the university is in recess. Specifically, this behavior suggests that online audiences are only active when learning activities are ongoing. The targeted audience shifted their attention to other modes of communication that address issues affecting them in their immediate environment beyond their universities. Second, a more significant number of likes were observed on Instagram posts when people in close proximity to the targeted audience, such as fellow students, were deployed to be part of the campaign and their images were used as part of the social media posts. In other circumstances, posts mentioning student volunteers and those who had won prizes offered as incentives for participating in COVID-19 tests or vaccination pathways also attracted significant online engagement. This finding provides empirical evidence that the involvement of authoritative figures and popular local stakeholders, by either mentioning or tagging them on social media posts, contribute to the broader dissemination of risk communication messages and more community engagement in the health promotion initiative. Third, the engagement behavior of the target audience changes as the health communication practitioners change the type of health messages they disseminate. This was observed in messages with personal incentives attracting more likes from Instagram users. This means that messages used in risk communication could significantly enhance online engagement. For example, risk communication messages could include a call to action and sharing of social media posts by those who have been tagged online. Since the degree of online community engagement depends on the topic, health communication practitioners can achieve more outreach and online engagement based on their choice of message content.

Even though this study has theoretical and practical implications, it also has some limitations. First, the data analyzed in this study are only from one health communication campaign. Reviewing several RCCE online campaigns can provide a more illuminating data set, analysis, and recommendations. Second, we only performed content analysis on one social media platform. Analysis of data from more than one platform and utilizing several social media analytic approaches would provide a more in-depth evaluation of user engagement and reactions to RCCE campaigns and provide more insights into the effectiveness of RCCE strategies used by public health communication practitioners. Third, this study did not capture user metadata, such as demographics. These factors could have provided more information on user engagement with online RCCE interventions.

Informed by the findings of this study, we recommend further research to understand the impact of various digital platforms on adopting protective behavior. Specifically, research that delves into other factors besides Risk Communication and Community Engagement would be helpful. Still, findings from this study serve as a foundation for informing further theory development and empirical research to understand the effects of social and behavioral change communication on individuals across different demographics and regions. Such future endeavors can inform potential strategies and policy shifts to mitigate adverse consequences of global health epidemics and pandemics. Our study's findings can also have possible implications for the better design of online and offline RCCE interventions.

KEY TAKEAWAYS

1. Social media messaging via Instagram can be influential in garnering user engagement.

2. Social media messaging strategies should include more content about dispelling myths and misinformation about COVID-19.

3. Authoritative information sources such as posts by university administrators are especially vital in spreading messages related to health.

4. Infographics and animated images grab greater attention on social media and are thus more useful in spreading health-related messages.

5. A mix of active communication strategies focused on strategic health messaging that is inquisitive in nature can be highly engaging.

6. Deploying student volunteers such as public health liaisons leads to more participatory and sustainable public health campaigns targeting students.

DISCUSSION QUESTIONS

• How would you design your campaign if you were tasked with creating a Risk Communication and Community Engagement campaign against COVID-19 targeting students from higher learning institutions?

• What would you do the same or different from the campaign documented in this study, and why?

REFERENCES

Abrams, Elissa M., and Matthew Greenhawt. 2020. "Risk Communication during COVID-19." *In Practice: The Journal of Allergy and Clinical Immunology* 8, no. 6 (June): 1791–94. https://doi.org/10.1016/j.jaip.2020.04.012.
Auxier, Brooke. 2021. "Social Media Use in 2021." Pew Research Center, April 7, 2021. https://www.pewresearch.org/internet/2021/04/07/social-media-use-in -2021/.

Bao, Huanyu, Bolin Cao, Yuan Xiong, and Weiming Tang. 2020. "Digital Media's Role in the COVID-19 Pandemic." *JMIR mHealth and uHealth* 8, no. 9 (September). https://doi.org/10.2196/20156.

Blanchard-Boehm, R. Denise. 1998. "Understanding Public Response to Increased Risk from Natural Hazards: Application of the Hazards Risk Communication Framework." *International Journal of Mass Emergencies and Disasters* 16, no. 3 (November): 247–78. https://doi.org/10.1177/028072709801600302.

Catalani, Caricia, Eric Green, Philip Owiti, Aggrey Keny, Lameck Diero, Ada Yeung, Dennis Israelski, and Paul Biondich. 2014. "A Clinical Decision Support System for Integrating Tuberculosis and HIV Care in Kenya: A Human-Centered Design Approach." *PLOS ONE* 9, no. 8 (August): e103205. https://doi.org/10.1371/journal.pone.0103205.

CDC (Centers for Disease Control and Prevention). 2022. "Covid Data Tracker." US Department of Health and Human Services, CDC. https://covid.cdc.gov/covid-data-tracker/#datatracker-home.

Center for Biologics Evaluation and Research. 2023. "COVID-19 Vaccines for 2023–2024." US Food and Drug Administration. Last modified October 4, 2023. https://www.fda.gov/emergency-preparedness-and-response/coronavirus-disease-2019-covid-19/covid-19-vaccines-2023-2024.

Costantino, Claudio, and Daniel Fiacchini. 2020. "Rationale of the WHO Document on Risk Communication and Community Engagement (RCCE) Readiness and Response to the Severe Acute Respiratory Syndrome Coronavirus 2 (SARS-CoV-2) and of the Italian Decalogue for Prevention Departments." *Journal of Preventive Medicine and Hygiene* 61, no. 1 (March): e1–e2. https://doi.org/10.15167/2421-4248/JPMH2020.61.1.1502.

Dryhurst, Sarah, Claudia R. Schneider, John Kerr, Alexandra L. J. Freeman, Gabriel Recchia, Anne Marthe van der Bles, David Spiegelhalter, and Sander van der Linden. 2020. "Risk Perceptions of COVID-19 around the World." *Journal of Risk Research* 23, no. 7–8: 994–1006. https://doi.org/10.1080/13669877.2020.1758193.

Fang, David, Chen-Ling Fang, Bi-Kun Tsai, Li-Chi Lan, and Wen-Shan Hsu. 2012. "Relationships among Trust in Messages, Risk Perception, and Risk Reduction Preferences Based upon Avian Influenza in Taiwan." *International Journal of Environmental Research and Public Health* 9, no. 8: 2742–57. https://doi.org/10.3390/ijerph9082742.

Heydari, S. T., L. Zarei, A. K. Sadati, N. Moradi, M. Akbari, G. Mehralian, and K. B. Lankarani. 2021. "The Effect of Risk Communication on Preventive and Protective Behaviors during the COVID-19 Outbreak: Mediating Role of Risk Perception." BMC Public Health 21, article no. 54 (January 6). https://doi.org/10.1186/s12889-020-10125-5.

Huang, Xiao, Zhenlong Li, Yuqin Jiang, Xiaoming Li, and Dwayne Porter. 2020. "Twitter Reveals Human Mobility Dynamics during the COVID-19 Pandemic." *PLOS ONE* 15, no. 11 (November): e0241957. https://doi.org/10.1371/journal.pone.0241957.

Kashte, S., A. Gulbake, S. F. El-Amin III, and A. Gupta. 2021. "COVID-19 Vaccines: Rapid Development, Implications, Challenges and Future Prospects." *Human Cell* 34, no. 3: 711–33. https://doi.org/10.1007/s13577-021-00512-4.

Keni, Raghuvir, Anila Alexander, Pawan Ganesh Nayak, Jayesh Mudgal, and Krishnadas Nandakumar. 2020. "COVID-19: Emergence, Spread, Possible Treatments, and Global Burden." *Frontiers in Public Health* 8, no. 216 (May). https://doi.org/10.3389/fpubh.2020.00216.

Khan, M. Laeeq, Muhammad Ittefaq, Yadira Ixchel Martínez Pantoja, Muhammad Mustafa Raziq, and Aqdas Malik. 2021. "Public Engagement Model to Analyze Digital Diplomacy on Twitter: A Social Media Analytics Framework." *International Journal of Communication* 15: 1741–69.

Kratz, Molly M., Don Weiss, Alison Ridpath, Jane R. Zucker, Anita Geevarughese, Jennifer L. Rakeman, and Jay K. Varma. 2015. "Community-Based Outbreak of *Neisseria meningitidis* Serogroup C Infection in Men Who Have Sex with Men, New York City, New York, USA, 2010–2013." *Emerging Infectious Diseases* 21, no. 8 (August): 1379–86. https://doi.org/10.3201/eid2108.141837.

Liu, Jie, Wanli Xie, Yanting Wang, Yue Xiong, Shiqiang Chen, Jingjing Han, and Qingping Wu. 2020. "A Comparative Overview of COVID-19, MERS and SARS: Review Article." *International Journal of Surgery* 81:1–8. https://doi.org/10.1016/j.ijsu.2020.07.032.

Malabadi, Ravindra B., Kiran P. Kolkar, Neelambika T. Meti, and Raju K. Chalannavar. 2021. "Outbreak of Coronavirus (SARS-CoV-2) Delta Variant (B.1.617.2) and Delta Plus (AY.1) with Fungal Infections, Mucormycosis: Herbal Medicine Treatment." *International Journal of Research and Scientific Innovation* 8, no. 6 (June): 59–70. https://doi.org/10.51244/IJRSI.2021.8603.

Malik, Aqdas, M. Laeeq Khan, Anabel Quan-Haase. 2021. "Public Health Agencies Outreach through Instagram during the COVID-19 Pandemic: Crisis and Emergency Risk Communication Perspective." *International Journal of Disaster Risk Reduction* 61 (July). https://doi.org/10.1016/j.ijdrr.2021.102346.

Morrow-Howell, Nancy, and Ernest Gonzales. 2020. "Recovering from Coronavirus Disease 2019 (COVID-19): Resisting Ageism and Recommitting to a Productive Aging Perspective." *Public Policy & Aging Report* 30, no. 4: 133–37. https://doi.org/10.1093/ppar/praa021.

Nellis, Stephen, and Joseph Menn. 2020. "Demand for Video Calling Continues to Surge, Microsoft and Others Say." Reuters, April 9, 2020. https://www.reuters.com/article/us-health-coronavirus-software-idUSKCN21R2oP/.

Ngai, Cindy Sing Bik, Sabine Einwiller, and Rita Gill Singh. 2020. "An Exploratory Study on Content and Style as Driving Factors Facilitating Dialogic Communication between Corporations and Publics on Social Media in China." *Public Relations Review* 46, no. 1 (March): 1–11. https://doi.org/10.1016/j.pubrev.2019.101813.

Nicola, Maria, Zaid Alsafi, Catrin Sohrabi, Ahmed Kerwan, Ahmed Al-Jabir, Christos Iosifidis, Maliha Agha, and Riaz Agha. 2020. "The Socio-economic Implications of the Coronavirus Pandemic (COVID-19): A Review." *International Journal of Surgery* 78 (June): 185–93. https://doi.org/10.1016/j.ijsu.2020.04.018.

Nivette, Amy, Denis Ribeaud, Aja Murray, Annekatrin Steinhoff, Laura Bechtiger, Urs Hepp, Lilly Shanahan, and Manuel Eisner. 2021. "Non-compliance with

COVID-19–Related Public Health Measures among Young Adults in Switzerland: Insights from a Longitudinal Cohort Study." *Social Science & Medicine* 268:1–9. https://doi.org/10.1016/j.socscimed.2020.113370.

Otieno, A. W., J. Roark, M. L. Khan, S. Pant, M. J. Grijalva, and Scott Titsworth. 2021. "The Kiss of Death—Unearthing Conversations Surrounding Chagas Disease on YouTube." *Cogent Social Sciences* 7, no. 1. https://doi.org/10.1080/23311886.2020.1858561.

Prasad Singh, Jagajeet, Anshuman Sewda, and Dutt Gupta Shiv. 2020. "Assessing the Knowledge, Attitude and Practices of Students Regarding the COVID-19 Pandemic." *Journal of Health Management* 22, no. 2: 281–90. https://doi.org/10.1177/0972063420935669.

Rau, Gerald, and Yu-Shan Shih. 2021. "Evaluation of Cohen's Kappa and Other Measures of Inter-rater Agreement for Genre Analysis and Other Nominal Data." *Journal of English for Academic Purposes* 53:101026. https://doi.org/10.1016/j.jeap.2021.101026.

Snape, Matthew D., and Russell M. Viner. 2020. "COVID-19 in Children and Young People." *Science* 370, no. 6514: 286–88. https://doi.org/10.1126/science.abd6165.

Strekalova, Yulia A. 2017. "Health Risk Information Engagement and Amplification on Social Media: News about an Emerging Pandemic on Facebook." *Health Education & Behavior* 44, no. 2: 332–39. https://doi.org/10.1177/1090198116660310.

Thng, Zheng Xian, Marc D. De Smet, Cecilia S. Lee, Vishali Gupta, Justine R. Smith, Peter J. McCluskey, Jennifer E. Thorne, John H. Kempen, Manfred Zierhut, Quan Dong Nguyen, Carlos Pavesio, and Rupesh Agrawal. 2021. "COVID-19 and Immunosuppression: A Review of Current Clinical Experiences and Implications for Ophthalmology Patients Taking Immunosuppressive Drugs." *British Journal of Ophthalmology* 105, no. 3 (March): 306–10. https://doi.org/10.1136/bjophthalmol-2020-316586.

Timmis, Kenneth, and Harald Brüssow. 2020. "The COVID-19 Pandemic: Some Lessons Learned about Crisis Preparedness and Management, and the Need for International Benchmarking to Reduce Deficits." *Environmental Microbiology* 22, no. 6: 1986–96. https://doi.org/10.1111/1462-2920.15029.

UNESCO. 2021. "One Year into COVID-19 Education Disruption: Where Do We Stand?" UNESCO.org, March 19, 2021. https://www.unesco.org/en/articles/one-year-covid-19-education-disruption-where-do-we-stand.

US Census Bureau. 2019. "Census Bureau Reports Nearly 77 Million Students Enrolled in U.S. Schools." Census.gov, December 3, 2019. https://www.census.gov/newsroom/press-releases/2019/school-enrollment.html.

Varghese, Nirosha Elsem, Iryna Sabat, Sebastian Neumann-Böhme, Jonas Schreyögg, Tom Stargardt, Aleksandra Torbica, Job van Exel, Pedro Pita Barros, and Werner Brouwer. 2021. "Risk Communication during COVID-19: A Descriptive Study on Familiarity with, Adherence to and Trust in the WHO Preventive Measures." *PLOS ONE* 16, no. 4: 1–15. https://doi.org/10.1371/journal.pone.0250872.

WHO (World Health Organization). 2020. "Coronavirus Disease (COVID-19): Situation Report—107." World Health Organization. https://www.who.int

/docs/default-source/coronaviruse/situation-reports/20200506covid-19
-sitrep-107.pdf.

———. 2022. "WHO Coronavirus (COVID-19) Dashboard." World Health Organization. Last modified July 5, 2023. https://covid19.who.int/.

———. n.d. "United States of America: WHO Coronavirus Disease (Covid-19) Dashboard with Vaccination Data." World Health Organization. Accessed 2023. https://covid19.who.int/region/amro/country/us.

Yeshaswini, B. N. 2020. "Closure of Educational Institutions due to Covid-19: Study on Higher Education Students." *M S Ramaiah Management Review* 11, no. 2 (July–December): 28–35. https://doi.org/10.52184/msrmr.v11i02.31.

5

Facts and Faith Fridays

An Example of a Faith Community and Cancer Center's Revival
against COVID-19 Misinformation

KATHERINE Y. TOSSAS, ARNETHEA L. SUTTON, MARIA D. THOMSON,
MAGHBOEBA MOSAVEL, JESSICA GOKEE LAROSE, ELIZABETH
PROM-WORMLEY, TREMAYNE ROBERTSON, VANESSA B. SHEPPARD,
RUDENE HAYNES, F. TODD GRAY, AND ROBERT A. WINN

This chapter discusses the development, relevance, and impact of an academic partnership with a faith-based community, which partnership was formed at the onset of the COVID-19 pandemic—a time when faith and community leaders were seeking trustworthy, evidence-based, up-to-date information directly from a reliable source to keep their congregations and communities safe. We describe how the Facts and Faith Friday movement started and how it evolved, from the perspective of the moment in time, the people, the platform, the resources/networks, and the impact. We discuss its attributes within the context of the Community-Engaged Research and the Risk Communication frameworks. We end with some reflections on its policy impact, replicability, scalability, pitfalls, longevity, and future directions.

THE MOMENT IN TIME (*KAIROS*)

On March 11, 2020, the World Health Organization declared the COVID-19 outbreak a global pandemic. Two days later, the execution of a no-knock warrant based on unverified information (misinformation) claimed the life of Breonna Taylor, a 26-year-old African American emergency medical technician in Louisville, Kentucky. By the end of May, the disproportionate loss of African American (Black) and Hispanic/Latinx (Brown) bodies to both COVID-19 and law enforcement, most prominently the life of George Floyd, would lead to countrywide demonstrations, protests, and riots (Tate, Jenkins, and Rich 2021). These events, amidst a presidential administration with a chaotic pattern framed as "transactional federalism" (Bowling, Fisk, and Morris 2020; Mude et al. 2021), would fuel misinformation, medical mistrust, and general sociopolitical and racial unrest nationally.

In Richmond, Virginia, known once as the capital of the Confederacy, this unrest manifested no differently than in other places. Amidst what some called a triple pandemic of COVID-19, anti-Black violence, and digital capitalism, 14 of the initial 15 COVID-19 deaths in the city were Blacks (Eller 2020; Ziarek 2020). In fact, between February 16 and June 28, 2020, COVID-19 cases were far greater among Black and Brown residents (235 and 364 per 100,000, respectively) compared to White residents (80 per 100,000). Between March and June 2020, there were 1,024 Black and 1,190 Brown emergency department visits per 100,000 residents compared to 512 per 100,000 among White residents in the Richmond region (Virginia Department of Health 2020). Among the initial Black victims of COVID-19 was the prominent bishop Gerald Glenn (Kesslen 2020). His death was a foreboding that COVID-19 was a health crisis far more serious than previously experienced in our lifetime.

In a Richmond-area COVID-19 needs assessment survey conducted between August 4 and November 11, 2020, half (50%) of respondents expressed a need to learn about available resources should they become infected with COVID-19. This need was greater among non-White participants (i.e., Black, Brown, and Asian participants, 59%) compared to White participants (47%). Similarly, 15% of non-White participants and 9% of White participants felt they needed a COVID-19 test (Prom-Wormley et al. 2020). These trends emphasized a need for more knowledge and connection to COVID-19 resources and support across the Richmond region, particularly to reduce the burden of COVID-19 in underserved racial/ethnic minority communities. With so many questions percolating from the medical, scientific, secular, and religious communities, there was a need for an open forum to voice community concerns about COVID-19 in real time. Like other communities, Richmond needed a coordinated, comprehensive, and community-centered response.

Pastor F. Todd Gray would best describe this moment in time as *kairos*—a Greek word meaning the right, critical, or opportune moment, with the appropriate tone, structure, and time—a decisive moment when conditions are right for the accomplishment of a crucial action. More concisely, he summarizes it as "God's time." This kairotic time led a pastor, an attorney, and a doctor to form an alliance through dialogue and a passion for service that came to be known as "Facts and Faith Fridays" (FFF). Facts referred to the credible, timely and evidence-based information shared directly from the scientific community. Faith referred to the participation and leadership from the local Black churches, historically known as trusted institutions and safe hubs for community organizing, information dissemination, and propelling the civil rights movement (Gadzekpo 1997). Friday was considered an ideal day, chosen by the co-leaders, that provided a sense of closing the week with timely, fact-based information that could be shared with congregations over the upcoming week. Pastor Gray summed up the need for this partnership nicely: "At the beginning of the [COVID-19] pandemic, we were kind of guessing and getting information from anywhere, so to have a real-time connection to medical information from a trustworthy source was important."

Faith leaders in Richmond wanted to understand and act on the rapidly evolving data and public health safety recommendations related to COVID-19 by receiving summaries of research results, having discussions with public health leaders, answering questions from congregants and lay leaders, and being connected/directed to appropriate resources. Some of the FFF participants were familiar with Virginia Commonwealth University (VCU) through previous faith-based, community-facing partnerships (Prom-Wormley et al. 2020). However, engagement challenges before COVID-19 included issues related to any one church having the capacity to serve as a convening organization across a collaborative. The COVID-19 pandemic provided a new opportunity for faith-based organizations to re-explore collaborations under the mutually beneficial, common goal of learning about multiple aspects of COVID-19, including epidemiology, symptoms, treatments, vaccines, etiology, and public health prevention strategies, as requested by faith-based leaders. According to attorney Rudene Haynes, "it was relevant. We learned terms like *positivity rate, IRR, COVID testing reliability,* the difference between *effectiveness* and *efficacy.* We then broadened the conversation to start talking about social justice issues: how to protest safely, how to safely transition to bring people back to church, talked sensible sanitation protocols to make people safe. We also brought a series of doctors to talk about what happens if you are in the hospital with COVID. . . . We've covered everything under the sun related to COVID."

THE PEOPLE

The leaders: The FFF started with a simple conversation between a pastor, a lawyer, and a doctor in response to a real-life crisis—a global pandemic that was ravaging Black and Brown communities in Virginia. Importantly, all three individuals were Black, trusted community leaders, and known for their commitment to health equity. These individuals had "street credibility" among diverse groups of people throughout Richmond and had established connections with local and national stakeholders. Dr. Robert Winn was, at the time, the only Black director of a cancer center—the Virginia Commonwealth University Massey Comprehensive Cancer Center (MCCC)—designated by the National Cancer Institute. Rudene Haynes, a prominent attorney, wife to a faith leader, active Richmond community leader, and a member of the MCCC Advisory Board, thought it crucial to introduce him to members of the Black faith community, beginning with Pastor F. Todd Gray from the historic Fifth Street Baptist Church.

The participants: The conversation naturally moved toward the pandemic and how it was wreaking havoc in the congregations and the community. This led to a genuine offer by Dr. Winn to be a resource, providing updated information about COVID-19 and addressing questions/concerns from the Black community, with attorney Haynes and Rev. Gray as co-leaders and conveners. The initial target audience included faith-based leaders of Black churches in the Richmond area and surrounding communities. The original core group were faith leaders from approximately twenty-six churches, representing over 21,000 congregants (figure 5.1).

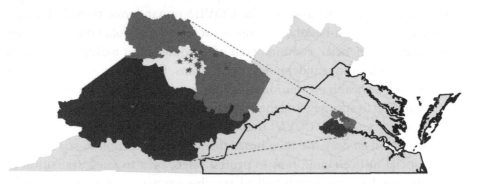

FIGURE 5.1. Map of the initial twenty-six "Facts and Faith Fridays" participating Black churches across five Virginia localities (Richmond City, Henrico County, Chesterfield County, Brunswick County, and James City). The bolded black line on the map represents the VCU Massey Cancer Center Catchment Area.

FFF attendance began to increase and diversify, based on needs and requests specifically raised by the Black faith leaders and the co-organizers. What once involved faith leaders, attorney Haynes, Dr. Winn, and a few MCCC leaders evolved to include other MCCC members and staff, leaders of the affiliated health system, and VCU faculty and staff, in addition to individuals and organizations active in the greater Richmond community. Many individuals who work in community outreach and engagement, both at the university and health system levels, participated in FFF to take information back to their respective communities. Organizers encouraged others to join. The number of participants in any given week ranged from 35 to 150. Participation fluctuated depending on the perceived relevance of the topics to individual participants and their availability. The maximum number of participants to date was approximately 12,000, which occurred when Dr. Anthony Fauci, then director of the NIH's National Institute of Allergy and Infectious Diseases, spoke to the group.

Other FFF presenters have included the First Lady of the United States; a US congressman; local elected officials; gubernatorial candidates Terry McAuliffe and Glenn Youngkin; US senators; Virginia General Assembly members; a superintendent of schools; and NIH, FDA, and CDC leaders.

THE PLATFORM

From phone to Zoom: FFF began as a three-way cellular phone call, progressed to a conference call, and evolved into a video conference (Zoom) call, mimicking the normalization of Zoom throughout the pandemic. Phone calls were the initial preferred method for faith leaders, as many of them, at the time, were unfamiliar with Zoom or did not know how to use it. The calls offered an intimate foundation for building trust and camaraderie. As time progressed, faith leaders were open to bringing more individuals to the calls because there was already a level of trust, community, and partnership cultivated in the early stages of FFF.

A platform to exchange reliable information/concerns in near–real time: FFF gave Black faith leaders a platform to ask questions and exchange information directly with thought leaders in medicine, implementation science, and advocacy. There was a direct exchange between decision-makers and faith leaders, which allowed faith leaders to receive credible, fact-based information directly from expert sources. Additionally, decision-makers received direct feedback from faith leaders, providing the opportunity to have real-time influence on identifying critical decisions in the war on COVID-19, including the timing of reopening facilities and vaccine prioritization.

The church as a platform to amplify a message and align faith and science: Historically, churches have been considered trusted social anchors, especially during precarious times when government trust is low (Clopton and Finch 2011). Early in the COVID-19 pandemic, due to the recognition of the constitutionally protected rights of religious freedom, churches were the only anchor institutions that remained open when other anchor institutions (e.g., schools, libraries, and local businesses) were closed. As such, centering the faith leaders within the FFF conversations was crucial to combating misinformation within Black and Brown communities. By creating a safe space and direct access to leading medical and public health experts, FFF equipped faith leaders with trustworthy information and resources to share with their congregants and others in their network. Consequently, FFF participants became amplifiers of the most up-to-date evidence and would come to exemplify how facts and science can be allies of faith.

THE RESOURCES/NETWORKS

Guidance for accessing additional support was also shared during these discussions. For example, the institution facilitated access to resources, infrastructure, and networks. MCCC leveraged established community-engaged efforts to provide and coordinate the conference (and later Zoom) calls, helped create electronic flyers to spread the word about the FFF discussions, and provided administrative support for organizing the calendar of speakers. MCCC and VCU also leveraged their relationships with local, state, and national thought leaders / decision-makers. At the same time, faith community partners augmented the partnership by leveraging their extensive local network of civic and legislative leaders and directed the topics discussed to ensure they were responsive to the everyday concerns of their congregants and communities.

THE IMPACT

FFF topic areas focused on COVID-19 included (a) addressing questions about how to mitigate the spread of COVID-19, (b) evolving CDC guidelines, (c) the testing and development of vaccines, (d) myths about the spread of COVID-19, (e) COVID-19 safety precautions while protesting, and (f) vaccine hesitancy and access. These discussions were empowering to the Black faith congregations as they facilitated bidirectional sharing of information. Conversations expanded from COVID-19 to address other issues, including ones having to do with social/racial justice. For example, there were conversations regarding wealth, health, and income disparities, housing and food insecurities, as well as discussions with leaders and political candidates regarding their aims for serving the people of Virginia with a particular focus on vulnerable communities.

To date, FFF has had a profound impact in numerous ways. First, *increased knowledge and informed decision-making:* FFF offered a space where faith leaders could learn about, discuss, interpret, and contextualize the latest science and public health guidance related to COVID-19, which helped them make appropriate decisions related to church activities and positively impact knowledge in their communities at large. Specifically, FFF members learned early on about the different COVID-19 tests (PCR versus antigen tests), the timing of each test with respect to exposure, where tests could be obtained, and quarantine and social distancing protocols. Second, *policy impacts:* Upon learning about the enduring and disproportionately high COVID-19 rates in the Black and Latinx communities, FFF members authored a petition to then-governor Ralph Northam, requesting a delay in reopening Richmond as part of the Forward Virginia initiative, until COVID-19 rates were lower, specifically in the Black and Latinx communities. They also met with the director of the Virginia Department of Health and advocated to be considered essential workers and prioritized for vaccination. In their role as faith leaders, they played a crucial role in visiting the sick and dying and learning firsthand about the impact of COVID-19. Their advocacy during FFF expanded awareness to consider including other at-risk categories for vaccine prioritization, such as funeral home directors and maintenance workers. Richmond was initially the only place in the country to have these groups included in this Phase 1b "essential workers" category. Third, *increased community access to vaccination:* FFF faith leaders were able to access resources that they could share with their parishioners. For example, in addition to vaccination priority for faith leaders, FFF participating churches, such as Pastor Hodges's Second Baptist Church, were some of the first sites to offer COVID-19 vaccines in their areas. Fourth, *advocacy:* FFF members had direct, personal, and consistent access to high-level leaders to discuss concerns beyond FFF meetings. For instance, the FFF participants had the opportunity to speak directly with decision-makers, such as leaders within the FDA and CDC, to talk about vaccine ingredients and manufacturing and discuss the difference between emergency and full vaccine approval. Furthermore, FFF members were able to identify and advocate for their community's collective needs to these leaders. For example, they spoke with leaders regarding school closings, voter mobilization (transportation, early voting, mail-in ballots), and rental assistance. More generally, Dr. Winn made himself available via phone calls to address any ad hoc needs from the FFF community.

FFF WITHIN THE CONTEXT OF EXISTING HEALTH PROMOTION FRAMEWORKS

This section details how key public health and health promotion frameworks were instrumental to the growth and success of the FFF movement and its eventual impact—including principles of community engagement, emergency risk communication, and the Community-to-Bench model of conducting scientific/medical research (CTSA Consortium 2011; WHO 2017; Tossas et al. 2020).

Utilizing principles of community engagement: Community engagement is a collaborative process where groups, connected by geography or shared interests, work together to address well-being issues and create ambitious visions for their common future. With an emphasis on collaborative efforts, the goal is to build trust, foster relationships, and achieve positive impacts for the community (CTSA Consortium 2011; Born 2012). Community engagement principles are essential for guiding leaders and organizations in establishing effective engagement processes and partnerships. These nine principles (table 5.1) can be categorized into three groups: factors to contemplate before engagement, essentials for engagement, and requisites for achieving successful engagement (Schlake 2015). At the onset of the pandemic, it was immediately evident that grassroots organizing and community engagement strategies would be critical for reducing the devastating impact of the virus (Holley 2016; Fedorowicz, Arena, and Burrowes 2020). Typically, most academic-community partnerships with faith or community-based organizations are initiated by the university partner and center on an issue aligned with the researcher's area of expertise, available funding, and perception of community need (Drahota et al. 2016; Noel et al. 2019). The COVID-19 pandemic changed everything, including the unidirectional nature of engagement solicitations. Indeed, in contrast to typical academic-community partnerships (Mosavel et al. 2019), the FFF partnership was initially developed in response to this community-driven and community-identified need—and made possible only because of essential existing and trusted relationships with the VCU MCCC.

TABLE 5.1. PRINCIPLES OF COMMUNITY ENGAGEMENT

Principle	Action
A) Factors to contemplate before engagement	
1. Engagement goals and targeted communities	Clearly express the intended goals of the community activity, whether it involves gathering facts, developing programs, or collectively addressing emerging issues through shared decision-making. Determine engaged participants based on factors such as geography, racial/ethnic group, age, or common interest. Collaborate with other organizations to contribute to shared efforts, recognizing that roles may evolve over time.
2. Community dynamics and perceptions	Conduct thorough research to understand the community's cultural, social, economic, and demographic aspects. Assess prior experiences with organizations, readiness for participation, and the perceived benefits or costs associated. This understanding is crucial for consensus building, effective communication, decision-making, and the establishment of meaningful partnerships.
B) Essentials for engagement	
3. Trust and support	Make engagement a collaborative process by involving community members in both the development and implementation stages. Initiate discussions with leaders and groups in their natural environments to identify concerns, issues, and barriers. Diversify the group composition and tailor it based on specific goals to build trust and secure ongoing support through shared goals and costs.
4. Collective self-determination	Prioritize the self-determination of both individuals and the community as a whole. Assist communities in identifying their issues, naming problems, developing action plans, implementing strategies, and evaluating outcomes. Successful engagement is more likely when community members identify with the issue, consider it important, exert influence, and contribute throughout the entire process.
C) Requisites for achieving successful engagement	
5. Collaborative change for health improvement	Emphasize the importance of equitable partnerships and of transparent discussions on power dynamics and decision-making. Collaborating individuals and organizations should identify co-learning opportunities and contributions that may benefit from the engagement partnership.
6. Community diversity in engagement	Acknowledge diversity related to economics, education, employment, or health and recognize culture defined by language, race, ethnicity, age, gender, literacy, or personal interests. Employ inclusive processes, strategies, and techniques to engage individuals, minimize barriers, and celebrate community cultures and norms.
7. Community engagement through asset mobilization	Utilize diverse community assets, including individual interests, skills, experiences, and social networks. Integrate these assets into the engagement process, collaborating with individuals and organizations to enhance skills for sustained long-term collaborations and outcomes.
8. Flexibility and shared control	Recognize that the community engagement process may lead to changes in individuals, organizations, alliances, social networks, and assets. Adapt and remain flexible to evolving community issues and needs to facilitate long-term collaboration.
9. Long-term commitment to community collaboration	While community engagement may initiate with a specific project, commit to establishing long-term partnerships for the greatest potential of successful outcomes addressing complex societal issues. Develop strategies to sustain collaborations and progress over time.

Source: Based on Schlake 2015.

While all nine principles of community engagement are central to partnership development, a few (shown in table 5.2) have particular relevance to FFF (CTSA Consortium 2011).

Importantly, these principles of community engagement (CTSA Consortium 2011) were upheld and honored as FFF grew—indeed, the Black faith leaders drove the agenda and priorities for FFF. As relationships and trust deepened, the shared agenda came to include combating vaccine misinformation and implementation barriers, as well as addressing the myriad health inequities exacerbated by the pandemic. These principles of community engagement provide a blueprint for developing and maintaining such critical relationships so that, when another public health crisis occurs, the necessary partnership structures and trust have already been developed with key community leaders.

TABLE 5.2. PRINCIPLES OF COMMUNITY ENGAGEMENT AND FFF COLLABORATION

Clear purpose and shared agenda	Immediately, this university-faith partnership coalesced around a clear purpose and a shared, urgent agenda to save lives by inviting the key leaders of the local faith-based community to gather each Friday afternoon to learn about the most updated, relevant, community-specific COVID-19 information to share with their congregants. As this partnership developed and members continued to witness research in action, a noticeable appreciation was developed for the significant lifesaving potential of clinical research.
Understanding community context	It was critical to integrate the centrality of faith as a guidepost to inform meeting procedures (e.g., starting and ending with prayer) and as recognition of the vast social capital of the religious leaders. In particular, the religious leaders were considered frontline leaders in the public health effort to combat the impact of COVID-19 on Black and Brown communities. Religious leaders shaped the FFF conversations by recommending topics, but more importantly, they trusted civic and community leaders. These conversations shed light on historical and present-day mistrust, providing a springboard for future collaborations to strengthen relationships and build trustworthiness.
Cultivating strong relationships	The egalitarian partnership among the FFF leadership, coupled with complete transparency and trust regarding their shared agenda, allowed them to highlight concerns particular to Black communities and advocate for strategies that recognized these concerns. Finally, the partnership demonstrated a solid and ongoing drive to reduce the devastating impact of COVID-19 on their congregants and the broader community. The FFF's partnership acknowledged the importance of developing cross-sector diverse partnerships and, as such, invited entities with considerable decision-making power who could address needs, for example, related to vaccine implementation.
Leveraging resources	All partners leveraged resources available to them to meet the needs of the FFF movement. This willingness to expend available capital reflects the mutual investment in the FFF mission and helped strengthen the partnership. Examples include: Attorney Haynes: • Relationships with community and civic leaders • Deep connections with Black clergy, including Pastor Gray Faith-based leaders: • Vast social capital and reach within their congregations • Relationships with civic and legislative leaders VCU Massey Comprehensive Cancer Center: • Relationships with local medical and public health leaders (e.g., Virginia Department of Health, housing authority) • Relationships with national leaders from CDC, FDA, and NIH • Practical and financial resources (e.g., Zoom, administrative support for meetings)

Risk communication framework: Risk communication is vital to guiding preparation and response for any public health emergency, crisis, or threat. Communication timeliness and continued information dissemination are essential for the public to perceive their risk and make informed decisions to protect themselves, their families, and their communities (Reynolds and Quinn 2008). Evidence-based frameworks for risk communication, such as the WHO's Risk Communication Guidance, aid emergency response professionals to develop a strategic approach for effective communication (WHO 2017). The WHO's Risk Communication Guidance is grounded in evidence-based principles and a systems-focused approach (Lin et al. 2014; WHO 2017). Key recommendations of this framework emphasize the importance of engaging with the affected communities to build trust; building capacity for risk communication within existing national and local response systems; and continuous practice of planning, messaging, engagement, monitoring, and evaluation of communication strategy, including content, timing, and audience (WHO 2017).

Table 5.3 describes how the FFF collaboration addressed these key components of emergency risk communication to successfully disseminate information, dispel misinformation, and provide communities with actionable, science-backed recommendations to help protect themselves, their families, and communities.

TABLE 5.3. WHO EMERGENCY RISK COMMUNICATION FRAMEWORK AND FFF COLLABORATION

Building trust and engaging the community Affected Clarity, timeliness, acknowledgment of uncertainty, and transparency are key to building trust. Collaborative and contextually appropriate decision-making support communities with actionable information able to promote evidence-based decisions.	FFF-directed communication and issues salient to the faith leaders and their communities were at the forefront of each meeting. Dr. Winn and guest speakers clarified what was known, what was unknown, and provided updates about changes in infection and testing rates, vaccination development, and availability. Faith leaders identified salient challenges and barriers and challenged FFF to work together to identify real-time solutions.
Integrating emergency communication into existing (health) systems Proximity of the system leaders to national response leaders to support integration of risk communication recommendations at local, regional, and national levels. Coordination of existing systems can be leveraged to support tailored risk communication and recommendations. Capacity building through coordination of groups, training, and preparation on what information to share and how.	Though not a health system, FFF leveraged existing faith community systems. We see this as an innovative and instrumental adaptation supporting the success of the FFF collaborative. Building on the existing faith leader networks allowed bidirectional communication with wide community reach. It also allowed capacity building as leaders learned new information and identified new channels for resource development and implementation, and led to wider appreciation of the importance of clinical research to communities. Finally, the FFF collaborative had a direct link to national leaders involved in multiple aspects of the pandemic response.

TABLE 5.3. WHO EMERGENCY RISK COMMUNICATION FRAMEWORK AND FFF COLLABORATION

(continued)

Emergency risk communication practice	FFF provided a platform for religious leaders to discuss the needs of their churches, their congregants, and their
Assessment of needs, coordinated implementation, and ongoing monitoring of public awareness and knowledge is required to enable responsiveness. Messaging should be in lay language, come from multiple and reputable sources, and recommend specific actions that can be readily performed.	surrounding communities. These discussions led to agenda items and provided an impetus for experts who joined the calls and provided information and resources for faith leaders to take back to their communities. These discussions included mask mandates and where to get masks, to vaccine rollout schedules, to COVID-19 protocol and safety recommendations for in-person church services and gatherings.

Community-bench bidirectional model: Most naturally fitting to the FFF structure was the Community-Bench Bidirectional Model (CBM). The unique CBM approach advocates for absolute integration of community intelligence into research by way of a level playing field of cyclical engagement, resting on three fundamental pillars: (a) community in-reach, (b) data democracy, and (c) flipped research (Tossas et al. 2020). While the FFF movement was not a research initiative, its development was a prime example of *community in-reach.* It represents the integration of external (community residents) and internal (academic partner) intelligence to co-inform and co-direct scientific inquiry and drive a common agenda. It also represents an exercise in *data democratization,* providing unfettered access to relevant, real-time scientific data through presentations, apps, websites, reports, and community convenings. Again, while not a research initiative, the FFF represented the "flipped research" pillar by decentralizing the execution of this initiative away from the academic institution (where research normally occurs, particularly in laboratories and clinics) and instead setting the FFF call in a neutral environment. In this manner, FFF challenged the traditionally episodic influence of the typical community advisory boards or community meetings, instead promoting co-leadership, cross-collaboration, and multi-level partnerships to maximize community impact.

LESSONS LEARNED

What Worked

- Snowball approach to increase reach and participation: Upon FFF's inception, Pastor Gray leveraged his network of local faith leaders to provide a launchpad for the first meetings. With time, these leaders tapped into their social and professional networks, expanding the reach beyond Richmond to include churches over seventy miles away, across urban and rural areas. This engagement approach was critical in expanding the reach of FFF, particularly as COVID was and still is negatively impacting Black communities and rural communities.

- Participant-informed agenda: An important aspect that allowed FFF to thrive is that the academic institution (the VCU MCCC) did not (and should not) monopolize the programming. The MCCC co-creates, facilitates, and organizes, while the FFF members orchestrate and decide on the topics for discussion. A flexible and community-driven agenda that is responsive to salient needs and concerns has been central to the success of FFF.

- Credible and trustworthy leaders: FFF simply would not have developed or grown to have the impact it has had if the individuals who began these conversations were not trusted leaders in the community. Their credibility and social capital were fundamental building blocks, and that existing trust and respect was then extended to the medical and scientific experts that presented to the group.

- Leveraging academic and community resources toward the same goal: The success of the FFF movement reflects both the MCCC's established partnerships resulting from their community-engaged efforts and the demonstrable influence and extensive network of the faith-based leaders through their congregations and relationships with civic and legislative leaders. This collaborative partnership and allowance for a shared network within the context of the urgent agenda of saving lives further strengthened the partnership (Belone et al. 2016).

What Didn't Work?

- Digital divide: One of the challenges that arose on the community side was related to the digital divide experienced by folks with differential access to a reliable cell phone or Wi-Fi signal, as well as those less adept with technology. One of the ways in which the group tried to address these pitfalls was by conducting sessions to teach people how to use their mobile hotspot or simply encouraging participants to join via the phone number provided by the Zoom platform. However, more could have been done.

- Transition from conference call to Zoom: We had some administrative missteps early on when the Zoom number changed frequently, so may

have lost or confused some people in the process. Participation did
rebound after this early phase.

- Limited reach beyond Baptist churches: FFF consists of predominantly
  Baptist churches, which may have made some other churches and
  faith communities feel excluded. Of note, COVID-19 has had a
  disproportionate impact on Black and Brown communities, many of
  whom are served locally through the Baptist churches represented in
  FFF. Thus, the overrepresentation of Black churches within FFF was
  understandable and even appropriate—but there is a common danger
  that any group can become a de facto closed group, in that only those
  connected to that circle will be included. Employing diverse methods
  to increase reach is therefore important, including regular invitations
  to potential new participants. One figure identified by an FFF member and participant in our research was the newly appointed dean at
  the Virginia Union University School of Theology, singled out for his
  role in the training of the next generation of faith leaders.

RECOMMENDATIONS FOR FUTURE PRACTICE

With the lofty goal of being a local model for national impact, the ideal future
for FFF is that it becomes a self-sustaining hub of trustworthy health resources,
providing information on cancer and other chronic diseases, informing public
health policies, and engaging in advocacy about such issues as access to frontline
drugs and other treatments, among other activities. The FFF could also serve
as an incubator to build, support, and strengthen health ministries, extending
beyond the walls of the church into the surrounding communities. The enumeration of short-term impacts above is evidence that this simple model of direct
community-expert interaction on a weekly basis both builds upon and supports
the extant power within communities. A critical deviation from existing frameworks, such as the risk communication framework discussed above, is that the
FFF is an example of the impact of an informed community working from its
own innate power, without needing to be "empowered" by an outside entity.

   With the dramatic impact of COVID-19 on cancer patients, a desire arose
for the FFF members to become partners in promoting cancer screening and
education, in order to mitigate the inevitable surge in late-stage cancer diagnoses due to care delays resulting from such events as COVID-19 closures
and stay-in-place orders. To be sustainable, this partnership would require
sustainable leadership as well as monetary and administrative resources.

With such positions and resources, FFF partners can help build and liaise with health ministries across churches, as this leadership should live within the churches. Most importantly, its sustainability would be directly dependent on its relevancy, credibility, accessibility, and flexibility/responsiveness. That is, FFF will remain viable as long as discussions remain grounded in issues relevant to participating communities, while leaders continue to bring in credible experts who speak with authority, scientific evidence, and accessible language and keep to an agenda that is flexible and responsive to emerging issues, rather than set on any one institutional goal. Dr. Robert A. Winn summarizes FFF's impact nicely:

> While on the surface the FFF might not seem to have direct benefit to the National Cancer Institute (NCI) comprehensive designation for Massey [Comprehensive Cancer Center] as a state institution, it is our moral obligation to serve. But in actuality, the FFF not only aligns with the NIH [National Institutes of Health] directives around COVID, but it is also one of the purest examples of community outreach and engagement [COE], critical to the NCI designation process. At its highest order, this is what COE should do—facilitate research and engagement not only at and for Massey but at the state level. Perhaps unthinkable pre-COVID 19, FFF become the perfect example of bidirectional engagement. The greatest things come out of trying to do the right thing first (prioritizing what's right). Part of the magic was not being so prescriptive at the beginning.

SUMMARY

The FFF partnership between Black faith leaders and MCCC is an exemplar of community-engaged research principles in action. Responding to the devastating toll of the COVID-19 pandemic, Black clergy sought out trusted sources of information to allow them to better serve their congregations. This community-driven need was the impetus for an academic-community partnership that has provided credible information and guidance from the very early days of the pandemic to the present day. The shared agenda, mutual respect and trust, and deep appreciation for context—all attributes of effective community-academic partnerships—were the pillars upon which the FFF partnership was built (Noel et al. 2019). The FFF partnership has grown and evolved, having galvanized a community and its leaders, and resulted in tangible public health and policy impacts.

DISCUSSION QUESTIONS

• One of the main drawbacks of prevention work is that it is intangible. In fact, successful prevention leads to an absence of events. What are some creative ways in which we can maintain or develop this kind of sustained community engagement, contributory to prevention, in the absence of triggering events?

• From the perspective of the academic institution: What are some ways we can incentivize academic institutions to participate in and support these kinds of bidirectional initiatives in a way that honors and respect the community's power? How do we balance the opportunities for academic rigor (planning and grounding work in existing frameworks, estimating "power," predicting/preventing attrition, measuring changes and impact over time) while respecting and responding to the changing needs of the community?

• From the perspective of the community partners: What does the partnership need to focus attention/effort on for particular preventive activities? How can it best facilitate the work of member organizations (churches and other religious entities, secular community groups, etc.)?

REFERENCES

Belone, Lorenda, Julie E. Lucero, Bonnie Duran, Greg Tafoya, Elizabeth A. Baker, Domin Chan, Charlotte Chang, Ella Greene-Moton, Michele A. Kelley, and Nina Wallerstein. 2016. "Community-Based Participatory Research Conceptual Model: Community Partner Consultation and Face Validity." *Qualitative Health Research* 26, no. 1 (January): 117–35. https://doi.org/10.1177/1049732314557084.

Born, Paul. 2012. *Community Conversations: Mobilizing the Ideas, Skills, and Passion of Community Organizations, Governments, Businesses, and People.* Toronto: BPS Books.

Bowling, Cynthia J., Jonathan M. Fisk, and John C. Morris. 2020. "Seeking Patterns in Chaos: Transactional Federalism in the Trump Administration's Response to the COVID-19 Pandemic." *American Review of Public Administration* 50, no. 6–7: 512–18. https://doi.org/10.1177/0275074020941686.

Clopton, Aaron Walter, and Bryan L. Finch. 2011. "Re-conceptualizing Social Anchors in Community Development: Utilizing Social Anchor Theory to Create Social Capital's Third Dimension." *Community Development* 42, no. 1: 70–83. https://doi.org/10.1080/15575330.2010.505293.

CTSA Consortium (Clinical and Translational Science Awards Consortium). 2011. *Principles of Community Engagement—Second Edition.* Bethesda, MD: National Institutes of Health.

Drahota, Amy, Rosemary D. Meza, Brigitte Brikho, Meghan Naaf, Jasper A. Estabillo, Emily D. Gomez, Sarah F. Vejnoska, Sarah Dufek, Aubyn C. Stahmer, and Gregory A. Aarons. 2016. "Community-Academic Partnerships: A Systematic Review of the State of the Literature and Recommendations for Future Research." *Milbank Quarterly* 94, no. 1 (March): 163–214. https://doi.org/10.1111/1468-0009.12184.

Dumenci, Frances. 2013. "Community Engagement Step by Step: Working Together to Improve Health." *VCU News,* November 1, 2013. Accessed October 13, 2021. https://news.vcu.edu/article/community_engagement_step_by_step.

Eller, Donnelle. 2020. "Fact Check: Black People Make Up Disproportionate Share of COVID-19 Deaths in Richmond, Virginia." *USA Today,* May 5, 2020. https://www.usatoday.com/story/news/factcheck/2020/05/05/fact-check-blacks-make-up-all-covid-19-deaths-richmond-virginia/3086558001/.

Fedorowicz, Martha, with Olivia Arena and Kimberly Burrowes. 2020. *Community Engagement during the COVID-19 Pandemic and Beyond: A Guide for Community-Based Organizations.* Washington, DC: Urban Institute. https://www.urban.org/research/publication/community-engagement-during-covid-19-pandemic-and-beyond.

Gadzekpo, Leonard. 1997. "The Black Church, the Civil Rights Movement, and the Future." *Journal of Religious Thought* 53/54, no. 2/1: 95–112. https://www.proquest.com/docview/222116831.

Holley, Kip. 2016. *The Principles for Equitable and Inclusive Civic Engagement.* Columbus: Kirwan Institute for the Study of Race and Ethnicity, Ohio State University.

Kesslen, Ben. 2020. "Bishop Who Preached 'God Is Larger than This Dreaded Virus' Dies of COVID-19." NBC News, April 18, 2020. https://www.nbcnews.com/news/us-news/bishop-who-preached-god-larger-dreaded-virus-dies-covid-19-n1183281.

Lin, Leesa, Elena Savoia, Foluso Agboola, and Kasisomayajula Viswanath. 2014. "What Have We Learned about Communication Inequalities during the H1N1 Pandemic: A Systematic Review of the Literature." *BMC Public Health* 14: 484. https://doi.org/10.1186/1471-2458-14-484.

Mosavel, Maghboeba, Jodi Winship, Valerie Liggins, Tiffany Cox, Mike Roberts, and Debra S. Jones. 2019. "Community-Based Participatory Research and Sustainability: The Petersburg Wellness Consortium." *Journal of Community Engagement and Scholarship* 11, no. 2: 54–66. https://doi.org/10.54656/VPOF1594.

Mude, William, Victor M. Oguoma, Tafadzwa Nyanhanda, Lillian Mwanri, and Carolyne Njue. 2021. "Racial Disparities in COVID-19 Pandemic Cases, Hospitalisations, and Deaths: A Systematic Review and Meta-Analysis." *Journal of Global Health* 11:05015. https://doi.org/10.7189/jogh.11.05015.

Noel, Lailea, Farya Phillips, Katherine Tossas-Milligan, Krista Spear, Nathan L. Vanderford, Robert A. Winn, Robin C. Vanderpool, and S. Gail Eckhardt. 2019. "Community-Academic Partnerships: Approaches to Engagement."

American Society of Clinical Oncology Educational Book 39:88–95. https://doi
.org/10.1200/EDBK_246229.

Prom-Wormley, Elizabeth C., Faisal Ilyas, De'Nisha Wilson, Danita Gregory,
Aquanetta Scott, Patricia Willaford, Laleta Fritz, Joanne Towles, Dyanne
Broidy, Helen Frye, et al. 2020. "A Participatory Group Process within a Health
Collaborative to Collect and Disseminate Needs Assessment Data." *Progress
in Community Health Partnerships: Research, Education, and Action* 14, no. 3
(Fall): 285–97. https://doi.org/10.1353/cpr.2020.0034.

Reynolds, Barbara, and Sandra Crouse Quinn. 2008. "Effective Communication
during an Influenza Pandemic: The Value of Using a Crisis and Emergency
Risk Communication Framework." *Health Promotion Practice* 9, no. 4 Supp.
(October): 13S–17S. https://doi.org/10.1177/1524839908325267.

Schlake, M. R. 2015. "Community Engagement: Nine Principles." *Cornhusker Economics,* June 3, 726.

Tate, Julie, Jennifer Jenkins, and Steven Rich. 2021. "Fatal Force: Police Shootings Database." *Washington Post.* Accessed August 24, 2021. https://communityresourcehub
.org/resources/police-shootings-database/.

Tossas, K. Y., K. S. Watson, G. A. Colditz, C. R. Thomas, J. H. Stewart, and R. A.
Winn. 2020. "Advocating for a 'Community to Bench Model' in the 21st Century." *EBioMedicine* 53, no. 102688 (March). https://doi.org/10.1016/j.ebiom
.2020.102688.

Virginia Department of Health. 2020. "COVID-19 in Virginia." https://www.vdh
.virginia.gov/coronavirus/.

WHO (World Health Organization). 2017. *Communicating Risk in Public Health
Emergencies: A WHO Guideline for Emergency Risk Communication (ERC) Policy and Practice.* Geneva, Switzerland: World Health Organization. https://
apps.who.int/iris/handle/10665/259807.

Ziarek, Ewa Plonowska. 2020. "Triple Pandemics: COVID-19, Anti-Black Violence, and Digital Capitalism." *Philosophy Today* 64, no. 4 (Fall): 925–30.
https://doi.org/10.5840/philtoday20201124377.

Part 3

ENVIRONMENTAL HEALTH

6

COVID and Environmental Health

MICHELE MORRONE

Just like public health, environmental health is key to both societal and individual well-being. When the environment is healthy, the public has a greatly increased chance to be healthy; the public cannot be healthy if the environment is not. Environmental health (EH) is more than just a critical component of public health practice; it is, in fact, the reason that public health exists as a profession. EH is one of the oldest approaches to protecting health and preventing disease. Historical accounts of public health document its foundation in using sanitation to improve environmental conditions. These approaches can be traced back to prehistoric societies through medieval periods, the Renaissance, and into modern times (Tulchinsky and Varavikova 2015). Diseases that later defined public health as a profession such as plague (spread by fleas), yellow fever (spread by mosquitoes), and cholera (spread by water) were managed with environmental health practices. Clean drinking water and sewage disposal that characterized the sanitary movement in the 1800s are identified as the "most important medical milestones" in history (Ferriman 2007).

In 1999, the Centers for Disease Control and Prevention (CDC) identified "ten great public health achievements" of the twentieth century (CDC 1999). It is notable that EH has a role in at least six of these: motor vehicle safety, safer workplaces, control of infectious diseases, safer and healthier foods, fluoridation of drinking water, and recognition of tobacco as a health hazard. Without EH professionals (EHPs) inspecting workplaces and food establishments, engaging in outbreak investigations, and monitoring the quality of our air and water, these achievements would not have been possible.

Today, EH is more essential than ever to public health at the local, state, national, and global levels. Registered environmental health specialists have earned a national credential based on their education and experience. This education is built on a strong foundation in science, including chemistry, physics, biology, epidemiology, and toxicology. Colleges and universities can become accredited by the National Environmental Health Science and Protection Accreditation Council when they comply with rigorous curriculum requirements. Students enrolled in and graduating from accredited programs are eligible to serve as commissioned officers in the US Public Health Service (USCC 2023). In many states, these students are also eligible to sit for the credentialing exam with less work experience than others because their course of study has prepared them to do so.

The COVID pandemic has transformed the responsibilities of most public health professionals, including EHPs. The transformation has not only come in shifting day-to-day activities; it has also redefined relationships with those who must comply with environmental laws and regulations and the public at large. This chapter discusses the environmental health aspects of the pandemic by first summarizing the connection between environmental conditions and the spread of the virus. Two case studies demonstrate the role of EH in the pandemic: wastewater-based epidemiology and cruise ship response. Following these cases, an overview of the EH workforce is presented, including some specific activities and concerns of EHPs during the pandemic. The chapter concludes with a discussion of the challenges and lessons learned from those who were in the field.

THE ENVIRONMENT AND COVID TRANSMISSION

If not the most important, the environment is one of the most important elements in how diseases spread. This includes infectious and communicable diseases as well as those that are not spread from person to person. If you think about some common illnesses such as colds, flu, and diarrhea, the environmental mechanisms for their transmission are obvious. Respiratory diseases disperse through the air and gastrointestinal diseases spread through water and food. Chronic noncommunicable diseases such as cancers are also often linked to environmental exposures, including radiation and chemicals, although causation is more difficult to establish for these conditions (NCI 2022). Even diabetes and heart disease are related to environmental conditions such as food security and the built environment. So it is no surprise that the environment played a significant role in COVID's scope, even leading some to label the pandemic as "a global environmental health issue" (Yang and Lo 2021).

In the case of COVID, environmental circumstances have both exacerbated and mitigated its extent and impact, especially in vulnerable populations. Environmental conditions generally contribute to inequities that lead to disparate health outcomes in specific populations. In the United States, these inequities and disparate impacts led to the creation of the environmental justice movement in the 1980s. This movement continues to document that people of color are more likely to be exposed to pollution and unsafe environmental conditions than any other group (Bullard et al. 2007). We have seen COVID spread more rapidly and cause greater health consequences in places that have poor environments, especially related to air quality (Isphording and Pestel 2021). While more research is needed, the disproportionate impacts of COVID on people of color and those of low socioeconomic status is an environmental justice issue.

To contextualize COVID as an environmental health issue and because COVID is an airborne virus, the best example of the role of the environment in its spread is examining both indoor and outdoor air quality. Indoor environments include institutional, residential, commercial, and workplace settings. Outdoor environments include neighborhoods, public spaces, and recreational facilities.

INDOOR AIR QUALITY

It took several months after the pandemic was raging for policy-makers to accept that COVID was airborne, even as scientists pleaded for this recognition. In July 2020, several hundred scientists signed a letter urging authorities to acknowledge that the virus could be spread in the air and to strengthen guidance on environmental controls (Morawska and Milton 2020). At this time, we were focusing on handwashing and social distancing, both important preventive measures, based on the belief that virus particles were too heavy to remain suspended in the air. Airborne transmission would mean extending public health protections well beyond personal hygiene into more expensive and comprehensive approaches. Controlling airborne pathogens requires environmental controls such as enhancing ventilation and providing air filters. Inadequate ventilation was implicated in some of the most heartbreaking outbreaks of COVID in nursing homes (de Man et al. 2021). The tragedy in the institutional outbreaks is that there were warnings for decades about the quality of the air inside many of our buildings that serve vulnerable people.

Indoor air quality (IAQ) became a significant environmental health issue at the US Environmental Protection Agency (EPA) as evidence mounted about its impact on health. The surgeon general took a major step in 2005 when he issued a health advisory on radon (HHS 2005). Radon is a naturally occurring radioactive gas present in some indoor environments. It exudes from underground geological formations and can seep into basements or groundwater. People can be exposed to radon by breathing air in their basements, taking a shower, or drinking ground water. The EPA identifies radon as the leading cause of lung cancer in nonsmokers but it has remained a relatively obscure public health issue.

Research related to radon was followed by studies suggesting that environmental conditions inside schools could affect learning and overall student health. When it became clear that indoor air quality had the potential to affect children's health, calls came for more attention to ventilation systems in schools (Mendell et al. 2013). In 2009, the EPA created an IAQ Tools for Schools Action Kit that offers schools a wealth of resources to ensure safe and healthy indoor environments (EPA 2022). The overall goal of this kit was to help schools identify and mitigate risks, generate policies, and create IAQ management plans.

Managing IAQ is an integrated approach that focuses on controlling the source of indoor air pollutants (including viruses), ensuring adequate ventilation, and maintaining temperature and humidity levels. Ventilation is the key to minimizing risk from most indoor contaminants, including COVID. Ventilation occurs when indoor air is exchanged with outdoor air; outdoor air comes into the building while indoor air exhausts to the outside. This air exchange can occur naturally, by opening a window for example, or mechanically through use of heating, ventilation, and air-conditioning (HVAC) systems. Many schools, nursing homes, offices, and other buildings do not have options for natural ventilation due to energy efficiency architecture. To control the cost of heating or cooling buildings, structures have been designed with windows that are not meant to be opened. This design strategy contributed to a public health situation known as "sick building syndrome" (SBS). SBS carries a range of health consequences, including respiratory illnesses and headaches. SBS is mainly the result of inadequate ventilation, particularly the inability to bring fresh air into learning, work, or living environments (Abdul-Wahab 2011).

The air exchange rate is the number of times the air in a room is replaced with outdoor air. It is important to controlling air contaminants inside environments, reducing SBS, and creating healthy indoor spaces. Natural ventilation is preferred by many, but it might not provide sufficient airflow and exchange rates to minimize the spread of pathogens. Natural ventilation is also limited by uncontrollable weather conditions, building design, and institutional policies. Even with its limitations, small amounts of natural ventilation can effectively reduce infection risk when used in combination with masks and mechanical ventilation (Park et al. 2021). When windows cannot be opened, properly functioning HVAC systems are essential to reducing the spread of airborne pathogens. The leading authority on ventilation is the American Society of Heating, Refrigerating, and Air-Conditioning Engineers and they have been the source for COVID ventilation guidance. Their core recommendations focus on ventilation, filtration, air cleaning, and maintaining and operating HVAC systems (ASHRAE 2021).

As cases of COVID began climbing, most school districts shut down, an administrative control that probably saved many lives. However, administrative controls must be accompanied by environmental and behavioral strategies to maximize prevention. To address environmental controls in schools, it quickly became obvious that minimizing COVID transmission would require substantial investments to improve outdated and poorly maintained mechanical ventilation systems. In June 2020, the US Government Accountability Office (GAO) examined a representative sample of school districts and estimated that 41% of them needed to replace HVAC systems in at least half of their buildings (about 36,000 buildings) (GAO 2020). The GAO conducted surveys, visited districts, and walked through many school buildings. In their review, they found serious limitations with HVAC systems, including one school in Rhode Island that had HVAC components that were at least a hundred years old.

Inspecting schools, nursing homes, hospitals, correctional facilities, and other institutional settings is a routine component of EH practice. These inspections are guided by local ordinances, which are based on state laws and regulations. An institutional inspection involves examining all systems, including air handling, water supply, food safety, and waste management, along with the presence of chemical and biological contaminants. While it is rare to shut down institutions due to environmental concerns, inspections document conditions that could lead to poor health. Some examples of these circumstances in institutions include high levels of mold, lead, asbestos, and radioactive materials. Even with documented problems, schools are constrained in their ability to implement solutions due to inadequate resources. In many cases, school districts were likely aware of their weaknesses in managing the indoor environment after decades of deferred maintenance but were powerless to do anything about them.

One reason that the indoor environments of so many school buildings are marginal at best, and dangerous at worst, is because many school districts rely on local funding for capital improvements. While some states do allocate money for capital projects, there has been a long erosion of school infrastructure, which raises serious questions about safety inside schools during a pandemic. Recognizing the need to address school building conditions, federal legislation provided billions of dollars to local districts to help schools respond to the pandemic. Local school districts were given flexibility to determine how to use the funds. Activities to improve indoor air quality, including improvements in their HVAC systems, were allowable expenses (OESE 2023). However, in a review of how states are using this funding, it does not look like many are prioritizing improvements to HVAC systems (LePage and Jordan 2021).

OUTDOOR AIR QUALITY

Air quality in indoor environments is of great concern to minimizing the spread of COVID, but we cannot overlook the conditions in the outside environment. Research emerging during the pandemic suggests that outdoor air quality, specifically levels of particulate matter (PM), is associated with the incidence of COVID as well as the mortality rate from the virus (Wu et al. 2020; Vali et al. 2021). PM consists of microscopic particles less than ten microns in diameter, smaller than the diameter of a strand of human hair. Mainly associated with urban environments, PM can affect the overall air quality of large regions. This pollutant is a public health concern because biological and chemical contaminants can adhere to particles that can be inhaled deep inside the lungs. PM has long been associated with high rates of asthma and other respiratory diseases. Now there is evidence that exposure to PM while infected with COVID leads to an increased likelihood of death, especially in older populations (Isphording and Pestel 2021). In addition, outdoor air quality contributes to the inequities that create some of the health disparities that have come to light during the COVID pandemic (Rozenfeld et al. 2020).

On the other hand, one residual impact of COVID and global lockdowns is that some areas have seen significant improvements in air quality. In some ways, this was like impacts that were seen in Atlanta, Georgia, during the 1996 Olympics. As commuter travel decreased during the Olympics, so did levels of some air pollutants, resulting in a decrease in the severity of asthma in the city (Friedman et al. 2001). Numerous studies have examined the impact of reductions in commuter, recreational, and commercial travel, manufacturing, and construction on air quality during the pandemic. In most cases, air quality did improve during lockdowns, but these improvements varied based on geography and policy (Islam and Chowdhury 2021). Lockdowns and restrictions are not sustainable solutions to addressing environmental health, even with some evidence of how reductions in air pollution can improve public health (Liu, Wang, and Zheng 2021).

COVID presented researchers with a rare opportunity to examine the public health implications of policies that directly affect the environment. It also put a spotlight on the role of environmental health in preventing virus transmission. COVID also presented EHPs with unique opportunities to demonstrate how they could influence the trajectory of the pandemic by using tried and true environmental health techniques, as the cases below demonstrate.

EH PRACTICE MEETS COVID

Ensuring compliance with local, state, and federal health regulations is a sizable component of EH. These regulations are related to food safety, water sanitation, waste management, vector control, pools and spas, and safe buildings, among others. In many local public health agencies, the largest element of EH practice is inspecting facilities such as food retail establishments, schools, hotels, and nursing homes. The pandemic changed the inspection landscape in many ways. For example, one immediate impact was that it created a need for enhanced inspections at food service operations. While many food retail establishments were forced to shut down, others shifted from in-person dining to carry out and delivery. These new modes of food service require a different type of oversight by EHPs and a new way of conducting inspections (Brown and Pepper 2021).

During the pandemic, the importance of environmental health became clear for its role in affecting the severity and spread of the virus. The two cases below demonstrate the importance of EH in managing COVID by employing the essential services of environmental health (CDC 2023a). The case of wastewater-based epidemiology involves essential services related to research and monitoring. The cruise ship case highlights the essential services of diagnosing and investigating environmental health problems, mobilizing partnerships, and linking people to environmental health services.

WASTEWATER-BASED EPIDEMIOLOGY

Wastewater can be comprised of sewage generated in residences, institutions, or commercial establishments. It can also be effluent that comes from manufacturing, electricity generation, or other industries. Hospital wastewater is of particular concern because it can contain high levels of infectious agents, including SARS-CoV-2, and if not managed appropriately can contribute to community outbreaks (Achak et al. 2021). Wastewater monitoring was a tool during the pandemic to predict local virus activity, referred to as wastewater-based epidemiology (WBE). WBE involves obtaining samples of untreated wastewater, analyzing them in a laboratory, and using epidemiological methods to draw conclusions about the incidence and prevalence of pathogens, in this case COVID, in specific geographic areas (Patel et al. 2021). This approach exemplifies how environmental health can play a role in predicting local outbreaks so that authorities can be more prepared to respond to changing circumstances.

Wastewater is handled either in public treatment facilities or private systems. Publicly owned treatment works (POTWs) manage wastewater that is collected in sewers. Sewage managed at POTWs is "municipal wastewater" (EPA 2023). On the other hand, residences and other facilities that are not connected to sewers treat wastewater mainly in septic systems or other on-lot operations. These private systems are managed by individuals, facilities, and organizations. The EPA (2021) estimates that about 20% of all households in the country rely on private systems for wastewater management. Private systems are mainly in rural areas, so while WBE could be a worthwhile tool in many communities, it excludes rural places in which outbreaks of COVID can also be widespread and pervasive.

Regardless of its source, wastewater contains microbiological organisms, radioactive elements, and chemical contaminants. POTWs operate under permits mandated in the Clean Water Act, which sets standards for amounts of specific contaminants allowable in treated water. The wastewater treatment train begins with the collection system that transmits sewage to the treatment plant. This raw, untreated, sewage includes constituents that can tell the story of the place from which it is collected. The presence of pharmaceuticals, bacteria, and viruses in wastewater can be indicators of personal and community behaviors (EPA 2004).

To apply WBE, a water sample needs to be taken before it enters the treatment process, because once water goes through a treatment plant it is technically and legally clean enough to be released back into the environment. To use WBE, sampling sometimes takes place at the treatment plant, but these samples would provide a snapshot of a large area such as multiple neighborhoods in one city. When possible, it is more useful to sample from smaller areas, such as individual buildings, to pinpoint where outbreaks are occurring. This sampling approach requires specific protocols to ensure chain of custody as the sample goes from the field to the laboratory.

In areas without sewers, untreated wastewater may be a greater concern, especially if COVID prevalence is high. If the virus can survive in wastewater, people might be exposed to the virus in the same way that they might be exposed to legionella. Legionella is a bacterium that can become airborne in running water and is periodically responsible for outbreaks of pneumonia, especially in people over fifty (CDC 2021a). Untreated wastewater is not thought of as a great concern in developed countries, even though there are still places in the US that use so-called "straight pipes" that take sewage from homes directly to streams or rivers. These straight pipe areas exist for many reasons, including historical development, discrimination, and a lack of resources for improvements (Maxcy-Brown et al. 2021). Research connecting the airborne spread of COVID to untreated sewage is evolving, with calls for focused efforts to examine the relationship (Wathore et al. 2020).

In response to promising information from WBE, the Centers for Disease Control and Prevention launched the National Wastewater Surveillance System. At the time of this writing, the CDC was monitoring approximately 1,200 sites around the country. Data are submitted to the CDC from local health departments, which gather samples at POTWs. The CDC cautions that wastewater sampling for SARS-CoV-2 is only part of a more comprehensive approach to disease surveillance due to its many limitations (CDC 2023b). Wastewater-based epidemiology can serve as a warning that a specific place may be heading into a change in COVID prevalence, which can then lead to additional education, testing, and local preparations to manage a surge.

CRUISE SHIPS

As the discussion below indicates, one of the first major trouble spots related to the spread of COVID developed on cruise ships. Under normal circumstances, cruise ships are public health priorities because of the multiple ways in which people can be exposed to pathogens. Food is available around the clock, often in buffet settings, waste management is paramount to minimizing pests, clean potable water is vital, and thousands of people from across the globe are living in close quarters. In addition, many passengers are vulnerable because of age and medical supplies and personnel are limited. Public health professionals in the CDC's Vessel Sanitation Program (VSP) are charged with ensuring health and safety on cruise ships (CDC

2023c). Specifically, Environmental Health Officers (EHOs) conduct sanitation inspections, monitor the spread of illnesses, train crew on preventive protocols, and respond to outbreaks. EHOs are part of the US Public Health Service and are commissioned officers who work under the surgeon general.

The *Diamond Princess* was the first cruise ship to gain COVID notoriety after a symptomatic passenger tested positive for the virus on January 25, 2020. Cases on the ship continued to climb and by February 25 there were 691 confirmed cases on board, making it the "largest cluster of COVID-19 cases outside mainland China" (Moriarty et al. 2020). The *Diamond Princess,* which ultimately docked in Japan, is the most studied of the COVID cruise ship outbreaks, even though outbreaks were occurring on other vessels at the same time (Kordsmeyer et al. 2021).

In March 2020, the VSP was faced with a new challenge as the *Grand Princess* cruise ship was heading toward California, after multiple stops in Mexico, with sick passengers and crew on board (Wittry and Kincaid 2021). Before EHOs from the VSP could even begin the task of conducting an environmental assessment of the ship, they encountered the first test of their response capacity. San Francisco refused to allow the ship to land in its harbor, so it had to dock in Oakland. The Oakland port is not a passenger terminal and it does not have facilities for passengers to disembark. This meant that the ship stayed in the bay while arrangements were made to ensure the health and safety of passengers as they came ashore. Shelter and hygiene facilities had to be available and port logistics required the coordination of multiple agencies at all levels of government. After the ship docked, EHOs were responsible for ensuring dock worker safety, monitoring sanitation facilities, assisting first responders, and working with the ship's medical team on disinfection and onboard quarantine.

When the situation with the *Grand Princess* began to unfold, there were no mask mandates and the CDC was focusing protocols largely on minimizing the spread of the virus by promoting hand washing and surface disinfection. However, as the situation continued to develop, new information was published in the *New England Journal of Medicine* suggesting that the virus could be spread person to person by aerosols (van Doremalen et al. 2020). The EHOs thus had to shift some of their activities to focus on PPE and training workers on how to use N95 respirators.

The environmental assessment (EA) of the *Grand Princess* demonstrates the breadth of responsibility that environmental health professionals have daily. The EA included monitoring compliance with quarantine protocols, developing cleaning and disinfection protocols, and addressing issues with garbage, pests, laundry, food, and drinking water. As those who were directly involved in the response tell it, environmental health was foremost in preventing the virus from spreading both on the ship and into the community. They also detail the immense amount of planning and coordination that was necessary. More than one year after the response to the *Grand Princess,* the EHOs identified lessons learned. For example, while inspections and compliance usually follow well-established procedures and regulations, they realized the importance of maintaining some flexibility because there were so many unknowns. In addition, it was and is imperative to address mental health and ethical issues when people are isolated on board a ship (Nakazawa, Ino, and Akabayashi 2020).

EHOs are one component of the environmental health workforce, and their jobs were exceptionally important during the pandemic. They work at the national level and can be deployed where they are most needed. However, much environmental health is local and, as the section below shows, the pandemic has underscored some of the weaknesses in the EH workforce.

EH WORKFORCE AND COVID

Despite its importance to protecting public health, EH is facing numerous challenges that have had some bearing on its role in the COVID response and beyond. Graduates of EH programs are declining, and the current workforce is aging. Due to low salaries, many qualified EH graduates avoid working in public health agencies, choosing instead to seek employment in the more lucrative private industry (NEHSPAC 2020). While public health offers numerous benefits that the private sector often does not, such as pensions and standard work schedules, health departments are the settings for some of the most stressful scenarios. During the pandemic, public health practitioners were both praised and villainized. Some professionals were threatened, others have just walked away from their careers in frustration. The longer-term impacts of the pandemic on the public health workforce remain to be seen, and at this point we do not know if these impacts will be mostly positive or negative.

Working as an EHP in a local health department is demanding under normal circumstances because of their broad responsibilities and lack of resources. Prior to COVID, there were serious challenges with the current state of EH practice arising from an expanding portfolio of duties (Brooks et al. 2019). Added to daily tasks is the reality that EH personnel are also part of emergency response and outbreak investigation teams.

Even with the state of the workforce, EHPs were exceptionally qualified to tackle COVID due to their experience with emergency response, epidemiology, communication, data, and technology. EHPs are often first responders during disasters; this includes natural disasters such as hurricanes and anthropogenic disasters such as the September 11 attacks. During a disaster, basic sanitation measures are critical and clean drinking water, safe food, and sanitary facilities are often planned and managed by EH units. Effective communication is probably the most important element of disaster management and EHPs are generally experienced with this. In many ways, COVID has been a long-term disaster scenario that has involved rapidly changing conditions that EHPs are trained to deal with as part of their normal job duties.

A significant part of the job of many EHPs is investigating outbreaks. These include large-scale incidents such as the nationwide outbreak of *E. coli* in spinach in 2016 and local occurrences such as botulism at a church supper. An outbreak investigation involves a team with multiple skills and EHPs are experienced with basic epidemiology approaches as well as environmental assessments and monitoring. We have seen local health departments become the front line for COVID response and prevention. They have been responsible for educating the public, enforcing mask mandates, and implementing large-scale vaccination opportunities. This has often necessitated shifting responsibilities, as many have taken an "all hands on deck" approach; EHPs have served multiple roles in many local health departments.

In 2020 the National Environmental Health Association conducted two needs assessments to understand the impact of COVID on the EH workforce. The first was completed in May and the second in October (NEHA 2020). They used a convenience sample to gather information quickly from environmental health practitioners across the United States. The results indicated that the job responsibilities in EH units had shifted to strengthen the local public health response to the pandemic. Most respondents indicated that they became more heavily involved in duties that are not necessarily part of their regular work. As the COVID pandemic continued to grow, EHPs became critical members of an integrated public health response. They served numerous roles that are both within and outside of their routine responsibilities. These roles included ones that specifically related to three core public health functions: assessment, policy development, and assurance (Rodrigues et al. 2021). For example, EH professionals were needed for public relations and communications as well as contact tracing and participating on local taskforces or emergency response committees. The experience with COVID has underscored the fact that EHP skills are essential to managing a pandemic.

The pandemic strained many EH units. According to several local health commissioners in Ohio, this strain led to high levels of exhaustion and overall mental health concerns (Brown and Pepper 2021). One health commissioner said that "even answering phones became overwhelming." In some cases, long-standing relationships with local businesses suffered because of zero tolerance in complying with state COVID guidelines. Local health departments had no experience operating under a statewide and state-declared public health emergency and in places where COVID was surging they struggled to keep up with rapidly evolving conditions. Added to shifting assignments was the fact that school districts, businesses, and healthcare facilities needed guidance while constituents were debating mask mandates and vaccine requirements (Brown and Pepper 2021).

LESSONS LEARNED: EH IS ESSENTIAL

The COVID pandemic underscored the power of EH in many ways. The ten essential services that EH practitioners provide (CDC 2023a) routinely mean they are indispensable members of a pandemic response team. The need to monitor, diagnose, and investigate environmental health problems is evident in controlling the spread of the virus. Their experience with educating the public, mobilizing partnerships, and developing policies and plans means that EH personnel have the skills to contribute to prevention actions. In addition, the capacity to enforce laws and link people to needed services allows EH practitioners to serve key roles in encouraging changes in community health behaviors. Overall, since EHPs are generalists, they can fulfill multiple roles in handling a pandemic.

Even as they have had an intensive impact in public health practice during the pandemic, it has not been without challenges. One of these is that relationships with partners and operators have been redefined. Prior to the pandemic, EH inspections relied on positive communications with food service managers, nursing home administrators, pool operators, school principals, and others. EHPs do not approach inspections in a punitive way. Rather, their goal is to identify weaknesses or noncompliance with regulations and provide education and support to improve operations. During the pandemic, as compliance with mandates became more urgent, relationships that were built over years became strained. The urgency was because even minor deficiencies in compliance with COVID regulations could lead to community-wide outbreaks. Before COVID, a food service facility might be responsible for a few people suffering from gastrointestinal illness if it had minor violations of basic sanitation measures such as employee handwashing. During COVID, those same minor violations could lead to an outbreak that involved hundreds of people who had never set foot in the facility.

Just as with many other health professionals, the mental health issues experienced by EHPs were real. As we saw nightly news coverage of doctors and nurses struggling with their mental health, the public health workforce was also struggling, with much less visibility and in a somewhat different way. People rallied around hospital workers, referring to them as frontline personnel. It was rare to see the same support for public health workers, also frontline personnel. In some cases, public health professionals were vilified for their preventive approaches and guidance to stop the spread (Hegyi 2020). As the pandemic wore on and additional surges started, the criticism of public health professionals only seemed to grow. It got to the point that policies focused more on protecting the "rights" of people who refused to follow public health guidance rather than of those who would. Politicians around the country stoked the ire toward public health professionals as they passed legislation to restrict basic preventive measures such as mask wearing and social distancing. While all public health professionals were dealing with expanded responsibilities during the pandemic, some were also dealing with people who disparaged them and even threatened them for doing their jobs to protect the public (CDC 2021b).

As some politicians and members of the public lambasted public health, the evolving scientific information during the pandemic meant that EHPs had to be flexible and innovative. It is not possible to conduct inspections from home under lockdown, so many EHPs were not able to conduct a major part of their regular work. Students who needed internships to complete their degrees were unable to work in the field. The National Environmental Health Association and the CDC offered students access to their online training materials, which allowed students to earn credit in place of their internships, but this was no substitute for real-world experience. The results of the modified internship requirement are likely to be minor overall, but there is little doubt that they led to many students having difficulty in finding a job and experiencing delay in passing credentialing exams. The EH workforce will have suffered as a consequence.

The pandemic has both highlighted and changed environmental health. While the highlighting may lead to more understanding of the importance of EH, the changes it brought may not be temporary. One of the best things that we can do to help environmental and public health professionals adjust to the new realities is provide opportunities to enhance communication skills throughout their education. This includes embedding conflict resolution, public participation, and educational approaches in the entire college curriculum. It could also include ongoing training for those already in the workforce in dealing with difficult people while still getting their preventive messages to the public. Our environmental health workforce is highly skilled at managing environmental problems, but many may have been caught off guard when it comes to the techniques and skills needed to manage engaging and guiding the public in this difficult new era.

DISCUSSION QUESTION

- Explain the role of environmental health practitioners in managing the COVID pandemic. What specific responsibilities did they have? Discuss the value of EH in public health in the context of COVID.

REFERENCES

Abdul-Wahab, Sabah A., ed. 2011. *Sick Building Syndrome in Public Buildings and Workplaces.* Heidelberg: Springer.

Achak, Mounia, Soufiane A. Bakri, Younes Chhiti, Fatima E. M. Alaoui, Noureddine Barka, and Wafaa Boumya. 2021. "SARS-CoV-2 in Hospital Wastewater during Outbreak of COVID-19: A Review on Detection, Survival and Disinfection Technologies." *Science of the Total Environment* 761:143192. https://doi.org/10.1016/j.scitotenv.2020.143192.

ASHRAE (American Society of Heating, Refrigerating, and Air-Conditioning Engineers). 2021. "Core Recommendations for Reducing Airborne Infectious Aerosol Exposure." *ASHRAE,* October 19, 2021. https://www.ashrae.org/file library/technical resources/covid-19/core-recommendations-for-reducing-airborne-infectious-aerosol-exposure.pdf.

Brooks, Bryan W., Justin A. Gerding, Elizabeth Landeen, Eric Bradley, Timothy Callahan, Stephanie Cushing, Fikru Hailu, Nancy Hall, Timothy Hatch, Sherise Jurries, et al. 2019. "Environmental Health Practice Challenges and Research Needs for U.S. Health Departments." *Environmental Health Perspectives* 127, no. 12 (December): 125001. https://ehp.niehs.nih.gov/doi/10.1289/EHP5161.

Brown, Chad, and Jack Pepper. 2021. Interview by author. June 21.

Bullard, Robert D., Paul Mohai, Robin Saha, and Beverly Wright. 2007. *Toxic Wastes and Race at Twenty, 1987–2007: A Report Prepared for the United Church of Christ Justice & Witness Ministries.* Cleveland, OH: United Church of Christ. https://www.nrdc.org/sites/default/files/toxic-wastes-and-race-at-twenty-1987-2007.pdf.

CDC (Centers for Disease Control and Prevention). 1999. "Ten Great Public Health Achievements—United States, 1900–1999." *Morbidity and Mortality Weekly*

Report (MMWR) 48, no. 12 (April 2): 241–43. https://www.cdc.gov/mmwr /preview/mmwrhtml/00056796.htm.

———. 2021a. "*Legionella:* About the Disease." Centers for Disease Control and Prevention. Last modified March 25, 2021. https://www.cdc.gov/legionella /about/index.html.

———. 2021b. "Symptoms of Depression, Anxiety, Post-traumatic Stress Disorder, and Suicidal Ideation among State, Tribal, Local, and Territorial Public Health Workers during the COVID-19 Pandemic—United States, March–April 2021." *Morbidity and Mortality Weekly Report (MMWR)* 70, no. 26 (July 2): 947–52.   https://www.cdc.gov/mmwr/volumes/70/wr/mm7026e1.htm?s_cid= mm7026e1_w#contribAff.

———. 2023a. "Environmental Public Health and the 10 Essential Services." Centers for Disease Control and Prevention. Last modified January 27, 2023. https://www.cdc.gov/nceh/ehs/10-essential-services/index.html.

———. 2023b. "National Wastewater Surveillance System (NWSS)." Centers for Disease Control and Prevention. Last modified March 14, 2023. https:// www.cdc.gov/healthywater/surveillance/wastewater-surveillance/wastewater -surveillance.html.

———. 2023c. "Vessel Sanitation Program." Centers for Disease Control and Prevention. Last modified May 26, 2023. https://www.cdc.gov/nceh/vsp/default.htm.

de Man, Peter, Sunita Paltansing, David S. Y. Ong, Norbert Vaessen, Gerard van Nielen, and Johannes G. M. Koeleman. 2021. "Outbreak of Coronavirus Disease 2019 (COVID-19) in a Nursing Home Associated with Aerosol Transmission as a Result of Inadequate Ventilation." *Clinical Infectious Diseases* 73, no. 1: 170–71. https://doi.org/10.1093/cid/ciaa1270.

EPA (US Environmental Protection Agency). 2004. *Primer for Municipal Wastewater Treatment Systems.* EPA bulletin 832-R-04–001. Washington, DC: US Environmental Protection Agency. https://www.epa.gov/sites/default/files/2015-09 /documents/primer.pdf.

———. 2021. "Septic Systems Overview." US Environmental Protection Agency. Last modified January 19, 2021. https://19january2021snapshot.epa.gov/septic /septic-systems-overview_.html.

———. 2022. "Indoor Air Quality Tools for Schools Action Kit." US Environmental Protection Agency. Last modified December 13, 2022. https://www.epa.gov/iaq -schools/indoor-air-quality-tools-schools-action-kit.

———. 2023. "Municipal Wastewater." US Environmental Protection Agency. Last modified July 24, 2023. https://www.epa.gov/npdes/municipal-wastewater.

Ferriman, Annabel. 2007. "*BMJ* Readers Choose the 'Sanitary Revolution' as Greatest Medical Advance since 1840." *British Medical Journal* 334:111. https:// doi.org/10.1136/bmj.39097.611806.DB.

Friedman, Michael S., Kenneth E. Powell, Lori Hutwagner, LeRoy M. Graham, and W. Gerald Teague. 2001. "Impact of Changes in Transportation and Commuting Behaviors during the 1996 Summer Olympic Games in Atlanta on Air Quality and Childhood Asthma." *JAMA* 285, no. 7 (February): 897–905. http:// dx.doi.org/10.1001/jama.285.7.897.

GAO (Government Accountability Office). 2020. "K–12 Education: School Districts Frequently Identified Multiple Building Systems Needing Updates or Replacement." Report to Congressional Addressees GAO-20-494 (June). https://www.gao.gov/assets/gao-20-494.pdf.

Hegyi, Nate. 2020. "Public Health Officials Discuss Why They Quit during the COVID-19 Pandemic." National Public Radio, August 6, 2020. https://www.npr.org/2020/08/06/899679894/public-health-officials-discuss-why-they-quit-during-the-covid-19-pandemic.

HHS (US Department of Health and Human Services). 2005. "Surgeon General Releases National Health Advisory on Radon." US Department of Health and Human Services Press Office, January 12, 2005. http://www.adph.org/radon/assets/surgeon_general_radon.pdf.

Islam, Md. Saiful, and Tahmid Anam Chowdhury. 2021. "Effect of COVID-19 Pandemic-Induced Lockdown (General Holiday) on Air Quality of Dhaka City." *Environmental Monitoring and Assessment* 193:343. https://doi.org/10.1007/s10661-021-09120-z.

Isphording, Ingo E., and Nico Pestel. 2021. "Pandemic Meets Pollution: Poor Air Quality Increases Deaths by Covid-19." *Journal of Environmental Economics and Management* 108:102448. https://doi.org/10.1016/j.jeem.2021.102448

Kordsmeyer, Ann-Christin, Natascha Mojtahedzadeh, Jan Heidrich, Kristina Militzer, Thomas von Münster, Lukas Belz, Hans-Joachim Jensen, Sinan Bakir, Esther Henning, Julian Heuser, et al. 2021. "Systematic Review on Outbreaks of SARS-CoV-2 on Cruise, Navy and Cargo Ships." *International Journal of Environmental Research and Public Health* 18, no. 10 (May): 5195. https://doi.org/10.3390/ijerph18105195.

LePage, Brooke, and Phyllis W. Jordan. 2021. "With an Influx of COVID Relief Funds, States Spend on Schools." *FutureEd,* January 3, 2021. https://www.future-ed.org/with-an-influx-of-covid-relief-funds-states-spend-on-schools/.

Liu, Feng, Meichang Wang, and Meina Zheng. 2021. "Effects of COVID-19 Lockdown on Global Air Quality and Health." *Science of the Total Environment* 755, part 1 (February): 142533. https://doi.org/10.1016/j.scitotenv.2020.142533.

Maxcy-Brown, Jillian. Mark A. Elliott, Leigh A. Krometis, Joe Brown, Kevin D. White, and Upmanu Lall. 2021. "Making Waves: Right in Our Backyard—Surface Discharge of Untreated Wastewater from Homes in the United States." *Water Research* 190:116647. https://doi.org/10.1016/j.watres.2020.116647.

Mendell, M. J., E. A. Eliseeva, M. M. Davies, M. Spears, A. Lobscheid, W. J. Fisk, and M. G. Apte. 2013. "Association of Classroom Ventilation with Reduced Illness Absence: A Prospective Study in California Elementary Schools." *Indoor Air* 23, no. 6 (December): 515–28. https://doi.org/10.1111/ina.12042.

Morawska, Lidia, and Donald K. Milton. 2020. "It Is Time to Address Airborne Transmission of Coronavirus Disease 2019 (COVID-19)." *Clinical Infectious Diseases* 71, no. 9 (November): 2311–13. https://doi.org/10.1093/cid/ciaa939.

Moriarty, Leah F., Mateusz M. Plucinski, Barbara J. Marston, Ekaterina V. Kurbatova, Barbara Knust, Erin L. Murray, Nicki Pesik, Dale Rose, David Fitter, Miwako Kobayashi, et al. 2020. "Public Health Responses to COVID-19

Outbreaks on Cruise Ships—Worldwide, February–March 2020." *Morbidity and Mortality Weekly Report (MMWR)* 69, no. 12 (March 27): 347–52. http://dx .doi.org/10.15585/mmwr.mm6912e3.

Nakazawa, Eisuke, Hiroyasu Ino, and Akira Akabayashi. 2020. "Chronology of Covid-19 Cases on the Diamond Princess Cruise Ship and Ethical Consider- ations: A Report from Japan." *Disaster Medicine and Public Health Preparedness* 14, no. 4: 506–13. https://dx.doi.org/10.1017/dmp.2020.50.

NCI (National Cancer Institute). 2022. "Cancer-Causing Substances in the Envi- ronment." National Cancer Institute. Last modified June 17, 2022. https://www .cancer.gov/about-cancer/causes-prevention/risk/substances.

NEHA (National Environmental Health Association). 2020. "How Covid-19 Is Im- pacting the EH Workforce." National Environmental Health Association. Last updated October 30, 2020. https://emergency-neha.org/covid19/eh-workforce -reports/.

NEHSPAC (National Environmental Health Science & Protection Accredita- tion Council). 2020. "2019–2020 Update of Accredited Programs." National Environmental Health Science & Protection Accreditation Council. https:// www.nehspac.org/wp-content/uploads/2020/09/2020_9_11_-Annual-Update -Report-FINAL.pdf.

OESE (Office of Elementary & Secondary Education). 2023. "Elementary and Sec- ondary School Emergency Relief Fund." US Department of Education. Last modified May 17, 2023. https://oese.ed.gov/offices/education-stabilization-fund /elementary-secondary-school-emergency-relief-fund/.

Park, Sowoo, Younhee Choi, Doosam Song, and Eun Kyung Kim. 2021. "Natural Ventilation Strategy and Related Issues to Prevent Coronavirus Disease 2019 (COVID-19) Airborne Transmission in a School Building." *Science of the Total Environment* 789:147764. https://doi.org/10.1016/j.scitotenv.2021.147764.

Patel, Manvendra, Abhishek K. Chaubey, Charles U. Pittman Jr., Todd Mlsna, and Dinesh Mohan. 2021. "Coronavirus (SARS-CoV-2) in the Environment: Oc- currence, Persistence, Analysis in Aquatic Systems and Possible Management." *Science of the Total Environment* 765:142698. https://doi.org/10.1016/j.scitotenv .2020.142698.

Rodrigues, Matilde A., Manuela V. Silva, Nicole A. Errett, Gayle Davis, Zena Lynch, Surindar Dhesi, Toni Hannelly, Graeme Mitchell, David Dyjack, and Kirstin E. Ross. 2021. "How Can Environmental Health Practitioners Contrib- ute to Ensure Population Safety and Health during the COVID-19 Pandemic?" *Safety Science* 136:105136. https://doi.org/10.1016/j.ssci.2020.105136.

Rozenfeld, Yelena, Jennifer Beam, Haley Maier, Whitney Haggerson, Karen Bou- dreau, Jamie Carlson, and Rhonda Medows. 2020. "A Model of Disparities: Risk Factors Associated with COVID-19 Infection." *International Journal for Equity in Health* 19:126. https://doi.org/10.1186/s12939-020-01242-z.

Tulchinsky, Theodore H., and Elena A. Varavikova. 2015. *The New Public Health.* 3rd ed. San Diego: Academic Press. https://doi.org/10.1016/C2010-0-68514-2.

USCC (US Commission Corps). 2023. "Officer and Student Training Programs." US Department of Health and Human Services. https://www.usphs.gov/students/.

Vali, Mohebat, Jafar Hassanzadeh, Alireza Mirahmadizadeh, Mohammad Ho-
    seini, Samaneh Dehghani, Zahra Maleki, Fabiola Méndez-Arriaga, and Haleh
    Ghaem. 2021. "Effect of Meteorological Factors and Air Quality Index on the
    COVID-19 Epidemiological Characteristics: An Ecological Study among 210
    Countries." *Environmental Science and Pollution Research* 28:53116–26. https://
    doi.org/10.1007/s11356-021-14322-6.

van Doremalen, Neeltje, Trenton Bushmaker, Dylan H. Morris, Myndi G. Hol-
    brook, Amandine Gamble, Brandi N. Williamson, Azaibi Tamin, Jennifer
    L. Harcourt, Natalie J. Thornburg, Susan I. Gerber, et al. 2020. "Aerosol and
    Surface Stability of SARS-CoV-2 as Compared with SARS-CoV-1." *New En-
    gland Journal of Medicine* 382:1564–67. https://www.nejm.org/doi/full/10.1056
    /nejmc2004973.

Wathore, Roshan, Ankit Gupta, Hemant Bherwani, and Nitin Labhasetwar. 2020.
    "Understanding Air and Water Borne Transmission and Survival of Coronavi-
    rus: Insights and Way Forward for SARS-CoV-2." *Science of the Total Environ-
    ment* 749:141486. https://www.ncbi.nlm.nih.gov/pmc/articles/PMC7402210/.

Wittry, Beth, and Erin Kincaid. 2021. "CDC COVID-19 Response: Grand Prin-
    cess." Unpublished presentation at National Environmental Health Associa-
    tion Annual Education Conference, June 2021.

Wu, X., R. C. Nethery, M. B. Sabath, D. Braun, and F. Dominici. 2020. "Air Pollu-
    tion and COVID-19 Mortality in the United States: Strengths and Limitations
    of an Ecological Regression Analysis." *Science Advances* 6, no. 45 (November):
    eabd4049. https://doi.org/10.1126/sciadv.abd4049.

Yang, Xi, and Kevin Lo. 2021. "Environmental Health Research and the COVID-19
    Pandemic: A Turning Point towards Sustainability." *Environmental Research*
    197:111157. https://doi.org/10.1016/j.envres.2021.111157.

7

Pandemic Plastic

An Environmental Health Perspective on PPE Littering

KUJANG LAKI, IMAN IKRAM, AND GRACE OFORIWA SIKAPOKOO

The advent of the COVID-19 pandemic has exacerbated the complexities of addressing plastic waste management. In an effort to respond to the ongoing pandemic, the Centers for Disease Control and Prevention (CDC) recommended the use of personal protective equipment (PPE), including disposal masks, surgical gloves, hand sanitizers, and face shields, to decrease exposure to and transmission of COVID-19 (Jenco 2020.) The increased use of single-use PPE by healthcare professionals and the mandated use of facemasks by the public to contain the spread of the disease has altered the dynamics of plastic waste production (Vanapalli et al. 2021). Further, the view of the hygienic superiority of single-use plastics over other options has shifted consumer preference in support of plastic packaging (Scaraboto, Joubert, and Gonzalez-Arcos 2020). In turn, this preference necessitates adopting safe and proper disposal of plastic waste to reduce the detrimental effects of plastic pollution on the environment. This chapter traces the challenges hindering the safe and proper disposal of plastic waste, highlights strategies that have reduced its harmful impact on the environment, and provides recommendations to further reduce the impact of PPE pollution in the future.

The heightened use of PPE has negatively impacted the environment, with the proliferation of PPE littering adding to existing plastic waste management issues. Literature states that the sheer mismanagement of plastic as a resource is a major part of what makes it toxic to the environment (Vanapalli et al. 2021; Fadare and Okoffo 2020). Single-use masks with layers of plastics combined with other materials threaten the environment since they cannot be recycled (Tenenbaum 2020). The increased use of PPE raises the risk of viral infection without appropriate sterilization. Moreover, improper PPE disposal leads to it entering waterways, adding to pollution and impacting life in both freshwater and marine environments, causing aquatic animals to choke and die in some cases (Fadare and Okoffo 2020). Plastic pollution is a pertinent issue that requires sustainable solutions for future prevention and outbreak response to infectious diseases. This review examines PPE littering associated with the COVID-19 pandemic, identifying salient issues and topics that could influence policy outcomes and training curricula for environmental practitioners. The chapter aims to inform dialogue and facilitate policies to promote proper and safe PPE disposal to safeguard the environment. Furthermore, it seeks to address knowledge gaps regarding PPE pollution associated with COVID-19 and other potentially airborne pandemics, highlight current mitigation efforts, and provide suggestions for improved waste management and legislation.

THE EMERGENCE OF CORONAVIRUS (COVID 19) PANDEMIC

The World Health Organization (WHO) identified a novel coronavirus as the contributing agent of a new-found type of pneumonia. Subsequently named COVID-19, it was first reported as the source of respiratory disease in December 2019 in Wuhan, Hubei Province, China (Okuku et al. 2021; Tabish et al. 2021). The initial cases of infection occurred among a group of patients with pneumonia of an unknown cause the majority of whom had visited the city's Huanan (South China) Seafood Wholesale Market. At the time of this writing, COVID-19, a type of coronavirus, is the third-largest epidemic that began in Asia, after severe acute respiratory syndrome (SARS) and Middle East respiratory syndrome (MERS) (Tabish et al. 2021).

Coronaviruses are large gram-positive single-stranded RNA viruses belonging to a family of viruses called Coronaviridae existing in alpha-, beta-, gamma-, and delta-subfamilies commonly linked to animals (Jenco 2020; Ahn et al. 2020; Okuku et al. 2021). The alpha and beta subfamilies originated from bats, while gamma and delta originated from birds and pigs. These viruses are prevalent worldwide in animals, but very few strains have been known to affect humans. In humans, they cause respiratory infections ranging from the common cold to more severe diseases such as SARS, MERS, and

COVID-19 (Jenco 2020). COVID-19 is triggered by a beta coronavirus sub-family called severe acute respiratory syndrome coronavirus (SARS-CoV-2), which affects the lower respiratory tract and occurs in humans as pneumonia. In the context of COVID-19, SARS-CoV-2, rampant in several mammalian species also butchered and sold in the Wuhan seafood market mentioned above, first spread to humans there and manifested clinically as pneumonia (Joseph and Fagbami 2020; Okuku et al. 2021; Liu et al. 2020).

Existing literature on coronavirus suggests that the dense population of Wuhan, convenience, and accessibility to the marketplace that sells live animals contributed to the emergence of the outbreak (Tabish et al. 2021). Thus, the ease of access and openness of the market and the frequent interaction between humans and animals contributed to the initial cases of exposure and transmission. Moreover, the paucity of early containment due to failure to trace the detailed exposure history within the first series of patients contributed to the rapid rate of spread in Wuhan. A report by the World Health Organization (2020) explains that it declared an endemic of viral pneumonia on January 30, 2020. On March 11, COVID-19 was upgraded to a pandemic by the WHO (2020) due to the global logarithmic growth of outbreaks in more than 114 countries. Therefore, a national emergency was declared by the CDC in the United States on March 13. By mid-April, there were more than 1.8 million COVID-19 cases confirmed worldwide along with a continuing upward trend (Okuku et al. 2021).

From the onset of COVID-19, travel-related exportation led to its spread throughout the world from person to person through respiratory droplets. According to the CDC (2020), these droplets can land on objects while talking, coughing, or sneezing and people encountering them can become infected with COVID-19. The disease symptoms vary from mild to severe and, in some cases, with no illness representation. Symptoms include fever, cough, shortness of breath or difficulty breathing, headache, nasal congestion, muscle pain, sore throat, loss of smell or taste, and diarrhea. Hence, the CDC (2020) recommended everyday preventive actions that include washing hands often, wearing a mask, covering coughs and sneezes, cleaning and disinfecting frequently touched surfaces daily, practicing social distancing, staying at home, and, eventually, vaccination. As an initial or short-term response to the virus, most countries immediately enforced lockdown or stay-at-home measures and the wearing of disposable masks in public. Overall, these measures proved to be highly effective. Additional measures adopted by several countries were travel restrictions, isolation, and minimizing or banning large public or even smaller crowded gatherings.

The persistent COVID-19 pandemic aggravated the use of single-use plastics such as PPE worldwide (De-la-Torre et al. 2021; Patrício Silva et al. 2021; Prata et al. 2020). Single-use plastics include gloves, protective medical suits, masks, hand sanitizer bottles, takeout plastics, food and polyethylene goods packages, and medical test kits (Benson, Bassey, and Palanisami 2021). The pandemic has presented new challenges to conventional waste management as a result of the massive production, use, and disposal of PPE (De-la-Torre et al. 2021; Vanapalli et al. 2021). This increased use of PPE is a startling and inadequately understood form of plastic pollution that raises significant concerns.

COVID-19 AND PPE

As a part of COVID-19 containment, treatment, and protective measures, the WHO and CDC have recommended using personal protective equipment such as facemasks, splashproof garments, surgical gloves, face shields, hand sanitizers, and wipes by both frontline healthcare workers and the general public. While single-use plastics and PPE such as face masks were primarily made for the protection of healthcare workers to prevent occupational hazards, nonmedical professionals adopted the use of facemasks during the outbreak of SARS in 2003 and H1N1 in 2009 (Fadare and Okoffo 2020). These preventive methods proved to be effective and were recommended once more to combat the COVID-19 pandemic. Researchers have also advocated for the use of face masks because, apart from their efficacy in preventing direct inhalation of virus particles, they have been shown to significantly reduce the risk of infection posed by the number of times a person touches their face, mouth, and nose with unwashed hands (Fadare and Okoffo 2020). The adoption of face masks by the larger public created an upsurge in demand and a consequent global shortage of face masks for frontline healthcare workers. The WHO (2020) estimated a monthly order of 89 million masks, 76 million pairs of gloves, and 1.6 million goggles by healthcare workers alone. As a result, countries like China and Japan increased their PPE production efforts.

All of these factors led to a vastly increased amount of waste generated from single-use plastic worldwide. Based on projections as of the end of 2020, an estimated 3.4 billion single-use facemasks or face shields were being discarded daily across the globe. Asia, with the highest population, was estimated to be producing 1.8 billion discarded facemasks per day, followed by Europe (445 million), Africa (411 million), Latin America and the Caribbean (380 million), North America (244 million), and Oceania (22 million).

Taking into account COVID-19 policies in specific countries at the time, re-searchers set the estimated daily use of facemasks in China (1.4 billion popu-lation) at 702 million, India (1.3 billion population) at 386 million, the United States (331 million inhabitants) at 219 million, Brazil (212 million people) at 140 million, Nigeria (206 million population) at 75 million, and the United Kingdom (67 million population) at 45 million (Benson, Bassey, and Pala-nisami 2021). If actual use was anything even approaching these estimates, single-use plastics and PPE have dramatically exacerbated existing plastic pollution problems and constitute an impending threat to our collective ex-istence and the survival of marine organisms.

Ironically, the initial impacts of COVID-19 were positive for the environ-ment. Early studies revealed a reduction of nitrogen oxide (NO2) concen-trations in China; a drop in greenhouse gas emissions in France, Germany, Spain, and Italy; and cleaner beaches due to reduced waste generation by tourism activities (Okuku et al. 2021). Other studies showcased ecosystem recovery from reduced air and water pollution, slowed depletion of ground-water levels, and alleviation of other issues caused by human activities. Nonetheless, the significant increase in discarded PPE items prompted by their mandatory use and increased voluntary demand has resulted in grave environmental concerns due to incorrect disposal in public places and the natural environment (Okuku et al. 2021). Despite the magnitude of the prob-lem, there are no clear instructions and disposal mechanisms (De-la-Torre et al. 2021). In addition, this is expected to worsen the current plastic pollution challenges generated by millions of tons of plastic that endanger our oceans, marine organisms, and collective environmental health (Canning-Clode et al. 2020; De-la-Torre et al. 2021). Moreover, the production of facemasks has increased more than ten times in the initial ten months as new virus variants have been introduced and continue to surge. As a result, many PPE items are stranded on the coastlines, beaches, rivers, and littering cities (De-la-Torre et al. 2021; Canning-Clode et al. 2020).

PPE LITTERING

The COVID-19 crisis exemplifies the central role of plastic in everyday life. More specifically, it highlights a relatively rare positive value of single-use plas-tic, by controlling the spread of the virus (Okuku et al. 2021). Still, although PPEs are a safe option for many functions, they are an environmental liabil-ity due to their new role as a primary supplier of plastic pollution during air-borne disease pandemics. Personal protective equipment has developed into a new category of litter invading countless distinct public spaces, including indoor spaces such as shopping centers and outdoor spaces such as roadsides, car parking areas, parks, and beaches (Thiel et al. 2021). A report released by Ocean Conservancy in 2021 revealed that volunteers had removed 107,219 individual pieces of PPE from beaches and waterways in 2020. A World Wildlife Fund report stated that even if 1% of masks were being disposed of incorrectly, up to 10 million masks were polluting the environment each month (World Wildlife Fund 2020).

While some in the general public have embraced the use of PPE to contain the spread of COVID-19, new environmental challenges persist. PPE waste has been and in many parts of the world still is a leading contributor to the vast plastic waste in the environment. As we experience resurgences of COVID-19 and the arrival of other pandemics, we will undoubtedly see consequent rises in PPE waste. In response to the rise in COVID-19 cases worldwide, waste management's energy and environmental impacts rose exponentially (Tabish et al. 2021; Fadare and Okoffo 2020). Since coronaviruses may remain infectious and transmittable for several days on surfaces, there are concerns about SARS-CoV-2 transfer via the management of discarded PPE (Thiel et al. 2021). There are significant hazardous waste management concerns due to the need to ensure the elimination of residual pathogens in household and medical wastes. PPE waste has been increasingly identified in freshwater and marine ecosystems, adding even more microplastics to aquatic environments. Studies show that improper disposal of biomedical waste (PPE exposed to the virus) may result in the transmission of disease via sewage, water bodies, and groundwater (Shammi, Behal, and Tareq 2021). In 2020, numerous facemasks were found on highways and in drainages globally (Fadare and Okoffo 2020). To exemplify, in February 2020, Ocean Asia, an organization dedicated to activism and research on marine pollution, reported the incidence of PPE littering, namely "face masks of different types and colours," in the ocean off Hong Kong (Fadare and Okoffo 2020).

Numerous countries have developed and implemented recommendations about handling potentially contaminated waste with the increased health risk associated with discarded PPE. However, coordinated strategies are needed to mitigate the adverse effects of PPE littering on the environment. Currently, no regulations exist regarding microplastic pollution management strategies in many parts of the world (Fadare and Okoffo 2020). This situation may contribute to pathogens' long persistence and transmission, including of SARS-CoV-2, resulting in future disease outbreaks. The lack of internationally unified plastic regulation and pollution management can be seen as largely due to a conflict in economic interests. Within the United States, plastic lobbyists seized the opportunity presented by COVID-19 to advocate for single-use plastics as the ultimate resource for maintaining hygiene as well as longer shelf life for fresh produce (Vanapalli et al. 2021). Without proper regulations, planning, and mandatory policy interventions, the surge in plastic use is likely to prompt a new global public health crisis (Vanapalli et al. 2021).

ENVIRONMENTAL IMPACT OF PLASTIC POLLUTION

An N95 mask and a disposable surgical mask contain, respectively, an estimated 11 and 4.5 grams of polypropylene, polystyrene, polycarbonate, and/ or polyacrylonitrile (Khoironi et al. 2020). The thermoplastic polymer fraction of these plastic substances breaks into smaller particles known as microplastics due to numerous factors, such as UV exposure, high temperature, hydrophobicity, and change in pH (Khoironi et al. 2020). Gloves also pose an environmental threat as they are made of latex plastic and contain harmful addictive chemicals. Moreover, polypropylene does not degrade or mineralize readily due to its extraordinarily resilient nature, high molecular weight, hydrophobic properties, and elevated surface roughness (Jiang 2018). In sum, polypropylene settles in the environment in the form of microplastics, posing a threat to marine ecosystems and further intensifying plastic pollution.

Prior to the pandemic, plastic waste management was already considered a major environmental problem because of rising fears about contamination in terrestrial and marine ecosystems (Tabish et al. 2021). The extensive use of face masks has further increased the number of microplastics entering the environment. Microplastics present severe adverse outcomes, including the threat to aquatic life, which comprises a key portion of the food web and support of human survival (Fadare and Okoffo 2020). Plastic particles are a growing concern in maintaining global food safety standards as more microplastics are getting into food products intended for human consumption (Fadare and Okoffo 2020). In the realm of public health, discarded PPEs pose an environmental and health risk as they are made from nonbiodegradable plastics that are already found in seafood, which is a major source of protein for many countries globally. Marine organisms such as birds, sea turtles, fish, and whales and other marine mammals are at risk of entanglement by and ingestion of latex gloves, leading to severe injuries and death (Benson, Bassey, and Palanisami 2021). The presence of plastics in the natural environment has also been credited as a contributing factor in climate change, owing to the significant carbon emissions involved in their production. Further, microplastics in the environment are potential routes of pathogens at varying levels. They enable the settlement of several pathogenic microorganisms (bacteria, viruses, fungal filaments, and spores) in aquatic ecosystems, leading to transmission of diseases already present or even new to these environments.

Meanwhile, the pandemic led to the deferrals of bans on single-use plastics and recycling systems in the United States, as a mitigation measure to limit the risk of spreading COVID-19 in recycling facilities (Okuku et al. 2021; Vanapalli et al. 2021). As of this writing, there is a provisional relaxation on single-use plastic bag bans in several states in the United States, such as New Hampshire, New York, and Massachusetts, which is likely to have protracted adverse outcomes on consumer behavior (Patrício Silva et al. 2021; Prata et al. 2020; Vanapalli et al. 2021).

Like most plastic litter, PPEs are mostly composite materials made of different synthetic nondegradable polymers (De-la-Torre et al. 2021; Fadare and Okoffo 2020). Plastic polymers can be positively, neutrally, or negatively buoyant in the water system. High-density polymers, such as polyester (PEST), polyvinyl chloride (PVC), and polyvinyl alcohol (PVA), are likely to sink and reach bottom marine sediments. Most 3-ply surgical masks are made of polypropylene (PP), while others may include different materials like polycarbonate (PC), polyethylene (PE), and PEST (De-la-Torre et al. 2021). Regarding gloves, the most commercially available materials are PVC, latex, and nitrile. Face shields are manufactured from various materials, including polyethylene terephthalate glycol (PETG), PC, acetate, and PVC (De-la-Torre et al. 2021).

Owing to the multiple materials that constitute standard PPE, along with their non-degradability and persistence in the environment, it is deducible that their fate will vary depending on specific characteristics. As observed with other plastic pollutants, some PPE items remain in the environment for long periods, with many of them potentially carried long distances by surface oceanic currents. In contrast, others may become buried in riverine and ocean sediment, ultimately becoming part of the geological record (De-la-Torre et al. 2021). Currently, microplastics are widely known for their ubiquitous presence in the environment, bioavailability to organisms of all taxa, and detrimental effects on the environment (De-la-Torre et al. 2021). These substances can interfere with the reproductive systems of aquatic organisms, consequently reducing their growth rate. PPE items may also be ingested entirely by marine megafauna and apex predators, such as whales, sharks, turtles, marine mammals, or seabirds. Marine fauna can also become entangled with the elastic cords of face masks and some face shields (De-la-Torre et al. 2021).

The use of PPE and other plastic medical items in the home poses its own class of environmental challenges. Contaminated masks, gloves, medicine bottles and the medicines themselves, and other items can easily mix with household garbage, thus perpetuating the risk of coronavirus and other infections (Tabish et al. 2021). Residual pathogens in household waste are an area of serious concern and one that is difficult to address. For instance, waste materials associated with the pandemic and other medical sources should be kept separate from other flows of household waste and collected by municipal specialists or waste management operators, treated as hazardous waste, and disposed of separately (Tabish et al. 2021). However, these materials are generally only disposed of properly by health facilities, not at the community level, while it is impossible to monitor and ensure their appropriate handling by households.

Single-use plastic has been necessary in managing the virus, even though, in most other applications, it is generally seen as an environmental problem. This is best exhibited by the tremendous use of plastic packaging materials, drinking bottles, and fast-food takeout containers as leading sources of microplastics globally (Fadare and Okoffo 2020). Meanwhile, prevention or reduction steps across the globe have greatly increase the amount of plastic waste. Consumers see single-use plastics as a convenient option for hygienic safeguards against the spread of COVID-19. Lockdown initiatives have also resulted in a rise in the quantity of packaging used to produce and distribute food (Tabish et al. 2021).

PPE littering will continue to intensify environmental issues with plastics that already existed before the pandemic took place. While this rise is inevitable, communication efforts are needed to educate the public on best practices to protect the environment. Existing literature states that microplastic particles invade almost every ecosystem. A significant portion ends up in freshwater bodies, finally reaching the marine environment. Fadare and Okoffo (2020) examined the degradation of face masks used in the environment and found traces of polypropylene in the outer layer and polyethylene in the inner layer. Their findings suggest that plastic particles may accrue in the environment quickly. Similar results regarding polypropylene and polyethylene were previously reported from eight sandy beaches and four sea surface stations along the coastline of Qatar (Abayomi et al. 2017).

In 2017, the WHO authorized the incineration of PPE and additional infectious/hazardous waste, notably of plastic accumulated before the pandemic. As a consequence, the mandate expanded the load on incineration facilities and the current infrastructure could not keep up with the immense rise in plastic waste production with the onset of the pandemic. The estimated amassed medical waste of 240 tons per day in Wuhan, China, exceeded the province's incineration capability (49 t/d) (Vanapalli et al. 2021). Ineffective and under-maintained systems with only nominal air pollution control equipment, along with open burning of plastic waste in many parts of the world, lead to the release of hazardous gases like dioxins and furans. Plastic waste handled by incineration alone emitted approximately 5.9 million metric tons of carbon dioxide (CO_2) in the United States and 16 million metric tons of greenhouse gases in 2015 globally (Vanapalli et al. 2021). A separate CO_2 assessment of nonrecyclable plastics showed that landfills cause fewer CO_2 emissions (253 g per kg) than incineration (673–4605 g per kg) (Patrício Silva et al. 2021). Thus, it is imperative to consider prevailing mitigation measures and offer better methods to deter future plastic pollution challenges.

MITIGATION STRATEGIES

Previous long-term strategies such as "reduce, reuse, and recycle" designed to combat and lessen plastic pollution are no longer effective (Patrício Silva et al. 2021). Although the strategy made initial gains, it is no longer sufficient to curtail the rapid growth of plastic waste in our ecosystems, considering low recycling rates that are just 9% globally (Geyer, Jambeck, and Law 2017). The COVID-19 pandemic has disrupted plastic pollution mitigation efforts due to the excessive use of plastic-based medical material to prevent and control the escalation of the coronavirus disease. In the realm of environmental health, researchers have documented some ecological implications and consequences of plastic pollution. Consequently, numerous countries recognized the latent health risk of discarded PPE and developed and implemented mitigation measures, such as dedicated PPE waste bins and better management of municipal waste (Selvaranjan et al. 2021). PPE bins have been put in place in Montreal, Canada, and Guimarães, Portugal, which has aided in the separation of PPE waste for specific treatment using incineration and recycling methods (Prata et al. 2020). In South Korea, special safe waste management measures were put in place for COVID-19 waste (Selvaranjan et al. 2021). These included not keeping COVID-19 waste for more than twenty-four hours, and instead having the waste incinerated on the day of collection at a temperature above 1,100 degrees Celsius. They also used steam at high temperatures to disinfect the waste.

The National Oceanic and Atmospheric Administration promotes awareness of plastic pollution through public education programs (Li, Busquets, and Campos 2020). Countries like Ireland have placed levies on consumers of single-use bags. Countries such as South Africa and China have combined both bans and levies on retailers. Other effective mitigation strategies include exploring eco-friendly alternatives and social mobilization concerning and awareness of COVID-19 globally. Last, Fadare and Okoffo (2020) underscore that we must find a sustainable solution through environmental health literacy that safeguards the environment through the reduction, elimination, and proper management of PPEs.

A thermochemical process for recycling PPE is another potential solution to reduce the impact of PPE littering (Rakib et al. 2021). The process entails converting PPE waste into gas and liquid fuels through pyrolysis, which is the breaking down of plastics using heat (Aragaw 2020). Using degradable plastics such as bio-based or biodegradable plastics is emerging as a preferred sustainable solution (Patrício Silva et al. 2021). This would decrease PPE's contribution to the devastating effects of our current, almost total reliance on synthetic (petroleum-based) plastics. However, the market for this type of disposable mask is quite limited, although they are currently commercially available (Selvaranjan et al. 2021). Other possible solutions include 100% reusable, recyclable, or compostable PPE, which could mitigate concerns regarding reusable PPE with the use of proper hygiene and sterilization (Patrício Silva et al. 2021).

RECOMMENDATIONS

The COVID-19 pandemic has led to the use of a wide range of tools to communicate health recommendations and government regulations to the general public and more specific audiences. Future communication efforts should move beyond solely emphasizing wearing face masks, washing hands, and social distancing—their most common focus—to include messages on the proper disposal of masks. Moreover, with high rates of discarded PPE on beach shores, several environmental health scholars have recommended providing PPE-related signs and waste bins, establishing strict waste disposal regulations, and improving enforcement (Thiel et al. 2021). The novelty and severity of COVID-19 has demonstrated the need for educational campaigns that advocate proper use and disposal of face masks, litter prevention, and reduction of single-use waste to deter the negative impacts of PPE littering on the environment, in the context of COVID-19 or any other future epidemics.

Such measures form part of the most important recommendation for the management of PPE disposal: providing guidelines for individuals and communities. There are structures and policies in place for medical and chemical waste, but almost nowhere are comparable policies and practices in place for the generic disposal of PPE outside medical facilities. A robust strategy for sterilization and disinfection of surgical gowns and masks—and now PPE—is carried out by healthcare workers. Stakeholders, policy-makers, and governments need to develop a green solution that includes the three *Rs* (reduce, reuse, recycle) as a feasible solid-waste management approach to the use of PPEs by the general public (Benson, Bassey, and Palanisami 2021).

At the government level, the guidance issued by the Ocean Conservancy (March 2021) to address plastic pollution should be incorporated into executive-level action plans. In the United States, robust funding should be provided for the EPA and National Oceanic and Atmospheric Administration to tackle waste management challenges related to PPE. The government could also create waste-producer responsibility programs for the private sector, to establish its responsibility for the full life cycle of plastic products. Public awareness programs on disposal as well as proper use of PPE should be implemented (Prata et al. 2020). Fadare and Okoffo (2020) propose sensitization of the general population on effective litter management, enlisting them in providing sustainable solutions to waste management. Advertising campaigns underlining the importance of proper disposal of PPE and the adverse effects of improper disposal should be carried out (Prata et al. 2020). Members of the community and university and college students can be encouraged and helped to advocate for waste segregation (Shammi, Behal, and Tareq 2021), including through social media, which already plays a vital role in promoting public awareness and executing campaigns. Facilities like grocery stores, restaurants, and malls should have appropriate bins for proper disposal of PPE used by employees and customers (Prata et al. 2020). Deliberate and inadvertent flushing of PPE results in the transportation of PPE and contaminated wastewater as a key source of freshwater and marine plastic pollution (De-la-Torre et al. 2021; Patrício Silva et al. 2021; Shammi, Behal, and Tareq 2021), so there is a need for improved plumbing systems in healthcare facilities and homes, among other places, to avoid this often overlooked risk point (Shammi, Behal, and Tareq 2021).

Some of the individual-level recommendations suggested by Ocean Conservancy (March 2021) include cutting the ear loops of masks, because intact ear loops pose an entanglement risk to wildlife. Other recommendations include disposing of PPE responsibly at home, using trash bags that are sealed and kept in cars or carried out for safe disposal at drop-off locations or through municipal waste services. Certainly, when a family member is sick or recovering from communicable disease all PPE should be treated this way, but it should also be done in the course of everyone's daily life during an epidemic. Additionally, not flushing sanitizing wipes and following health authority guidelines for the use of reusable PPE are responsible measures that individuals can take.

The surging demand for PPE in the healthcare sector requires conservation strategies that further support the proper sterilization and disinfection of surgical gowns and masks. The US FDA has also suggested the employment of reusable surgical gowns instead of disposable single-use PPE to act as a barrier to microbial and fluid transmission during surgical procedures. However, these strategies should be carried out keeping in mind the guidelines aimed at reducing COVID-19 risk for both healthcare workers and patients (Patrício Silva et al. 2021). Reusable alternatives for use in healthcare applications as well as for the public should be produced and financially incentivized at the industrial-sector level (Patrício Silva et al. 2021).

LIMITATIONS

This chapter focused on how PPE littering has contributed to plastic pollution, reviewed current mitigation strategies, and provided recommendations for behavior change approaches. While the chapter presents vital information on factors affecting PPE and other plastic pollution sources, there are several limitations. The chapter does not cover PPE disposal, reusable PPE, and the disposal of biomedical and other contaminated waste in specific economic sectors, such as the chemical and pharmaceutical industries. Second, the chapter employed secondary data. Primary data obtained from in-depth interviews and focus group discussions would have generated detailed firsthand accounts, which could offer insight into other contributing factors in relation to PPE and plastic pollution. Future researchers might consider organizing in-depth interviews with stakeholders at various levels to better understand the challenges to proper disposal of PPEs. The same applies to community-based participatory approaches with the general public and environmental groups.

CONCLUSION

The COVID-19 pandemic has exerted tremendous pressure on current conventional solid-waste management practices. The massive quantities of PPE plastic waste generated worldwide have been generally mishandled, with inappropriate disposal, landfill, and/or incineration techniques that end up polluting aquatic ecosystems (De-la-Torre et al. 2021). Disease outbreaks are increasingly prone to raise immense environmental concerns and adverse effects. The pandemic has impacted all aspects of our environmental challenges, and its effects on the environment will and should shape our discourse on environmental issues.

The long-term harmful effects can be seen in living organisms dwelling in freshwater, marine, and terrestrial habitats. However, it is possible to identify, establish, and expand the use of timely and necessary prevention and control measures, as well as to advocate, enact, and support changes in public and private behavior, so we can work together to avoid such consequences in the future. By addressing salient issues related to PPE littering and exploring topics that could influence both governmental policy and training curricula for environmental practitioners, researchers and scholars can help enable future prevention and response efforts to curb environmental impacts from health outbreaks. It is critical that, in doing so, we highlight the need for and importance of working with all stakeholders in addressing PPE and plastic pollution.

Future reviews can further explore attempts to change behaviors through communication efforts such as PPE anti-littering campaigns. Vital research insights can be specifically used to train and build the capacity of environmental communication professionals. Key findings may be incorporated in the design and dissemination of information, education, and communication toolkits to address PPE littering, and can be used to revise existing environmental communication materials. There is also a need to identify successful uses of the advisories, fines, and mitigation strategies put in place in various states that may serve as models that other states may adopt in addressing PPE littering.

The work of scholars and public health professionals can also support the planning and implementation of local litter clean-up activity. By identifying the causes of increased PPE littering, ways to remedy those causes, and short-term mitigation strategies in dealing with their effects, research and information shared can support the deployment of government and private resources and the mobilization of community participants in cleaning up the discarded gloves, masks, wipes, face shields, and hand sanitizer bottles that we have seen littering stores, parking lots, parks, sidewalks, public transport, gutters, and streets during periods of wide-scale use of PPE during the height of the COVID-19 pandemic, and which will threaten to return whenever we experience similar conditions.

The long-term goals of the overview provided here are to inform dialogue, facilitate policies, and develop sustained communication interventions to promote proper and safe PPE disposal to safeguard the environment. There are many others doing scholarly work toward the same goals, some of whom we have cited. This growing body of work could be used to advocate and support the necessary review of existing guidelines for managing garbage and recycling at the international, national, state, and county levels. Results can be shared with organizations such as the WHO, the CDC, the American Public Health Association, Johns Hopkins and other universities with research departments active in public health and related spheres, the Solid Waste Association of North America, public and private waste management companies, community and environmental groups, and elected officials at all levels to inform policy, practices, curricula, and environmental health literacy in the broader population.

DISCUSSION QUESTION

- As environmental health scholars and practitioners, what are some immediate and effective health communication strategies to reduce waste and eliminate the spread of disease?

REFERENCES

Abayomi, Oyebamiji Abib, Pedro Range, Mohammad Ahamd Al-Ghouti, Jeffrey Philip Obbard, Saeed Hashim Almeer, and Radhouane Ben-Hamadou. 2017. "Microplastics in Coastal Environments of the Arabian Gulf." *Marine Pollution Bulletin* 124, no. 1: 181–88. https://doi.org/10.1016/j.marpolbul.2017.07.011.

Ahn, Jin Young, Yujin Sohn, Su Hwan Lee, Yunsuk Cho, Jong Hoon Hyun, Yae Jee Baek, Su Jin Jeong, Jung Ho Kim, Nam Su Ku, Joon-Sup Yeom, et al. 2020. "Use of Convalescent Plasma Therapy in Two COVID-19 Patients with Acute Respiratory Distress Syndrome in Korea." *Journal of Korean Medical Science* 35, no. 14: e149. https://doi.org/10.3346/jkms.2020.35.e149.

Aragaw, Tadele Assefa. 2020. "Surgical Face Masks as a Potential Source for Microplastic Pollution in the COVID-19 Scenario." *Marine Pollution Bulletin* 159:111517. https://doi.org/10.1016/j.marpolbul.2020.111517.

Benson, Nsikak U., David E. Bassey, and Thavamani Palanisami. 2021. "COVID Pollution: Impact of COVID-19 Pandemic on Global Plastic Waste Footprint." *Heliyon* 7, no. 2 (February): e06343. https://doi.org/10.1016/j.heliyon.2021.e06343.

Canning-Clode, João, Pedro Sepúlveda, Sílvia Almeida, and João Monteiro. 2020. "Will COVID-19 Containment and Treatment Measures Drive Shifts in Marine Litter Pollution?" *Frontiers in Marine Science* 7:691. https://doi.org/10.3389/fmars.2020.00691.

De-la-Torre, Gabriel Enrique, Carlos Ivan Pizarro-Ortega, Diana Carolina Dioses-Salinas, Justine Ammendolia, and Elvis D. Okoffo. 2021. "Investigating the Current Status of COVID-19 Related Plastics and Their Potential Impact on Human Health." *Current Opinion in Toxicology* 27:47–53. https://doi.org/10 .1016/j.cotox.2021.08.002.

Fadare, Oluniyi O., and Elvis D. Okoffo. 2020. "Covid-19 Face Masks: A Potential Source of Microplastic Fibers in the Environment." *Science of the Total Environment* 737:140279. https://doi.org/10.1016/j.scitotenv.2020.140279.

Geyer, Roland, Jenna R. Jambeck, and Kara Lavender Law. 2017. "Production, Use, and Fate of All Plastics Ever Made." *Science Advances* 3, no. 7 (July): e1700782. https://doi.org/10.1126/sciadv.1700782.

Jenco, Melissa. 2020. "CDC Updates Guidance on PPE for Health Care Personnel; COVID-19 Declared a Pandemic." American Academy of Pediatrics, March 11, 2020. https://publications.aap.org/aapnews/news/8021/CDC-updates-guidance -on-PPE-for-health-care.

Jiang, Jia-Qian. 2018. "Occurrence of Microplastics and Its Pollution in the Environment: A Review." *Sustainable Production and Consumption* 13:16–23. https:// doi.org/10.1016/j.spc.2017.11.003.

Joseph, A. A., and A. H. Fagbami. 2020. "Coronaviruses: A Review of Their Properties and Diversity." *African Journal of Clinical and Experimental Microbiology* 21, no. 4: 258–71. https://doi.org/10.4314/ajcem.v21i4.2.

Khoironi, Adian, Hadiyanto Hadiyanto, Sutrisno Anggoro, and Sudarno Sudarno. 2020. "Evaluation of Polypropylene Plastic Degradation and Microplastic Identification in Sediments at Tambak Lorok Coastal Area, Semarang, Indonesia." *Marine Pollution Bulletin* 151:110868. https://doi.org/10.1016/j.marpolbul .2019.110868.

Li, Chaoran, Rosa Busquets, and Luiza C. Campos. 2020. "Assessment of Microplastics in Freshwater Systems: A Review." *Science of the Total Environment* 707:135578. https://doi.org/10.1016/j.scitotenv.2019.135578.

Liu, Kui, Yuan-Yuan Fang, Yan Deng, Wei Liu, Mei-Fang Wang, Jing-Ping Ma, Wei Xiao, et al. 2020. "Clinical Characteristics of Novel Coronavirus Cases in Tertiary Hospitals in Hubei Province." *Chinese Medical Journal* 133, no. 9 (May): 1025–31. https://doi.org/10.1097/CM9.0000000000000744.

Morens, David M., and Jeffery K. Taubenberger. 2018. "Influenza Cataclysm, 1918." *New England Journal of Medicine* 379:2285–87. https://doi.org/10.1056 /NEJMp1814447.

Ocean Conservancy. 2021. *Pandemic Pollution: The Rising Tide of Plastic PPE.* Washington, DC: Ocean Conservancy.

Okuku, Eric, Linet Kiteresi, Gilbert Owato, Kenneth Otieno, Catherine Mwalugha, Mary Mbuche, Brenda Gwada, et al. 2021. "The Impacts of COVID-19 Pandemic on Marine Litter Pollution along the Kenyan Coast: A Synthesis after 100 Days Following the First Reported Case in Kenya." *Marine Pollution Bulletin* 162:111840. https://doi.org/10.1016/j.marpolbul.2020.111840.

Patrício Silva, Ana L., Joana C. Prata, Tony R. Walker, Armando C. Duarte, Wei Ouyang, Damià Barceló, and Teresa Rocha-Santos. 2021. "Increased Plastic Pollution Due to COVID-19 Pandemic: Challenges and Recommendations." *Chemical Engineering Journal* 405:126683. https://doi.org/10.1016/j.cej.2020.126683.

Prata, Joana C., Ana L. P. Silva, Tony R. Walker, Armando C. Duarte, and Teresa Rocha-Santos. 2020. "COVID-19 Pandemic Repercussions on the Use and Management of Plastics." *Environmental Science & Technology* 54, no. 13: 7760–65. https://doi.org/10.1021/acs.est.0c02178.

Rakib, Md. Refat Jahan, Gabriel E. De-la-Torre, Carlos Ivan Pizarro-Ortega, Diana Carolina Dioses-Salinas, and Sultan Al-Nahian. 2021. "Personal Protective Equipment (PPE) Pollution Driven by the COVID-19 Pandemic in Cox's Bazar, the Longest Natural Beach in the World." *Marine Pollution Bulletin* 169:112497. https://doi.org/10.1016/j.marpolbul.2021.112497.

Scaraboto, Daiane, Alison M. Joubert, and Claudia Gonzalez-Arcos. 2020. "Using Lots of Plastic Packaging during the Coronavirus Crisis? You're Not Alone." *The Conversation,* April 27, 2020. https://theconversation.com/using-lots-of -plastic-packaging-during-the-coronavirus-crisis-youre-not-alone-135553.

Selvaranjan, Kajanan, Satheeskumar Navaratnam, Pathmanathan Rajeev, and Nishanthan Ravintherakumaran. 2021. "Environmental Challenges Induced by Extensive Use of Face Masks during COVID-19: A Review and Potential Solutions." *Environmental Challenges* 3:100039. https://doi.org/10.1016/j.envc .2021.100039.

Shammi, Mashura, Arvind Behal, and Shafi M. Tareq. 2021. "The Escalating Biomedical Waste Management to Control the Environmental Transmission of COVID-19 Pandemic: A Perspective from Two South Asian Countries." *Environmental Science & Technology* 55, no. 7: 4087–93. https://doi.org/10.1021/acs .est.0c05117.

Tabish, Mohammad, Aisha Khatoon, Saad Alkahtani, Abdullah Alkahtane, Jawahir Alghamdi, Syed Anees Ahmed, Snober S. Mir, et al. 2021. "Approaches for Prevention and Environmental Management of Novel COVID-19." *Environmental Science and Pollution Research* 28, no. 30: 40311–21. https://doi.org/10 .1007/s11356-020-10640-3.

Tenenbaum, Laura. 2020. "The Amount of Plastic Waste Is Surging Because of the Coronavirus Pandemic." *Forbes,* April 25, 2020. https://www.forbes.com/sites /lauratenenbaum/2020/04/25/plastic-waste-during-the-time-of-covid-19/.

Thiel, Martin, Diamela de Veer, Nuxia L. Espinoza-Fuenzalida, Camilo Espinoza, Camila Gallardo, Ivan A. Hinojosa, Tim Kiessling, et al. 2021. "COVID Lessons from the Global South—Face Masks Invading Tourist Beaches and Recommendations for the Outdoor Seasons." *Science of the Total Environment* 786:147486. https://doi.org/10.1016/j.scitotenv.2021.147486.

Vanapalli, Kumar Raja, Hari Bhakta Sharma, Ved Prakash Ranjan, Biswajit Samal, Jayanta Bhattacharya, Brajesh K. Dubey, and Sudha Goel. 2021. "Challenges and Strategies for Effective Plastic Waste Management during and post COVID-19 Pandemic." *Science of the Total Environment* 750:141514. https://doi .org/10.1016/j.scitotenv.2020.141514.

World Wildlife Fund. 2020. "Nello smaltimento di mascherine e guanti serve responsabilita" [In the disposal of masks and gloves, responsibility is required]. World Wildlife Fund. April 29. https://www.wwf.it/scuole/?53500%2FNello -smaltimento-di-mascherine-e-guanti-serve-responsabilita.

Part 4

GLOBAL HEALTH SUCCESS
WITH OTHER PANDEMICS

8

Improving Global Pandemic Response

A History of Success and Challenges with Disease Outbreaks

SONYA PANJWANI, KOBI V. AJAYI, KRISTEN M. GARCIA,
TYRA MONTOUR, AND WHITNEY R. GARNEY

While COVID-19 has emerged as one of the most significant pandemics of the last century, disease outbreaks have occurred throughout history (WHO 2020a). In response, individuals and societies have attempted to prevent the rapid spread of disease through early detection and adequate treatment for those infected, more frequently focusing on the latter. Regardless of the approach adopted, these efforts have shared the same motivations, such as minimizing loss and reducing harm to life, and focus on the same goal: disease outbreak containment. The capacity to address these outbreaks has changed throughout history, especially with the emergence of healthcare technologies (St. Louis 2012). However, regardless of our increased capabilities in addressing disease outbreaks, we are not immune from their negative effects. Furthermore, as more frequent cross-cultural interactions occur with the ease of travel, we experience additional challenges in containing outbreaks within one country's borders (Lim, Hamilton, and Jiang 2015; Lindahl and Grace 2015). In light of COVID-19, it is evident that we need to look at historical perspectives on infectious disease outbreak response efforts with a critical eye. A retrospective study could prove useful for future emerging disease outbreak planning and response efforts.

In this chapter, we will examine some of the most influential disease outbreaks that have occurred throughout history through the lens of the World

Health Organization's (WHO) Integrated, People-Centered Health Services
(IPCHS) Framework (WHO, n.d.). The framework proposes restructuring
health systems with a focus on improving efficiency and functioning by building local capacity to address public health emergencies, among other health-
related issues. This discussion commences with a brief overview of disease
outbreaks throughout history, with variations in disease outbreak response
from ancient history to the modern era, followed by an in-depth look at the
WHO's IPCHS Framework and its application to disease outbreak response
efforts. To illustrate how this framework can be applied to disease outbreak
response, we present four of the most significant disease outbreaks, analyze
them through the strategies outlined in the WHO's framework, and relate the
analysis to the COVID-19 response. We conclude with a set of lessons learned
and recommendations for future practice, followed by an application to the
COVID-19 pandemic. The information presented will equip future public
health practitioners with the strategies and lessons learned from previous
outbreaks to help support and coordinate efforts to mitigate future disease
outbreaks.

DISEASE OUTBREAKS THROUGHOUT HISTORY

Disease outbreaks are not merely interesting events that help fill historical
texts; rather, these occurrences shape our civilizations and society. Throughout history, pandemics and epidemics have resulted in sizable reductions in
the world's populations, as shown in table 8.1. In some cases, these outbreaks
have resulted in the collapse of history's great civilizations, such as the Byz-
antine Empire. From a modern perspective, outbreaks continue to occur,
and despite their seeming to be anomalies as we experience them, they are
not unique from a historical perspective.

TABLE 8.1. SELECTED NOTABLE DISEASE OUTBREAKS THROUGHOUT HISTORY

Ancient, medieval, and early modern eras

Disease outbreak	Description
Plague of Athens, 430 BCE	During the Peloponnesian War, a plague hit Athens after the disease passed through Libya, Ethiopia, and Egypt. Most of the population was infected within three years, and possibly as many as 75,000 to 100,000 people, 25% of the city's population, died. The symptoms included fever, thirst, bloody throat and tongue, diarrhea, rash, and lesions. Physicians and scholars have identified the disease as either smallpox or typhus (Littman 2009).

Antonine Plague, 165 CE	The Antonine Plague began among the Huns, then infected the Germans, who transmitted it to the Romans. Symptoms reported lead researchers to think that the Antonine Plague was caused by smallpox. They included fever, sore throat, diarrhea, and pus-filled sores for some. It had a strong impact on military enlistment, the agricultural and urban economies, and consumption of state resources. There is limited reporting of events during the plague; historians and researchers estimate 7 to 8 million people were killed (Sabbatani and Fiorino 2009).
Plague of Cyprian, 249–70 CE	Named after bishop Cyprian of Carthage, the Plague of Cyprian included symptoms such as eye pain, high fevers, throat ulcers, and ailment of all limbs. Carthaginians helped disperse the disease, which passed through northern Africa into Egypt, then to Rome, Greece, and Syria. It is estimated that there were about 5,000 people killed a day in Rome due to this plague (Harper 2015).
Justinian Plague, 541–54 CE	The Justinian Plague began in Egypt, moving through the eastern Roman Empire and its surrounding nations, killing about 100 million people in the Roman Empire alone. It is also said to have contributed to the collapse of the Byzantine Empire. The most significant vector for the plague was fleas associated with wild rodents (Piret and Boivin 2020).
Black Death, 1347–51	The Black Death originated in East Asia and swept across Central Asia into Europe. This pandemic was ultimately responsible for the death of one-third of the world population, killing 200 million people. It had a major impact on medieval Europe's socioeconomic development, culture, art, religion, and politics (Piret and Boivin 2020).
Columbian Exchange, 1492 and beyond	The Columbian Exchange resulted in diseases being transferred between the New World (the Americas) and the Old World (Europe, North Africa, and the Middle East). Europeans brought deadly viruses and bacteria, such as smallpox, measles, typhus, syphilis, and cholera, to previously isolated communities. The exact magnitude is unknown; some regions lost an estimated 80% of their populations (Nunn and Qian 2010).
Great Plague of London, 1665–66	The Great Plague of London led to the loss of about 20% of London's population, with a total of 68,596 officially reported deaths (Shannon and Cromley 1980). Estimates by historians put the figure at approximately 100,000. This plague resulted from the transmission of disease from fleas on rats to humans.

Industrial era

Cholera pandemics: First 1817–24 Second 1827–35 Third 1839–56 Fourth 1863–75 Fifth 1881–86 Sixth 1899–1923	Cholera outbreaks have resulted in a total of seven pandemics, six during this specified time period. Cholera began in the Ganges delta of India and spread throughout the rest of the world to varying extents. Pandemics one through four were widespread; each subsequent pandemic occurred to a lesser extent in more developed countries due to advances in sanitation and public health response. Cholera is a waterborne bacteria that, when ingested, causes diarrhea, vomiting, thirst, and leg cramping in most of those affected. Combined, the first six cholera pandemics led to at least 8 million deaths; the total is probably greater, since in several countries case reports are suspected to be inaccurate or incomplete (Ramamurthy and Ghosh 2021).
Russian Flu, 1889–94	The Russian Flu is generally accepted to have been an influenza virus that initially spread rapidly over four months and continued thereafter. In the first year, 360,000 people died, with a total of about 1 million dying by the pandemic's end (Piret and Boivin 2020).
Spanish Flu, 1918–19	The Spanish Flu was caused by an H1N1 influenza A virus. Originally an avian-borne flu, this outbreak resulted in nearly 100 million deaths worldwide, with most victims being young adults. There were long-lasting social consequences, specifically a decline in social trust. Early reports of a flu outbreak in Madrid in early 1918 led to the name (Aassve et al. 2021).

TABLE 8.1. SELECTED NOTABLE DISEASE OUTBREAKS THROUGHOUT HISTORY (*cont.*)

Modern era

Asian Flu, 1957–59	The Asian Flu was caused by an H2N2 influenza A virus that began in Hong Kong and quickly spread throughout mainland China. There were 100,000 cases in Taiwan by mid-May 1957 and over a million in India by June 1957. In England, 14,000 people died within half a year. The next year, there was an estimated 1.1 million deaths globally, with 116,000 deaths in the United States (Jackson 2009). Estimates for total deaths over the course of the pandemic range as high as 4 million.
Seventh Cholera Pandemic, 1961–present	The seventh cholera pandemic began in Indonesia and has since dispersed through much of the world. Cholera has periodically surfaced in Zimbabwe (2008), Haiti (2010), Sierra Leone (2012), Mexico (2013), South Sudan (2014), Ghana (2014), and Yemen (2016). It is difficult to gauge the exact number of cholera deaths and cases due to underreporting. However, between 2008 and 2012 alone, there were an estimated 1.3–4 million cases per year and 95,000 deaths. In 2019, the WHO reported 923,037 cases and 1,911 deaths in 31 countries (Piret and Boivin 2020).
HIV/AIDS, 1981–present	The first cases of HIV/AIDS were reported in June 1981. The largest impact of the epidemic was among men who have sex with men (MSM) and among racial/ ethnic minorities, with increases in the number of cases among women and of cases attributed to heterosexual transmission. According to the most recent UNAIDS report, there are approximately 39 million people living with HIV globally and an estimated 1.3 million new HIV infections. Globally, 40.4 million people have died of AIDS-related illnesses since the beginning of the epidemic (UNAIDS 2023).
SARS, 2002–3	Severe acute respiratory syndrome (SARS) originated in Guangdong Province, China. It has been postulated that bats were the possible reservoir. SARS was reported in 29 countries in North America, South America, Europe, and Asia. A total of 8,437 cases were reported with 813 SARS-related deaths. SARS is a flu-like syndrome causing respiratory issues, fatigue, and high fever. Less common symptoms are nausea, vomiting, and diarrhea (Piret and Boivin 2020).
Swine Flu, 2009–10	Swine flu emerged in Mexico through person-to-person transmission, not from pigs to humans as its name implies (Parmar et al. 2011). The virus then spread globally over a mere six weeks. The WHO reported 18,631 laboratory-confirmed deaths. However, it is estimated that between 148,000 and 249,000 deaths occurred, based on calculations of excess death due to respiratory illness. Symptoms include fever, cough, sore throat, body aches, headache, chills, and fatigue (Burkardt 2011).

HISTORY OF DISEASE OUTBREAK RESPONSE

Ancient, Medieval, and Early Modern Eras

Just as in many ancient cultures, medieval societies drew a connection between the passage of time and the presence or absence of disease symptoms. During this time, mandatory isolation was established (Huremović 2019). After observation, individuals without symptoms of an illness were assumed not to be affected—and therefore, if in fact they were infected, might spread the disease upon reentering the community. Even so, beginning in the fourteenth century, some measure of safety was gained through the growing use of quarantine as a disease-control strategy, along with sanitary barriers, bills of health issued to ships, fumigation, disinfection, and regulation of groups who might be disseminating the illness or disease. Many communities blocked strangers, particularly traveling merchants and minority groups, from entering their towns during plagues. Some goods and merchandise would be thrown away, required continuous ventilation, or were doused in water for forty-eight hours. Forty days was a common standard for the isolation period (Tognotti 2013).

Industrial Era

Sanitary barriers and maritime quarantine were used against cholera in the nineteenth century. Maritime barriers helped protect smaller island communities, and items would be disinfected at borders. There was frequent opposition to the quarantine strategy, and many people did not take proper precautions. In the nineteenth and twentieth centuries, international prophylaxis regimes were introduced against cholera, plague, and yellow fever (Tognotti 2013).

Modern Era

Quarantine is a significant component of today's disease response along with the use of border controls, contact tracing, hygiene promotion, and surveillance, all of which may reduce the spread of diseases. In the beginning of the twentieth century, physicians began encouraging physical distancing in social settings and respiratory hygiene. Vaccines for seasonal influenza outbreaks became available, as well as antimicrobial drugs to treat ailments as appropriate. Control measures such as closures of businesses and bans on public gatherings have also been implemented (Tognotti 2013).

THE WHO'S INTEGRATED, PEOPLE-CENTERED HEALTH SERVICES FRAMEWORK

Resilient health systems, including public health responsiveness, are at the core of improving human health and responding to disease outbreaks. While significant progress has been made in health and life expectancy over time, relative improvements have been unequal among and within countries. Contributing factors include varying access to health services, shortages of health workers, and weak health systems. Where healthcare is accessible, care is often fragmented or of poor quality and, as a result, health system responsiveness and satisfaction with care remains low in many countries, often including a significant level of distrust of medical and governmental responses (WHO 2015). These factors are endemic in many societies and augmented during disease outbreaks. For example, fragile and poorly integrated health systems as well as popular lack of confidence in them were contributors to the spread of Ebola virus in West Africa (WHO, n.d.). Continued lack of implementation of international health standards, advisories, and regulations result in poor capacity to address outbreaks and leave many countries vulnerable. In response, the WHO has proposed a framework for strengthening health systems through the integration of health services with an emphasis on improving healthcare delivery at the community level (WHO, n.d.).

Model Description

In 2016, the WHO published the IPCHS Framework (see figure 8.1). The framework is the culmination of work guided by a consortium of leading research institutions and reviewed by member states, experts from the donor community, civil society representatives, and the WHO Secretariat. There are two key features of this framework: integrated health services and people-centered care. Integrated health services are defined as health services that (a) are managed and delivered for the continuum of health promotion, disease prevention, diagnosis, treatment, and disease management; (b) provide rehabilitation and palliative care services; (c) are coordinated across multiple levels and sites within and beyond the health sector; and (d) are delivered according to patients' needs throughout the course of their lives. A people-centered approach to care incorporates the perspectives of individuals, families, caregivers, and communities as participants in and users of trusted health systems. These systems are organized around the comprehensive needs of people rather than individual diseases. They respect social norms and provide education and support for patients to make decisions and actively participate in their own care. A people-centered approach should not only focus on patients' clinical encounters and person-centered care, however. It also brings attention to people's health as part of their communities and to the role of communities in helping shape health policy and health service provision (WHO, n.d.).

As noted, the IPCHS Framework promotes the strengthening of health systems and for health services to become more integrated and people-centered. In particular, it calls for the reorientation of health services to be responsive to the needs of individuals, families, caregivers, and communities, and for care that is coordinated both within and beyond the health sector, regardless of a country's

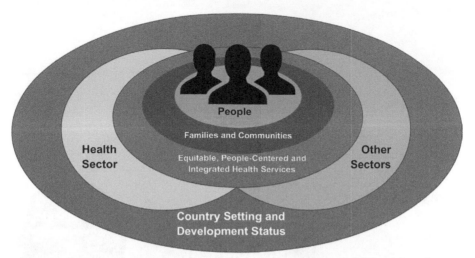

FIGURE 8.1. Integrated, People-Centered Health Services Framework (adapted from the WHO-HQ Global Strategy on people-centered and integrated health services, 2015).

development status. The model focuses on the idea that access to healthcare is a basic right, without distinction of ethnicity, religion, gender, age, disability, political belief, and economic or social condition as part of a human rights approach that ensures adequate and comprehensive care for all (WHO, n.d.).

KEY DOMAINS

The IPCHS Framework proposes five key interdependent strategies essential to improving health systems and access to care. These include:

(1) Empowering and engaging people and communities;
(2) Strengthening governance and accountability;
(3) Reorienting the model of care;
(4) Coordinating services within and across sectors; and
(5) Creating an enabling environment.

A schematic of the model by domain is included in figure 8.2. Due to their interdependence, lack of progress in one area could affect progress in other areas.

Strategy 1: Empowering and Engaging People and Communities

Empowering and engaging people and communities calls for the provision of opportunities, skills, and resources needed to empower users of health services and advocates for a reformed health system. At its core, it seeks to reveal

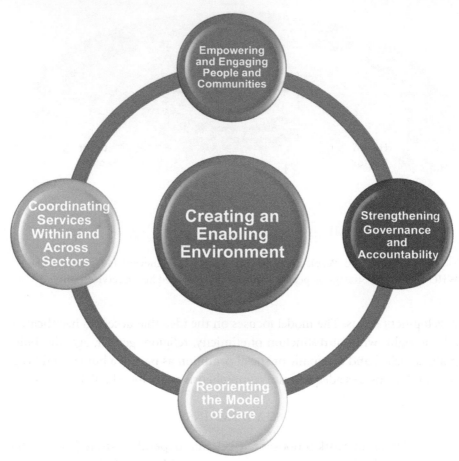

FIGURE 8.2. Integrated, people-centered health services model key domains (adapted from the WHO-HQ Global Strategy on people-centered and integrated health services, 2015).

community and individual resources for action at all levels. Furthermore, it supports the active engagement of communities in co-producing healthy environments and provides informal caregivers with the tools needed, including necessary education, to enhance their performance and with support to continue their role. Most importantly, this strategy requires the involvement of underserved and marginalized groups to guarantee universal access to quality services that are produced in conjunction with others to meet their specific needs (WHO, n.d.).

Strategy 2: Strengthening Governance and Accountability

In order to strengthen governance and accountability from the macro level (i.e., policymaking level) to the micro level (i.e., clinical intervention level), a participatory approach must be taken for policy formulation, decision-making, and performance evaluation. Good governance practices are transparent, inclusive, invulnerable to corruption, and efficient in their use of available resources and information to ensure the best possible results. They are bolstered by a robust system of accountability among policy-makers, managers, providers, and users and incentivize a people-centered approach. In order to build a shared vision and a joint approach to achieving it, this strategy calls for the establishment of a strong policy framework along with a compelling narrative for reform (WHO, n.d.).

Strategy 3: Reorienting the Model of Care

Reoriented models of care ensure that efficient and effective healthcare services are designed and provided through innovative care models that prioritize primary and community services and the co-production of health. To achieve this, a shift must occur from inpatient and curative care to outpatient and preventive care. Reoriented models of care require investment in holistic and comprehensive care that includes health promotion and prevention strategies that support people's overall health and well-being. Finally, they incorporate gender and cultural preferences in the design and operation of health services (WHO, n.d.).

Strategy 4: Coordinating Services within and across Sectors

In order to coordinate services within and across sectors, services should be built around the needs and demands of people. This is achieved through the integration of health service providers within and across healthcare settings, referral systems development and networks among levels of care, and the creation of linkages between health and other sectors. At the community level, such coordination requires intersectoral action to address social determinants of health and optimize the use of scarce resources, including partnerships with the private sector. Coordination of services does not require a prescribed approach to structures, services, or workflows; rather, it focuses on improving healthcare delivery through alignment of process and information and coordination among different services (WHO, n.d.).

Strategy 5: Creating an Enabling Environment

The creation of an enabling environment is at the center of the IPCHS Framework. This is accomplished by bringing together all stakeholders to engage in transformational change. This complex task requires the involvement of a diverse set of processes to bring about the necessary changes in leadership and management, information systems, quality improvement methods, workforce reorientation, legislative frameworks, financial arrangements, and incentives (WHO, n.d.).

APPLICATION TO DISEASE OUTBREAK RESPONSE

So how does this framework translate to disease outbreak response? With a comprehensive, intersectoral approach to healthcare delivery, the IPCHS Framework provides potential advantages for response efforts in the face of community and national outbreaks of highly infectious diseases and their transmission. These advantages include primary care and patient risk-level assignment at first contact, multidisciplinary teams for high-risk patients, vertical and horizontal integration of different types of providers and care, and integrated telehealth access facilities and services (Gong et al. 2021). Drawing on the strategies outlined above, tailored approaches for disease outbreak response could prove effective for community transmission containment. For example, efforts that focus on enhancing the public health workforce within a community could assist in infectious disease monitoring and information dissemination. Additionally, thorough facilitation at the government level and integration of resources, including health financing, across communities and regions could ensure timely medical testing and sufficient human capital to treat patients. Last, a joint approach to health information management systems, including symptoms tracking and disease surveillance, is essential to developing an infrastructure prepared to track and mitigate the spread of diseases (Natukunda et al. 2020).

In the following section, we outline some of the most impactful disease outbreaks that have occurred over the last two centuries and assess response efforts through the lens of the IPCHS Framework.

CASE STUDIES

Cholera

Cholera is caused by bacteria; most of those infected will have mild or no symptoms and recover without medical intervention (WHO 2021a). While cholera is reported back many centuries, numerous outbreaks and pandemics of cholera have occurred around the world, particularly over the last two hundred years (Pollitzer 1954; Samal 2014). These outbreaks have collectively led to some notable advancements in public health that formed the building blocks of response efforts. Advancements in sanitation and basic public health measures are effective in mitigating the spread of cholera throughout much of the world, but more localized epidemics still persist (History.com 2020).

The origins of cholera can be traced to the Ganges delta in India, but in 1817, cholera began to spread throughout the region along European trade routes. By 1820, it had spread throughout other parts of Asia, and 1821 marked its entry into Europe through passage on ships (Pollitzer 1954). The second cholera pandemic (1829–37) led to continued spread throughout Europe and into the Americas (Chan, Tuite, and Fisman 2013). Great Britain's first outbreak brought on some of the earliest documented public health measures to combat cholera, including the establishment of local boards of health and implementation of quarantines. The outbreaks in Great Britain also show the effects of media on public health efforts, as widespread distrust of doctors and inaccurate public perceptions were fueled by media coverage (History .com 2020).

The third pandemic (1846–60) affected Asia, Africa, Europe, and North America and resulted in the most deaths of any of the cholera pandemics (Pollitzer 1954; Samal 2014). One of the most notable resulting public health advancements came from the surveillance and tracking done in London by Dr. John Snow to identify the source of the outbreak. These efforts led to the simple action of removing the pump handle on a contaminated well, which significantly reduced disease spread (History.com 2020).

Advances in public health and sanitation reduced the spread of cholera in much of Europe and North America for the fourth and all subsequent cholera pandemics (History.com 2020). The fourth pandemic mostly occurred throughout Asia, Africa, and eastern and southern Europe. Cholera appeared in western Europe and North America, but to a lesser extent than was experienced in previous years (Pollitzer 1954). This period was also marked by advancements in microbiology when Robert Koch isolated the *Vibrio cholerae* bacterium, which led to a shift in governmental policy (Lee 2001).

The fifth pandemic (1881–96) was prominent throughout much of Asia and areas of Europe, as well as into Africa and South America, but progress in public health measures prevented the spread in North America (Pollitzer 1954). Advancements in microbiology continued during this period, resulting in more knowledge of cholera bacteria. The sixth cholera pandemic (1899–1923) was notable throughout India, the Middle East, Russia, and northern Africa, and similarly, the seventh cholera pandemic (1961–present) spread throughout Asia, the Middle East, and Africa (History.com 2020).

Since the beginning of the seventh pandemic, isolated outbreaks have occurred in various parts of the world, but greater understanding of the disease, prevention and treatment efforts, and mitigation through sanitation and basic public health practices have largely kept cholera at bay. The preventable and treatable nature of cholera has allowed it to become a model for coordinated efforts and prevention through public health practices on a world scale. Below is a synopsis of how lessons learned from cholera response fit within the WHO's IPCHS Framework and also how the lessons learned apply to COVID-19 pandemic response.

Strategy 1: Empowering and Engaging People and Communities

John Snow's work in tracing the 1852 London cholera outbreak empowered community-centered decision-making to halt the spread of cholera at the source (History.com 2020). This sort of environmental approach was successful in reaching all affected persons, including those who were underserved or marginalized and may not have been able to access care. This is comparable to the population-level contact tracing that was attempted with COVID-19 with varying results. With COVID-19, new technological, app-based tracing methods were used in addition to more traditional methods of contact tracing (Mbunge 2020).

Strategy 2: Strengthening Governance and Accountability

Discovery of the bacteria source in London brought about action to minimize infection through removing the pump handle on an infected well (History .com 2020). This was a first step in learning how to prevent and manage future cholera outbreaks. Additionally, the establishment of local boards of health, as was implemented in London during the second cholera pandemic, is an example of strengthening local governance in response to a pandemic (History.com 2020). The practice of controlling pandemics through governmental regulation persists today, as seen during COVID-19 in the implementation of lockdown and quarantine measures (Douglas et al. 2020).

Strategy 3: Reorienting the Model of Care

Advancements and knowledge of treatment have significantly reoriented societal response to cholera from one that was largely distrusting of medical approaches during early cholera pandemics to one where very basic medical care can treat cholera for a full and quick recovery (History.com 2020; WHO 2021a). With COVID-19, there was a concerted effort to establish a model of care early on, but research timelines delayed having definitive answers regarding optimal treatment measures.

Strategy 4: Coordinating Services within and across Sectors

As discussed above, cholera in many ways set the standard for public health response. Accordingly, the WHO has a comprehensive multisectoral plan for prevention of the spread of cholera. This plan specifically states a need for a "targeted multi-sectoral approach to prevent cholera recurrence: the strategy calls on countries and partners to focus on cholera 'hotspots,' the relatively small areas most heavily affected by cholera. Cholera transmission can be stopped in these areas through measures including improved [water, sanitation, and hygiene] and through use of [oral cholera vaccines]" (WHO 2021a). While there were barriers to smooth execution of the COVID-19 response, initial prevention was always intended to be multifaceted, through using methods such as contact tracing and isolation or quarantine, studying and establishing effective treatments for sick individuals, and development of effective vaccines.

Strategy 5: Creating an Enabling Environment

Higher standards for sanitation throughout much of the world have created an environment that largely enables elimination of cholera. However, these advancements are not prominent in less developed regions. Establishing a more disease free environment as the standard has been effective in ensuring prevention of cholera outbreaks, minimizing the need for response on a large scale. To minimize the future spread of COVID-19, accurate understanding of the disease mechanism and acceptance of prevention methods at the population level has been crucial and is constantly evolving as new developments occur.

1918 Influenza ("Spanish Flu")

The 1918 influenza pandemic, commonly referred to as the Spanish Flu, is the most widely compared to COVID-19. The Spanish Flu was caused by an H1N1 virus and spread globally from 1918 to 1919, although the pandemic persisted into 1920 (CDC 2019). In total, more than 50 million people died worldwide as a result (Parmet and Rothstein 2018). Below is an outline of how lessons learned from the 1918 influenza pandemic fit within the WHO's IPCHS Framework.

Strategy 1: Empowering and Engaging People and Communities

In the United States, the government called upon the American Red Cross to aid in providing substantial supplies, time, and other resources to fight the pandemic locally, offering a primary example of empowering local communities in public health response (Jones 2010). Because local chapters of the American Red Cross operated uniquely to address the pandemic in each city, comparisons could be made to exemplify best practices for community empowerment and volunteerism. The response to COVID-19 shed light on the differential experiences and needs of communities (Moore et al. 2020; Martinez-Juarez et al. 2020). various communities were less equipped to respond to outbreaks due to limited resources, high-risk jobs, information gaps, and other factors. For these reasons, a more localized, targeted response within communities could have alleviated later outcome disparities.

Strategy 2: Strengthening Governance and Accountability

The "Spanish Flu" was by no means the last of pandemics to be popularly referred to by its actual or supposed place of origin. In recent years, there has been increased recognition of the need for careful naming of diseases and pandemics to ensure that one group is not disproportionately blamed for disease spread and forced to carry an unfair burden of response. Naming based on the perceived source of a disease, whether it is a country, a region, or a social/demographic group can be extremely stigmatizing (Hoppe 2018).

With COVID-19, there were individuals and groups of people who insisted on referring to COVID-19 as the "China Virus" or "Wuhan Virus," resulting in stigmatization of certain groups of people (Budhwani and Sun 2020). A consequence of this was increased violence against individuals of Chinese descent (Hu et al. 2020). Stronger leadership and governmental response in focusing on pandemic response rather than blame could have potentially minimized some of these negative consequences.

Strategy 3: Reorienting the Model of Care

The 1918 influenza pandemic was characterized by few prevention efforts. Instead, much of the response was focused on nonpharmaceutical interventions (NPIs) such as quarantine or physical distancing in social situations (Greenberger 2018; Stern, Cetron, and Markel 2010). This pandemic shed light on the increased need for preparedness to prevent and quickly respond to future pandemics. Potential methods to accomplish this included testing, vaccination, and treatment protocols.

With COVID-19, there was an initial necessary focus on NPIs given a lack of immediate vaccination and treatment options (Hsiang et al. 2020). At the same time, a strong emphasis was placed on developing accurate diagnostic tests to identify cases, and many resources were put toward quickly developing and testing vaccines and treatments, although there were setbacks in their development and eventual acceptance of all three response protocols (Graham 2020; Koyama et al. 2020; Binnicker 2020).

Strategy 4: Coordinating Services within and across Sectors

Expanding on reorienting the model of care, the lessons learned from the 1918 influenza outbreak point to the need for a coordinated approach in the context of pandemics. Such an approach would involve prevention through vaccination as well as NPIs, development and propagation of optimal treatments, and a variety of public health approaches at all levels. In the area of prevention, NPIs should be thought of as a last resort and not the primary mechanism for disease control (Greenberger 2018). Quarantine and distancing can be effective, but efforts should be made to reduce dependency on measures that are not perceived well or seen as acceptable to the general population. With the COVID-19 response, there was extensive pushback to mask mandates, quarantines, and lockdowns, resulting in protests fed by a distrust of government already established in segments of society in the United States and globally. This distrust of government was a significant factor in vaccine distrust and other related issues (Joffe 2021; Latkin 2021).

Strategy 5: Creating an Enabling Environment

All of the previously mentioned lessons indicate the need to create an enabling environment through a coordinated, systemic approach. Although all of these elements are evident based upon lessons learned from the 1918 influenza pandemic, the reality is that many of them have not been consistently applied in the prevention of and response to pandemics, including COVID-19. This has been especially true where general governmental priorities have not matched public health priorities.

HIV/AIDS Pandemic

Human immunodeficiency virus (HIV) targets and weakens the immune system and progresses to acquired immunodeficiency syndrome (AIDS) at its most advanced stage. Individuals with HIV/AIDS have weakened CD4 cells (i.e., white blood cells), thereby putting them at an increased risk of a host of health problems, including infectious diseases (Greene 2007). AIDS was first recognized as a new disease in 1981, although some studies suggest that HIV began spreading between 1884 and 1924 in sub-Saharan Africa, many years before was previously thought (University of Arizona 2008). AIDS has since become a global health crisis, necessitating critical public health responses. Although there remains no cure for the illness to date, advancement in prevention and treatment efforts, such as early testing and antiretroviral (ARV) drugs, has led to a rapid decline in the spread of the virus (NPIN 2020). However, significant headway is needed to combat the persistent negative factors that have made it challenging to eradicate the transmission of the disease. Since 1981, HIV has caused approximately 36.3 million deaths, with over 37.7 million people living with HIV as of 2021. In 2020 alone, about 680,000 people died from HIV-related causes, and 1.5 million new HIV cases were reported the same year (PublicHealth.org, n.d.; Kaiser Family Foundation 2019). Over two-thirds (25.4 million or 67%) of people living with HIV are in sub-Saharan Africa (WHO 2021b; UNAIDS 2021). In the next section, we will discuss the HIV/AIDS pandemic response and how it fits into the WHO's IPCHS Framework around key periods.

Strategy 1: Empowering and Engaging People and Communities

At the time of the first reports of AIDS and the identification of HIV eight months later, the public relied almost entirely on mainstream news for information on this mysterious and frightening new disease. Because HIV/AIDS first spread among men who have sex with men, there was an immediate stigmatization attached to the disease and its chief victims, supported by misinformation and scaremongering. For quite a while, campaigns to respond to such attacks, channel reliable information, provide and point to services, and engage and empower individuals and the community arose almost entirely from activism within the community itself. With time, such campaigns were instated by other community organizations, certain government entities, and medical providers.

From the first diagnosis of HIV, there was increased mainstream news coverage to raise awareness to empower individuals, communities, formal and informal healthcare workers, and marginalized populations. Notable activities included research; advocacy; developing antiretroviral therapy; global, national, and regional programs; and convening an international conference on AIDS. Furthermore, funding opportunities increased for research efforts to better understand the spread of HIV/AIDS. In the latter years, global HIV-related deaths declined, but the number of new cases and deaths from HIV continued to increase in Africa. Calls for an HIV vaccine, in addition to greater focus on partnerships between regions, increased to raise funds for HIV and its associated comorbidities.

In the wake of COVID-19, there was an unprecedented level of health information disseminated across mainstream and alternative media, including social networking sites. In addition to and often using media outlets to spread the message, government agencies and leaders at all levels worked to engage the populace early on. Although targeting the general population, COVID-19 awareness campaigns put special emphasis on reaching individuals who were at heightened risk of contracting the virus (e.g., the elderly and those with preexisting health conditions). However, there was also a flood of hoaxes, conspiracy theories, and misinformation about the source, severity, credibility, and treatment of the virus across many media sources, but mostly on social networking sites. Unfortunately, these occurrences led to a considerable loss of lives due to the spread of misinformation (Tasnim, Hossain, and Mazumder 2020).

Strategy 2: Strengthening Governance and Accountability

During the early years of the HIV/AIDS pandemic, grassroots, local, and regional movements were established around the world. Examples include:

1. The Treatment Action Campaign, founded in 1998, is an HIV/AIDS activist organization based in South Africa that advocates for the availability of antiretroviral drugs in the country.

2. Project SIDA (Project AIDS) was a joint research project that began in the 1980s between Zaire, the United States, and Belgium to study AIDS in central Africa.

3. The United States President's Emergency Plan for AIDS Relief (PEPFAR) is the largest commitment by any nation to address a single disease in history. Since its inception in 2003, the US government has invested over $85 billion in global HIV/AIDS response in more than fifty countries around the world (HIV.gov 2021).

The WHO and the Joint United Nations Programme on HIV/AIDS (UNAIDS) issued guidance on "provider-initiated" HIV testing in healthcare settings. A global HIV forum with a focus on Africa and other regions was established. The Obama administration launched the Global Health Initiative, following up on PEPFAR, which had been established under the Bush presidency. Additionally, there was a growing focus on partnerships between the public and private sectors to curb local epidemics through the availability of a generic and single-pill HIV treatment regimen.

Similar partnerships between the public and private sectors, including between nonprofit and for-profit organizations, were and continue to be formed during the COVID-19 pandemic to aid in response efforts. One notable case was the donation of $250 million dollars to fight COVID-19 by the

Bill and Melinda Gates Foundation. The funds covered COVID-19 drugs and vaccines (Suzman 2020).

Strategy 3: Reorienting the Model of Care

Increased public health campaigns; prevention and treatment; testing and counseling; guidelines; and recommendations for individuals, communities, healthcare providers, and marginalized populations were established as part of the HIV/AIDS response effort. The first human vaccine trial in a developing country began in Thailand. With a better understanding of HIV, a global standard of care was also adopted. The WHO released new guidelines calling for earlier use of antiretrovirals for children under five with HIV, pregnant and breastfeeding women with HIV, and HIV-positive persons with uninfected sexual partners. The US issued revised recommendations for HIV testing in healthcare settings during the latter years.

Not surprisingly, the COVID-19 pandemic emerged with global health officials unprepared to manage its devastating impact. As the virus progressed and mutated, treatment protocols and guidelines were revised. Although, for the most part, the standard protocols remained unchanged, certain aspects of the COVID-19 protocols, particularly related to different population groups, were updated. For example, at the outset, there was limited information about the impact of COVID-19 on pregnant women and the fetus. Initial guidelines were cursory, suggesting that the virus could be similar to previous respiratory illnesses; however, as data became available, it was observed that the virus led to adverse birth outcomes (e.g., preterm birth) (Wastnedge et al. 2021).

Strategy 4: Coordinating Services within and across Sectors

The successful reduction of HIV-related deaths and increase in the use of antiretroviral therapy, testing, and guidelines speaks to the effectiveness of the multifaceted, integrated approach across nations that was developed at the time. Similar coordinated partnerships occurred during the COVID-19 pandemic, most notably between technological industries and the healthcare sector (WHO 2020b).

Strategy 5: Creating an Enabling Environment

Integrated local and grassroots movements continue to increase access to HIV treatment. Targeted public health education and the use of everyday people living with HIV as spokespeople for public health campaigns to destigmatize HIV are still prevalent today.

With COVID-19, several campaigns and messages were developed by grassroots movements to target diverse groups. For example, many individuals were hesitant about the COVID-19 vaccine, which resulted in their refusal to be vaccinated, and, by extension, weakened global efforts to reduce the virus spread and outcomes for those who contract it (Sallam 2021). To mitigate the issue, campaigns were developed to help curb vaccine hesitancy.

H1NI Swine Flu Pandemic

The 2009 H1N1 flu was first detected in the United States. It was initially called the "swine flu" because the virus had genes that resembled the North American swine lineage H1N1 and Eurasian swine lineage H1N1 influenza viruses. However, further investigations indicated that human cases were not linked to pigs, and the virus was circulating separately among humans and pig herds. The presence of a new virus prompted the WHO to declare the H1NI swine flu a public health emergency of international concern on April 25, 2009. Considering the virus's rapid spread to more than seventy countries, the WHO declared a pandemic on June 11, 2009. By the time the WHO declared an end to the pandemic in early August of 2010, it had spread to 214 countries and accounted for 18,449 deaths (WHO 2011; CDC 2010; CDC 2019). The rapid containment of the H1NI virus is indicative of the unparalleled global health efforts in eradicating the infectious disease. The following section will highlight the success of eliminating the H1N1 flu using the WHO IPCHS Framework.

Strategy 1: Empowering and Engaging People and Communities

The quick response of the US government and the WHO on surveillance, reporting, public health efforts, and campaigns was a key factor in the success of eradicating the H1N1 influenza virus. By April 26, 2009, over 39 million units of protective equipment (masks, gowns, gloves, and shields) and 11 million antiviral drug regimens were distributed across the United States. The WHO developed a rapid containment strategy comprising (a) recognition of the potential threat and severity of the virus; (b) drawing on experiences from SARS to contain the virus; and (c) localization of the virus through modeling, restricting movements, and provision of antiviral prophylaxis. The aim was to contain the virus in the initial stages of the outbreak.

In the initial stages of COVID-19, protective equipment was not readily accessible, even for healthcare workers. However, while high-income countries would eventually be able to easily source protective wear, low-and-middle-income countries (LMICs) suffered shortages (Staudenmaier 2020). Unfortunately, fake protective wear was produced by unethical companies that specifically targeted LMICs. While the situation improved, it highlights the disparities in access to healthcare services between LMICs and other regions.

Strategy 2: Strengthening Governance and Accountability

The launch of the H1N1 vaccine was a cornerstone in global health efforts. The WHO, governments, and industry accelerated efforts for the development and distribution of a vaccine and the first was commercially available for use in September 2009. Vaccine manufacturing in developing countries was an important strategy to meet the worldwide demand, and WHO efforts led to the acceleration of clinical trials to develop vaccines in Thailand and India.

Although COVID-19 continues to evolve, thus requiring continual epidemiologic monitoring and work on vaccines against its variants, the unusually speedy development of the initial vaccines was a remarkable feat that shows the effectiveness of concerted efforts by experts from a variety of disciplines. However, because of gaps in access to the COVID-19 vaccine in LMICs, initiatives such as COVID-19 Vaccines Global Access (COVAX) were developed as part of the global effort to ensure vaccine equity for vulnerable populations (UNICEF, n.d.).

Strategy 3: Reorienting the Model of Care

Swift changes were made in surveillance and reporting once it became evident that the H1N1 flu showed different markers from the 1918 flu. Among these changes, the United States shifted from reporting only confirmed cases to reporting both confirmed and probable causes.

From the time the spread of COVID-19 was declared a pandemic, countries focused on actively reporting confirmed cases and contact-tracing efforts. However, many countries underreported cases, either because of lack of testing infrastructure or to prevent damage to a country's reputation.

Strategy 4: Coordinating Services within and across Sectors

Multisectoral initiatives were formed between the WHO, regional organizations, public health institutions, ministries of health, and other key international agencies for the H1N1 outbreak response. The Global Outbreak Alert and Response Network, which was established in 2000 by the WHO, partnered with the World Organization for Animal Health, the Food and Agriculture Organization of the United Nations, and the Pan American Health

Organization, together with others, to provide coordinated infectious disease prevention measures that contributed to the successful eradication of the virus. There was also effective and rapid communication between countries, international agencies, technical experts, and the WHO. In the United States, a real-time PCR (polymerase chain reaction) test was developed less than two weeks after identification of the virus. As of May 1, 2009, the US CDC test kits were ready for shipping nationally and internationally.

Strategy 5: Creating an Enabling Environment

Effective and timely surveillance, compilation of epidemiological data, communication and information exchange, partnerships between countries and regions, and public health campaigns created an enabling environment to stop the spread of the disease and keep the pandemic at bay.

LESSONS LEARNED AND RECOMMENDATIONS FOR FUTURE PRACTICE

One of the key success factors across all the pandemics discussed is the need for accurate dissemination of public health messaging. This proved useful during the HIV/AIDS pandemic, for example, in regard to prevention and the use of antiretroviral therapy. Such messages must be tailored to marginalized communities and other subpopulations to ensure they are culturally relevant and acceptable, a key feature lacking in the HIV/AIDS pandemic response. Deficiencies in sanitary behaviors and conditions in the early cholera pandemics and the 1918 influenza pandemic highlight their importance for controlling the spread of disease. Significant headway has been made in this realm in developed countries, but further progress is needed among developing nations. Having public health institutions in place that advocate for prevention and disease control is also foundational to leading disease response efforts. Not only are they instrumental at the individual level for information dissemination and behavior change, but they are also crucial for advocacy efforts to communicate the need for policies and funding that support disease outbreak containment and response. These institutions could also be useful for holding government entities accountable: for example, by ensuring equitable access to adequate testing and treatment, especially for hard-to-reach populations such as those residing in rural areas. Another key success factor is the presence of collaborations and partnerships between international organizations, health systems, advocacy organizations, and governments. This proved to be the cornerstone for the rapid control of the H1N1 swine flu. Stakeholders must work together and share resources, such as protective equipment, testing kits, and vaccines, if available, during emergency situations to prevent the spreading of diseases across communities, nations, and the globe.

APPLICATION TO THE COVID-19 PANDEMIC

The COVID-19 pandemic brought to light inadequacies in our response efforts to control disease transmission, minimize loss of life, and reduce burdens on healthcare systems. It placed enormous financial, administrative, and logistical stress on health systems globally, revealing inefficiencies and setting back movements toward universal health coverage through disruptions in service provision and financial constraints (Neill et al. 2021). International health regulations governing health emergencies require national health systems to be equipped to prepare for, detect, and respond to emergencies. Building resilient health systems depends on a coordinated and integrated approach to health emergencies, employing evidence-based decision-making, knowledge integration in health systems, and the capacity to handle multiple moving parts at once. As described above, the most successful (this term is used loosely) disease outbreak responses employed multiple strategies outlined in the IPCHS Framework, suggesting that, if implemented to its full extent, this framework has the potential to support more coordinated efforts to better combat the next disease outbreak or pandemic that may arise.

DISCUSSION QUESTIONS

- Looking at the trends in disease outbreaks from ancient history to the present time, how have response efforts evolved?

- Knowing that disease outbreaks are inevitable, what further efforts are needed to help control their rapid spread and minimize loss of life?

REFERENCES

Aassve, Arnstein, Guido Alfani, Francesco Gandolfi, and Marco Le Moglie. 2021. "Epidemics and Trust: The Case of the Spanish Flu." *Health Economics* 30, no. 4 (April): 840–57. https://doi.org/10.1002/hec.4218.

Binnicker, Matthew J. 2020. "Challenges and Controversies to Testing for COVID-19." *Journal of Clinical Microbiology* 58, no. 11: e01695–20. https://doi.org/10.1128/jcm.01695-20.

Budhwani, Henna, and Ruoyan Sun. 2020. "Creating COVID-19 Stigma by Referencing the Novel Coronavirus as the 'Chinese Virus' on Twitter: Quantitative Analysis of Social Media Data." *Journal of Medical Internet Research* 22 no. 5 (May): e19301. https://doi.org/10.2196/19301.

Burkardt, Hans-Joachim. 2011. "Pandemic H1N1 2009 ('Swine Flu'): Diagnostic and Other Challenges." *Expert Review of Molecular Diagnostics* 11, no. 1: 35–40. https://doi.org/10.1586/erm.10.102.

CDC (Centers for Disease Control and Prevention). 2010. "The 2009 H1N1 Pandemic: Summary Highlights, April 2009–April 2010." Centers for Disease Control and Prevention. Last modified August 3, 2010. https://www.cdc.gov/h1n1flu/cdcresponse.htm.

———. 2019. "1918 Pandemic (H1N1 Virus)." Centers for Disease Control and Prevention. Last modified March 20, 2019. https://archive.cdc.gov/#/details?url=https://www.cdc.gov/flu/pandemic-resources/1918-pandemic-h1n1.html.

———. 2021. *Estimated HIV Incidence and Prevalence in the United States, 2015–2019.* HIV Surveillance Supplemental Reports, vol. 26, no. 1. https://www.cdc.gov/hiv/pdf/library/reports/surveillance/cdc-hiv-surveillance-supplemental-report-vol-26-1.pdf.

Chan, Christina H., Ashleigh R. Tuite, and David N. Fisman. 2013. "Historical Epidemiology of the Second Cholera Pandemic: Relevance to Present Day Disease Dynamics." *PLOS ONE* 8, no. 8: e72498. https://doi.org/10.1371/journal.pone.0072498.

Douglas, Margaret, Srinivasa Katikireddi, Martin Taulbut, Martin McKee, and Gerry McCartney. 2020. "Mitigating the Wider Health Effects of Covid-19 Pandemic Response." *BMJ* 369:m1557. https://doi.org/10.1136/bmj.m1557.

Gong, Fangfang, Guangyu Hu, Hanqun Lin, Xizhuo Sun, and Wenxin Wang. 2021. "Integrated Healthcare Systems Response Strategies Based on the Luohu Model during the COVID-19 Epidemic in Shenzhen, China." *International Journal of Integrated Care* 21:1–7. https://doi.org/10.5334/ijic.5628.

Graham, Barney S. 2020. "Rapid COVID-19 Vaccine Development." *Science* 368, no. 6494: 945–46. https://doi.org/10.1126/science.abb8923.

Greenberger, Michael. 2018. "Better Prepare than React: Reordering Public Health Priorities 100 Years after the Spanish Flu Epidemic." *American Journal of Public Health* 108, no. 11 (November): 1465–68. https://doi.org/10.2105/AJPH.2018.304682.

Greene, Warner C. 2007. "A History of AIDS: Looking Back to See Ahead." *European Journal of Immunology* 37, no. S1 (November): S94–S102. https://doi.org/10.1002/eji.200737441.

Harper, Kyle. 2015. "Pandemics and Passages to Late Antiquity: Rethinking the Plague of *c.* 249–270 Described by Cyprian." *Journal of Roman Archaeology* 28:223–60. https://doi.org/10.1017/S1047759415002470.

History.com. 2020. "Cholera." Last modified March 24, 2020. https://www.history.com/topics/inventions/history-of-cholera#section_2.

HIV.gov. 2021. "What Is PEPFAR?" US Department of Health & Human Services. Last modified June 28, 2021. https://www.hiv.gov/federal-response/pepfar-global-aids/pepfar.

Hoppe, Trevor. 2018. "'Spanish Flu': When Infectious Disease Names Blur Origins and Stigmatize Those Infected." *American Journal of Public Health* 108, no. 11 (November): 1462–64. https://doi.org/10.2105/ajph.2018.304645.

Hsiang, Solomon, Daniel Allen, Sébastien Annan-Phan, Kendon Bell, Ian Bolliger, Trinetta Chong, Hannah Druckenmiller, Luna Yue Huang, Andrew Hultgren, Emma Krasovich, Peiley Lau, Jaecheol Lee, Esther Rolf, Jeanette Tseng, and Tiffany Wu. 2020. "The Effect of Large-Scale Anti-contagion Policies on the COVID-19 Pandemic." *Nature* 584, no. 7820 (August): 262–67. https://doi.org /10.1038/s41586-020-2404-8.

Hu, Zhiwen, Zhongliang Yang, Qi Li, and An Zhang. 2020. "The COVID-19 Infodemic: Infodemiology Study Analyzing Stigmatizing Search Terms." *Journal of Medical Internet Research* 22 no. 11: e22639. https://doi.org/10.2196/22639.

Huremović, Damir. 2019. "Brief History of Pandemics (Pandemics throughout History)." In *Psychiatry of Pandemics: A Mental Health Response to Infection Outbreak,* edited by Damir Huremović, 7–35. Cham, Switzerland: Springer Nature, 2019.

Jackson, Claire. 2009. "History Lessons: The Asian Flu Pandemic." *British Journal of General Practice* 59, no. 565: 622–23. https://doi.org/10.3399/bjgp09X453882.

Joffe, Ari R. 2021. "COVID-19: Rethinking the Lockdown Groupthink." *Frontiers in Public Health* 9, no. 98: 625778. https://doi.org/10.3389/fpubh.2021.625778.

Jones, Marian M. 2010. "The American Red Cross and Local Response to the 1918 Influenza Pandemic: A Four-City Case Study." *Public Health Reports* 125, no. S3: 92–104. https://doi.org/10.1177/00333549101250S312.

Kaiser Family Foundation. 2019. "Global HIV/AIDS Timeline." Kaiser Family Foundation. Last modified July 20, 2019. https://www.kff.org/global-health -policy/timeline/global-hivaids-timeline/.

Koyama, Takahiko, Dilhan Weeraratne, Jane L. Snowdon, and Laxmi Parida. 2020. "Emergence of Drift Variants That May Affect COVID-19 Vaccine Development and Antibody Treatment." *Pathogens* 9, no. 5: 324. https://doi.org /10.3390/pathogens9050324.

Latkin, Carl A. Lauren Dayton, Grace Yi, Arianna Konstantopoulos, and Basmattee Boodram. 2021. "Trust in a COVID-19 Vaccine in the U.S.: A Social-Ecological Perspective." *Social Science & Medicine* 270:113684. https://doi.org /10.1016/j.socscimed.2021.113684.

Lee, Kelley. 2001. "The Global Dimensions of Cholera." *Global Change and Human Health* 2:6–17. https://doi.org/10.1023/A:1011925107536.

Lim, Keah-Ying, Andrew J. Hamilton, and Sunny C. Jiang. 2015. "Assessment of Public Health Risk Associated with Viral Contamination in Harvested Urban Stormwater for Domestic Applications." *Science of the Total Environment* 523 (August): 95–108. https://doi.org/10.1016/j.scitotenv.2015.03.077.

Lindahl, Johanna F., and Delia Grace. 2015. "The Consequences of Human Actions on Risks for Infectious Diseases: A Review." *Infection Ecology & Epidemiology* 5:30048. https://doi.org/10.3402/iee.v5.30048.

Littman, Robert J. 2009. "The Plague of Athens: Epidemiology and Paleopathology." *Mount Sinai Journal of Medicine* 76, no. 5 (October): 456–67. https://doi .org/10.1002/msj.20137.

Martinez-Juarez, Luis Alberto, Ana Cristina Sedas, Miriam Orcutt, and Raj Bhopal. 2020. "Governments and International Institutions Should Urgently Attend to the Unjust Disparities That COVID-19 Is Exposing and Causing." *eClinical Medicine* 23:100376. https://doi.org/10.1016/j.eclinm.2020.100376.

Mbunge, Elliot. 2020. "Integrating Emerging Technologies into COVID-19 Contact Tracing: Opportunities, Challenges, and Pitfalls." *Diabetes & Metabolic Syndrome: Clinical Research & Reviews* 14, no. 6 (November–December): 1631–36. https://doi.org/10.1016/j.dsx.2020.08.029.

Moore, Jazmyn T., Jessica N. Ricaldi, Charles E. Rose, Jennifer Fuld, Monica Parise, Gloria J. Kang, Anne K. Driscoll, et al. 2020. "Disparities in Incidence of COVID-19 among Underrepresented Racial/Ethnic Groups in Counties Identified as Hotspots during June 5–18, 2020—22 States, February–June 2020." *Morbidity and Mortality Weekly Report (MMWR)* 69, no. 33: 1122–26. https://doi.org/10.15585/mmwr.mm6933e1.

Natukunda, Julian, Bruno Sunguya, Ken Ing Cherng Ong, and Masamine Jimba. 2020. "Adapting Lessons Learned from HIV Epidemic Control to COVID-19 and future Outbreaks in Sub-Saharan Africa." *Journal of Global Health Science* 2, no. 2 (December): e21. https://doi.org/10.35500/jghs.2020.2.e21.

Neill, Rachel, Md. Zabir Hasan, Priyanka Das, Vasuki Venugopal, Nishant Jain, Dinesh Arora, and Shivam Gupta. 2021. "Evidence of Integrated Health Service Delivery during COVID-19 in Low and Lower-Middle-Income Countries: Protocol for a Scoping Review." *BMJ Open* 11, no. 5: e042872. http://dx.doi.org/10.1136/bmjopen-2020-042872.

NPIN (National Prevention Information Network). 2020. "HIV and AIDS Timeline." Centers for Disease Control and Prevention. Last modified October 21, 2020. https://npin.cdc.gov/pages/hiv-and-aids-timeline#1990.

Nunn, Nathan, and Nancy Qian. 2010. "The Columbian Exchange: A History of Disease, Food, and Ideas." *Journal of Economic Perspectives* 24, no. 2 (Spring): 163–88. http://www.doi.org/10.1257/jep.24.2.163.

Parmar, Saurabh, Nihar Shah, Megha Kasarwala, Madhavika Virpura, and Dharmeshkumar D. Prajapati. 2011. "A Review on Swine Flu." *Journal of Pharmaceutical Science and Bioscientific Research* 1, no. 1 (July–August): 11–17. http://www.jpsbr.org/index_htm_files/2.pdf.

Parmet, Wendey E., and Mark A. Rothstein. 2018. "The 1918 Influenza Pandemic: Lessons Learned and Not—Introduction to the Special Section." *American Journal of Public Health* 108, no. 11 (November): 1435–36. https://doi.org/10.2105/AJPH.2018.304695.

Piret, Jocelyne, and Guy Boivin. 2020. "Pandemics throughout History." *Frontiers in Microbiology* 11:631736. https://doi.org/10.3389/fmicb.2020.631736

Pollitzer, R. 1954. "Cholera Studies. 1. History of the Disease." *Bulletin of the World Health Organization* 10, no. 3: 421–61. https://pubmed.ncbi.nlm.nih.gov/13160764.

PublicHealth.org. n.d. "HIV and AIDS: An Origin Story." PublicHealth. Accessed January 4, 2024. https://www.publichealth.org/public-awareness/cancer/origin-story/.

Ramamurthy, Thandavarayan, and Amit Ghosh. 2021. "A Re-look at Cholera Pandemics from Early Times to Now in the Current Era of Epidemiology." *Journal of Disaster Research* 16, no. 1: 110–17. https://doi.org/10.20965/jdr.2021.p0110.

Sabbatani, Sergio, and Sirio Fiorino. 2009. "La peste antonina e il declino dell'Impero Romano. Ruolo della guerra partica e della guerra marcomannica tra il 164 e il 182 d.c. nella diffusione del contagio" [The Antonine Plague and the decline of the Roman Empire]. *Le infezioni in medicina* 17, no. 4: 261–75. https://www.infezmed.it/media/journal/Vol_17_4_2009_11.pdf.

Sallam, Malik. 2021. "COVID-19 Vaccine Hesitancy Worldwide: A Concise Systematic Review of Vaccine Acceptance Rates." *Vaccines* 9, no. 2 (February): 160. https://doi.org/10.3390/vaccines9020160.

Samal, Janmejaya. 2014. "A Historical Exploration of Pandemics of Some Selected Diseases in the World." *International Journal of Health Sciences and Research* 4, no. 2 (February): 165–69. https://www.ijhsr.org/IJHSR_Vol.4_Issue.2_Feb2014/26.pdf.

Shannon, Gary W., and Robert G. Cromley. 1980. "The Great Plague of London, 1665." *Urban Geography* 1, no. 3: 254–70. https://doi.org/10.2747/0272-3638.1.3.254.

St. Louis, Michael. 2012. "Global Health Surveillance." *Morbidity and Mortality Weekly Report (MMWR)* S61, no. 3: 15–19. https://www.cdc.gov/mmwr/preview/mmwrhtml/su6103a4.htm.

Staudenmaier, Rebecca. 2020. "Europe: Police Bust €15 Million Face Mask Scam." *Deutsche Welle*. Last modified April 14, 2020. https://www.dw.com/en/coronavirus-police-bust-massive-face-mask-scam/a-53123078.

Stern, Alexandra Minna, Martin S. Cetron, and Howard Markel. 2010. "The 1918–1919 Influenza Pandemic in the United States: Lessons Learned and Challenges Exposed." *Public Health Reports* 125, no. S3: 6–8. https://doi.org/10.1177/00333549101250S303.

Suzman, Mark. 2020. "Why We're Giving $250 Million More to Fight COVID-10." Gates Foundation. Last modified December 9, 2020. https://www.gatesfoundation.org/ideas/articles/coronavirus-funding-additional-250-million-suzman.

Tasnim, Samia, Md. Mahbub Hossain, and Hoimonty Mazumder. 2020. "Impact of Rumors and Misinformation on COVID-19 in Social Media." *Journal of Preventive Medicine and Public Health* 53, no. 3 (May): 171–74. https://doi.org/10.3961/jpmph.20.094.

Tognotti, Eugenia. 2013. "Lessons from the History of Quarantine, from Plague to Influenza A." *Emerging Infectious Diseases* 19, no. 2 (February): 254–59. https://doi.org/10.3201/eid1902.120312.

UNAIDS. 2021. *Global HIV & AIDS Statistics—Fact Sheet*. Geneva, Switzerland: UNAIDS Secretariat. https://www.unaids.org/sites/default/files/media_asset/UNAIDS_FactSheet_en.pdf.

UNAIDS. 2023. *Fact Sheet: Global HIV Statistics*. Geneva, Switzerland: UNAIDS Secretariat. https://www.unaids.org/sites/default/files/media_asset/UNAIDS_FactSheet_en.pdf.

UNICEF. n.d. "Coronavirus in West and Central Africa (COVID-19)." UNICEF. Accessed August 17, 2021. https://www.unicef.org/wca/coronavirus.

University of Arizona. 2008. "HIV/AIDS Pandemic Began around 1900, Earlier Than Previously Thought; Urbanization in Africa Marked Outbreak." ScienceDaily.com, October 2, 2008. https://www.sciencedaily.com/releases /2008/10/081001145024.htm.

Wastnedge, Elizabeth A. N., Rebecca M. Reynolds, Sara R. van Boeckel, Sarah J. Stock, Fiona C. Denison, Jacqueline A. Maybin, and Hilary O. D. Critchley. 2021. "Pregnancy and COVID-19." *Physiological Reviews* 101, no. 1: 303–18. https://doi.org/10.1152/physrev.00024.2020.

White House Office of National AIDS Policy. 2016. *National HIV/AIDS Strategy for the United States, Updated to 2020: Indicator Supplement.* Washington, DC: White House Office of National AIDS Policy. https://files.hiv.gov/s3fs-public /nhas-2020-indicators.pdf.

WHO (World Health Organization). 2011. "Pandemic Influenza A (H1N1)." World Health Organization. Last modified March 3, 2011. https://www.who.int/csr /resources/publications/swineflu/h1n1_donor_032011.pdf?ua=1.

———. 2015. *Tracking Universal Health Coverage: First Global Monitoring Report.* Geneva, Switzerland: World Health Organization. https://www.who.int /publications/i/item/9789241564977.

———. 2020a. "Rolling Updates on Coronavirus Disease (COVID-19)." World Health Organization. Last updated July 31, 2020. https://www.who.int /emergencies/diseases/novel-coronavirus-2019/events-as-they-happen.

———. 2020b. "COVID-19 and Digital Health: What Can Digital Health Offer for COVID-19?" World Health Organization. Last modified April 10, 2020. https://www.who.int/china/news/feature-stories/detail/covid-19-and-digital -health-what-can-digital-health-offer-for-covid-19.

———. 2021a. "Cholera." World Health Organization. Last modified February 5, 2021. https://www.who.int/en/news-room/fact-sheets/detail/cholera.

———. 2021b. "HIV/AIDS: Key Facts." World Health Organization. Last modified July 14, 2021. https://www.who.int/news-room/fact-sheets/detail/hiv-aids.

———. n.d. "Integrated People-Centred Care." World Health Organization. Accessed January 5, 2024. https://www.who.int/health-topics/integrated-people -centered-care#tab=tab_1.

COVID-19 and HIV

Similarities and Differences—What Have We Learned?

KATIE D. SCHENK AND JERRY OKAL

When COVID-19 emerged onto the global agenda in January 2020, it appeared to present novel challenges. But infectious disease experts already had a toolkit for responding to emerging infections, developed based on many years of experience responding to prior outbreaks of communicable disease. Building on a solid history of sharing lessons across experiences with other infectious pathogens (including SARS, MERS, Ebola, and polio), we seek to identify similarities and differences between SARS-CoV-2 (the virus that causes COVID-19) and HIV (the virus that causes AIDS) and derive lessons for prevention and mitigation, based on distilling lessons from the scientific literature and our own observations and reflecting on the state of the emerging science during the early days of the COVID-19 pandemic (Davtyan, Brown, and Folayan 2014; Drain 2015; Park, Thwaites, and Openshaw 2020). We affirm the critical importance of building on knowledge and tools gained fighting prior outbreaks to transfer lessons to the current global pandemic (Haseltine 2020).

Emerging in the early 1980s, HIV was identified as a retrovirus whose origins lie in zoonotic transmission from African primates (Hahn et al. 2000). The incubation period from initial infection to emergence of symptoms may be long, and untreated infection leads to death, so there is no widespread recovered population with immunity. As the virus is transmitted through mucosal contact with infected body fluids, HIV prevention strategies have focused on limiting or interrupting contact by addressing sexual behaviors and blood-borne exposures, especially among groups recognized as high risk. Initially without treatment, testing, or vaccine to directly address HIV, the role of non-pharmaceutical interventions in changing risk behaviors was recognized early as central to slowing the rapid spread of the virus through preexisting social networks (Kutscher and Greene 2020). Even as subsequent landmark scientific developments discovered and promoted powerfully successful roles for phar-maceutical interventions such as testing and treatment for HIV and AIDS, the continuing absence of a preventive vaccine for HIV suggests that limiting com-munity spread will continue to rely on prevention interventions to shift risk ex-posures among vulnerable groups, including both behavioral approaches (e.g., condom use, needle exchange) and biomedical approaches (e.g., PMTCT [prevention of mother to child transmission], PrEP [preexposure prophylaxis], VMMC [voluntary medical male circumcision]) (Ellenberg and Morris 2021).

In contrast, infection with SARS-CoV-2, identified as a coronavirus, is much more quickly acute than HIV, and there is growing awareness of long-term lingering symptoms among the recovered population. SARS-CoV-2 is transmitted through droplet and aerosol transmission, so behavioral preven-tion strategies rely on interrupting exposure through respiratory routes, in-cluding wearing a mask and social distancing. Exploring early responses to HIV through the lens of the similarities and differences between SARS-CoV-2 and HIV provides valuable lessons for slowing the spread and mitigating the impacts of SARS-CoV-2 (Carrasco et al. 2021).

In this chapter, we present lessons learned from past experiences with HIV and AIDS globally that were already apparent from the early days of the COVID-19 pandemic. We explore how to apply these early lessons to the ongo-ing threat posed by SARS-CoV-2, even as the state of the science of COVID-19 continued to evolve and emerge. We include lessons learned in the areas of:

1. science and technology,

2. politics,

3. public health communications,

4. sociobehavioral factors, and

5. intervention development.

By illustrating these lessons with extensive examples from experiences with both HIV and SARS-CoV-2, we highlight similarities and differences between these two global pandemics that were already apparent during the emergence of the COVID-19 pandemic. We conclude by offering perspectives on how to move forward with the development of evidence-based strategies for continued response to ongoing outbreaks during the evolving COVID-19 pandemic and prevention of the next pandemic.

LESSONS LEARNED

1. Science, Innovation, and Technologies

Establish a Widespread, Reliable Testing System

Throughout the global HIV pandemic, testing has been central to response efforts through strategic approaches including surveillance (population level), diagnostics (individual level) and targeting key vulnerable population groups. Early HIV diagnostic tests were slow and resource-intensive.[1] Subsequent improvements in testing technologies have led to the development of point-of-care testing delivering rapid results, facilitating the speedy initiation of antiretroviral treatment even in resource-limited settings (Drain 2015; Alexander 2016; Mateo-Urdiales et al. 2019; Strathdee et al. 2021). Current diagnostic frontiers now include promoting self-testing and at-home testing among at-risk populations (Ibitoye et al. 2014). Aggregating testing data can be used to (a) refine programming by targeting service delivery to specific audiences, (b) focus messaging according to risk groups, and (c) reduce ongoing transmission by prioritizing information for contact tracing (Carrasco et al. 2021).

Like HIV, testing is critical to the COVID-19 response, in order to identify those who have the virus, prevent continued transmission, and initiate treatment. Especially given the prevalence of asymptomatic transmission (see below), testing helps to determine risk and shape uptake of preventive behaviors (Carrasco et al. 2021). *Unlike HIV,* developing diagnostic tests to detect SARS-CoV-2 has been speedy. Benefiting from technological advances and learning from experiences with other infectious pathogens including SARS and MERS, scientists quickly sequenced the virus and developed molecular assays to identify active infection (Guan et al. 2020). Rapid deployment of increasingly sophisticated technologies (including point-of-care viral nucleic acid/PCR, antigen tests, and serologic testing) has enhanced prevention efforts by facilitating the immediate identification of those who need to isolate and the initiation of contact tracing to identify those who should quarantine (Babiker et al. 2020; Strathdee et al. 2021). Obstacles to global scale-up have forced the use of pooled testing strategies learned from experiences with HIV, especially in resource-limited settings (Sherlock et al. 1995; Boobalan et al. 2019; Strathdee et al. 2021). *Unlike HIV,* testing for SARS-CoV-2 requires coverage of a far wider population due to widespread exposures through respiratory transmission (Ellenberg and Morris 2021).

Acknowledge the Importance of Asymptomatic Transmission

An early study of the incubation period of HIV estimated its median incubation period at 9.8 years (Bacchetti and Moss 1989). During the incubation period, individuals are asymptomatic and most likely unaware that they are infected, but can still transmit infection. Recognizing this extended period of asymptomatic infection among people living with HIV (PLHIV) has been crucial to mitigating transmission (Carrasco et al. 2021). Interventions to promote HIV testing with "Know Your Status" campaigns have been instrumental in creating differentiated messaging based on serostatus, linking testing with prevention messaging, and facilitating early initiation of treatment (Carrasco et al. 2021), but the value of generalized HIV screening among asymptomatic populations is unproven (Chou et al. 2019).

Like HIV, initial responses to COVID relied on symptom-based approaches to case detection, isolation, and quarantine, reflecting perceived similarities with other respiratory viruses (Gandhi, Yokoe, and Havlir 2020). However, evidence (including from nursing homes) soon revealed the prominence of asymptomatic and presymptomatic transmission (He et al. 2020; Arons et al. 2020). Early estimates suggested an incubation period for SARS-CoV-2 of 2–14 days, during which time people who were unknowingly infected were transmitting SARS-CoV-2 infection (WHO 2020b). Thus, new prevention strategies are needed to promote testing—starting with the need to ramp up production of both PCR and rapid antigen tests and to communicate best practices for their use.

Recognize Interactions with Other Conditions

The global spread of HIV highlighted the importance of recognizing comorbidities (i.e., other conditions associated with the virus). Specific comorbidities commonly associated with HIV disease include TB, cardiovascular disease, and hepatitis (Lerner, Eisinger, and Fauci 2020; Anjorin et al. 2021). Experiences with HIV also highlight the importance of recognizing syndemics, which occur when biosocial conditions (e.g., gender-based violence, chronic malnutrition, mental health) combine with disease to exacerbate resultant poor health outcomes (Strathdee et al. 2021).

Like HIV, recognizing comorbidities and syndemics associated with SARS-CoV-2 will help us understand and address transmission dynamics.

Emerging evidence on specific comorbidities and wider syndemics associated with SARS-CoV-2 includes linkages to coinfection with malaria, HIV, and TB; comorbidity with preexisting noncommunicable diseases, including obesity, diabetes, and cardiovascular disease; and syndemics of substance abuse, mental health, and violence among disadvantaged and marginalized communities (Anjorin et al. 2021; Strathdee et al. 2021). While further evidence is sought for the different pathways reinforcing these linkages, separate impacts may combine to create a vicious cycle exacerbating vulnerability to negative outcomes and further contribute to racial and ethnic health disparities (Anjorin et al. 2021; Strathdee et al. 2021).

Clinical, Behavioral, and Implementation Science Research Play Critical Roles

Experiences with HIV have demonstrated the importance of establishing research networks to accelerate the development of HIV diagnostic and therapeutic technologies. The development of a preventive HIV vaccine has faced particular scientific challenges, which may be attributable in part to the speed of viral mutations (Haseltine 2020). However, even in the continuing absence of an HIV vaccine, significant advances in understanding immune responses have led to the development of the latest generation of antiretroviral therapies, helping individuals living with HIV to manage symptoms and keep the virus undetectable for extended periods (Strathdee et al. 2021). Beyond the headlines of biomedical bench research, important studies employing interdisciplinary methodologies grounded in the social and behavioral sciences, public health, and implementation science have advanced knowledge of how to treat, prevent, and mitigate the impacts of HIV and how to manage interventions outside laboratory settings by providing a strong evidence base to understand social determinants of HIV and drive the development of policies and programs.

Unlike HIV, the SARS-CoV-2 virus mutates relatively slowly, making it a far more accessible candidate for vaccine development. The development of proven efficacious vaccines for SARS-CoV-2 within a year from the identification of the virus represents an unprecedented acceleration of the typical vaccine research process, building on years of prior research, including the development of the mRNA platform (Fauci 2021). Vaccine development for SARS-CoV-2 has also benefited from innovations in HIV research, including the development of research infrastructure (e.g., pipelines, trials networks, clinical trial methodologies) (Haseltine 2020; Strathdee et al. 2021). *Like HIV,* research into how to implement strategies that slow the community spread of SARS-CoV-2 is enriched by the increasingly interdisciplinary research methodologies invoked by public health research questions, benefiting local partnerships to build research capacity (Kalbarczyk et al. 2019).

2. Politics

Avoid Politicization of Public Health Messaging

During the early days of the AIDS pandemic, understandings of HIV focused on exposures among specific at-risk groups in high-income countries (e.g., men who have sex with men, people with hemophilia), overlooking growing epidemiological evidence of widespread general population risks and impacts in lower-income countries (Halperin 2020). This imbalance gave rise to discriminatory views about AIDS taking root in public opinion (e.g., referring to AIDS as "the gay plague") and muting government action in order to avoid controversy (Halperin 2020; Olufadewa et al. 2021). However, despite initially slow governmental responses to HIV and AIDS worldwide and instances of flawed leadership,[2] both the United States and South Africa subsequently emerged as global leaders in AIDS response and activism, increasing funding for research and expanding access to antiretroviral treatment (Fassin 2013; Halperin 2020; Strathdee et al. 2021). As civil society activist groups began to play a more active role in shaping the HIV response, public perceptions eventually evolved to acknowledge risks felt throughout the general population and concrete commitments were made to address HIV on a global scale; for instance, the creation of the Special Program on AIDS at the World Health Organization in 1987, which later became UNAIDS (Knight 2008; Kim 2015; Olufadewa et al. 2021). However, critics allege that pressure to respond quickly to emerging health challenges at this time led to some costly or suboptimal decisions, including oversimplistic messaging, which were subsequently difficult to retract (Halperin 2020).

Like HIV, an initially disjointed, politicized, and oversimplified response to a public health challenge undermined clear and cohesive messaging across different jurisdictions and communication channels, including regarding guidance for social distancing and the use of masks. Political influence also negatively affected the uptake of COVID-19 vaccines among people who were receptive to messages questioning the safety and efficacy of this newly developed technology. For example, the late Tanzanian president John Magufuli dismissed the science and severity of COVID-19 on multiple occasions, encouraging vaccine hesitancy and reluctance to follow COVID-19 guidelines before his untimely death (Africanews 2021). *Like HIV,* the emergence of the SARS-CoV-2 virus illustrated the value of political communications in setting the tone and context of public health response. By making stigmatizing references to "the Chinese virus" and "Kung Flu," disparaging the use of facemasks to reduce transmission, and promoting the use of ungrounded strategies as cures (e.g., bleach, hydroxychloroquine), US president Donald Trump politicized and undermined crucial strategies for infection prevention and control and fostered stigma toward Asian and Asian American people (Moynihan and Porumbescu 2020; Olufadewa et al. 2021; Strathdee et al. 2021). As the political infighting continued, the popular media oversimplified debate to present arguments as a dichotomy between a stiflingly rigid lockdown and a reckless move to open up the economy (Halperin 2020). As COVID-19 spread across the globe, so too did speculation about its origins, including whether the virus had escaped from a lab or had been engineered as a bioweapon. *Like HIV,* the absence of clear leadership led to perfect conditions for the spread of conspiracy theories, guesswork, and propaganda.

Promote Global Cooperation and Responsibility

HIV was initially recognized among marginalized groups within wealthy countries, but by the mid-1980s the generalized population impacts in lower-income countries were being acknowledged. Due to chronic underfunding of health systems in sub-Saharan Africa, the global impacts of HIV and initial responses were highly inequitable, and lower-income countries required funding to mount an effective response (Hargreaves et al. 2020; Olufadewa et al. 2021, citing Mann 1987). Without international aid agreements, wealthy countries prioritized access to treatment and services for their own citizens, exacerbating prior inequalities in health and development (Hargreaves et al. 2020). Initial aid responses from wealthy countries led to bilateral agreements with AIDS-affected countries to boost health spending, but were plagued by duplications and inefficiencies. Experiences globally were increasingly highlighting the crucial role of partnerships with civil society groups in leading dialogue, mobilizing national response, and enabling outreach to marginalized and vulnerable communities (Berkman et al. 2005). Due to the speed at which HIV was spreading, coordinating a global response was seen as both ethical and mutually beneficial to donor and recipient countries, acknowledging that control of the AIDS pandemic in *any* country required it to be controlled in *all* countries. Coordinating a global response relied on recognizing that AIDS threatened to reverse prior gains in health and development throughout Africa, that developing a treatment or vaccine would require long-term commitment, and that service delivery required leverage through primary healthcare systems. Creating UNAIDS provided a pathway for creating strong strategic alliances to channel funding and expertise to national

AIDS programs and partner with civil society groups to prevent and control HIV (Mann 1987; Piot et al. 2004; Berkman et al. 2005; Piot et al. 2009; Olufadewa et al. 2021). These experiences with HIV illustrate the importance of global dialogue and cooperation in formulating a robust, effective public health response, implicating higher income countries with the responsibility to demonstrate global leadership and funding in addressing global inequities even between epidemic surges.

Like HIV, the spread of SARS-CoV-2 poses global challenges to equitable resource distribution. Initial governmental responses from wealthy countries prioritized their own citizens—for example, the United States purchased the entire global stockpile of the antiviral drug remdesivir, an early candidate treatment for COVID-19, also leading to fears that the US vaccine development program Operation Warp Speed would similarly deprive the rest of the world of access to prevention resources (Hargreaves et al. 2020; Strathdee et al. 2021). Following the development of efficacious vaccines to prevent SARS-CoV-2, controversies raged regarding their equitable distribution. The COVAX global initiative was intended to serve as a mechanism to enable national governments to put politics aside and prioritize saving lives through equitable global vaccine distribution (WHO 2020a). Both HIV and SARS-CoV-2 have illustrated global reliance upon a well-established system of research and development to accelerate the development of pharmaceutical interventions, but political and social obstacles have impeded progress. Global cooperation is required to galvanize effective responses.

Avoid Creating Stigma by Valuing Human Rights

From the early days of the virus, receiving an HIV-positive diagnosis was frequently associated with experiences of stigma and discrimination, including social isolation, gossip, and self-stigma, with widespread negative consequences—including reluctance to seek care—perpetuating virus transmission. For example, initial attempts to criminalize HIV transmission served as a barrier preventing individuals at high risk of HIV transmission from seeking care, and eventually failed to reduce disease transmission (Jürgens et al. 2009; Olufadewa et al. 2021). Pointing to the fact that stigma and discrimination toward PLHIV and marginalized high-risk populations present obstacles to pandemic response, HIV activists promoted a human rights–based approach that would recognize healthcare as a fundamental human right and thus facilitate opportunities to integrate HIV prevention and care services throughout primary healthcare systems (Olufadewa et al. 2021). With the subsequent arrival of effective HIV treatments, the human rights approach provided a paradigm for incorporating access to treatment into strategic plans to address HIV, even in countries with poorly developed health systems (Berkman et al. 2005).

Like HIV, strategies aimed at preventing transmission of SARS-CoV-2 also hold potential for creating stigma and possibly abusing human rights, by identifying key populations as vectors of the virus. For example, during the emergence of COVID-19 in Uganda, sex workers and truck drivers were openly targeted for transmitting disease and faced ridicule, exclusion, stigma, and discrimination (HealthGap Global Access Project 2020). Experiences with HIV have illustrated that the need for effective virus response measures is not incompatible with taking into account human rights and needs (for example, when restrictions on movement prevent people from earning income or accessing health services). As COVID-19 vaccination rolls out globally, messaging from local leaders and civil society could incorporate recognition that healthcare is a fundamental human right in order to hold governments accountable for respecting human rights and taking unique socioeconomic circumstances (e.g., hunger, extreme poverty) into account (Olufadewa et al. 2021).

3. Communications

Address Public Perceptions of Risk and Mitigation Measures

Early misunderstandings and fears about the threat posed by HIV led to the emergence of stigmatizing terminology and the scapegoating of certain groups perceived to be responsible or dangerous, including men who have sex with men (MSM), sex workers, and people who inject drugs (PWID). Rumors and misconceptions have a long history of affecting the delivery of public health services (Carrasco et al. 2021). For example, testing blood samples for HIV has historically been associated in Zambia with rumors of witchcraft or Satanism (Schenk et al. 2018). Deliberate disinformation has also played a role: Soviet authorities launched a campaign accusing the United States of creating HIV as part of biological weapons research (National Public Radio 2018; Olufadewa et al. 2021). Responding appropriately and effectively to misinformation or disinformation requires a sensitive approach toward building trust, clear communications, and community mobilization to action (Carrasco et al. 2021). Many early public information campaigns about HIV were designed to be frightening, leading many to believe that HIV represented a death sentence. The resulting fear and stigma encouraged people to avoid seeking HIV testing. Misunderstandings and fears about virus transmission also diverted the provision of health services toward people who were at lower risk (the "worried well"), who sought HIV tests after US basketball player Magic Johnson revealed his HIV-positive status (Halperin 2020). Experiences with HIV have demonstrated that promoting uptake of prevention and treatment services requires dispelling myths, addressing stigma, and being seen to respect privacy and confidentiality (Piot et al. 2009; Logie 2020).

Like HIV, SARS-CoV-2 has been susceptible to rumors and misinformation clouding public perceptions of risk and mitigation measures. Initial evidence about which individuals were most at risk of infection was initially unclear, and limited data led to widespread fear of severe outcomes (Halperin 2020). Social media readily amplified the rapid global spread of misinformation about SARS-CoV-2 through multiple channels (Carrasco et al. 2021). Preceded by a long history of vaccine hesitancy, promotion of the SARS-CoV-2 vaccines faced obstacles along predictable lines, with "anti-vaxxers" evoking familiar tropes of parental autonomy and fears for children's future fertility (Larson 2020). Responding to vaccine hesitancy requires efforts to provide reliable information about risk through trusted sources and sensitive community outreach through peer mobilizers and religious and community leaders (Carrasco et al. 2021; Strathdee et al. 2021).

Use Clear, Evidence-Based Communications to Create Cohesive Messaging

In the initial absence of clear guidance for HIV prevention and control, politicization and stigma fed public fear and drove potential clients away from seeking much-needed services for testing and care, perpetuating HIV transmission and underscoring the importance of stigma and discrimination as obstacles to accessing services (Piot et al. 2009; Drain 2015). In an atmosphere of pervasive uncertainty, fear, and even panic, the persecution of marginalized groups persisted, even as continued research advanced scientific knowledge about the virus (Halperin 2020). Clear communications informed by evidence and removed from political agendas are required in order to avoid fomenting distrust. Without public health guidance from trusted public health leaders or government agencies, the public was left to independently navigate risk decisions and behaviors (Arnold 2021). Subsequent advances in scientific understanding of transmission modes brought improved communication about prevention, demonstrating the value of health authorities being proactive in dispelling misinformation and partnering with media outlets to share clear, verified messages (Olufadewa et al. 2021). Successful HIV messaging campaigns have been those that identify and engage trusted sources and channels of information (including religious and community leaders, peer educators, and mass media) and that also respond flexibly to concerns changing over time and advancing scientific frontiers (Reed, Patel, and Baggaley 2018; Stankevitz et al. 2019; Atkins et al. 2020; Carrasco et al. 2021). HIV communications strategies have been particularly fraught due to sensitivities about sexual behavior and other taboo topics, highlighting the need for culturally sensitive communications that dynamically reflect local social mores (Berkman et al. 2005).

Like HIV, the early weeks of the COVID-19 pandemic were characterized by a charged atmosphere of pervasive anxiety and fear. While fear is understandable and can even be used positively to motivate behavior change (e.g., implementing social distancing), irrational fears can lead to suboptimal decision-making in the absence of clear guidance (e.g., incorrect use of personal protective equipment [PPE]) (Halperin 2020). Unclear messaging about SARS-CoV-2 bred suspicion and mistrust in health leadership and news media. Ready availability of multiple sources of contradictory information began to erode public trust in once-respected leadership authorities (Parmet and Paul 2020). The resultant discord discouraged many individuals from seeking care and adhering to prevention guidance, perpetuating disease transmission and slowing global mitigation efforts (Olufadewa et al. 2021). In a rapidly changing environment, effective public messaging requires trusted expertise that adapts to meet evolving needs for information and reflects real-time advances in scientific knowledge (Carrasco et al. 2021). As scientific knowledge advances, research may reveal updates to prior guidance, and clear communications are needed to convey that these are a natural, predictable consequence of extending the scientific knowledge base, not to be misconstrued as a policy reversal or "flip-flop."[3] For example, initial prevention strategies focused on minimizing the risks of virus transmission through surfaces (fomites); subsequent evidence called into question whether this was an overstatement relying too heavily on a transmission path responsible for only a small proportion of infections (Halperin 2020). Continuing debate about the origins of SARS-CoV-2 is another sensitive area requiring clear communications (Olufadewa et al. 2021).

4. Socioeconomic and Behavioral Factors

Recognize and Confront Disproportionate Inequities among Disadvantaged Groups

The HIV epidemic illustrated disproportionate impacts experienced by people who were already vulnerable, including those living in poverty or marginalized due to identity or behaviors. HIV exacerbated the impacts of preexisting health disparities among people lacking access to healthcare services, highlighting the role of social determinants of health in virus exposure and transmission and disease outcomes (Millett 2020; Hargreaves et al. 2020; Carrasco et al. 2021). Especially in low-income countries where already weakened and struggling healthcare systems were unable to protect the most disenfranchised people and communities, the AIDS pandemic directly exposed and worsened inequities in health outcomes (Kutscher and Greene 2020; Olufadewa et al. 2021). For example, vulnerable people experiencing limited access to healthcare services (e.g., HIV testing, treatment) include racial and ethnic minorities, MSM, people with disabilities, sex workers, truck drivers, prisoners, people who inject drugs (PWIDs), people who are trans, and many other individuals and communities facing a lack of socioeconomic opportunity, social exclusion, stigma, or other marginalization. Indicators reflecting inequitable outcomes include poor access and linkages to and retention in care, treatment initiation and adherence, and viral suppression (Strathdee et al. 2021).

Like HIV, the disproportionate effects of COVID-19 exacerbated preexisting health disparities among people who are impoverished or who lack access to essential services, and highlighted the crucial role of economic and racial disparities (Farquharson and Thornton 2020; Carrasco et al. 2021). Emerging US data already revealed the disproportionate mortality and morbidity burdens on communities of color and ethnic minorities, with health outcome disparities further reflected in access to testing and rates of hospitalization (Strathdee et al. 2021). Globally, evidence was growing that interventions to prevent and address the impacts of COVID-19 (including case identification and isolation, rapid testing and diagnosis, and contact tracing) remained inequitably distributed due to lack of resources in lower-income countries, a burden further exacerbated by disparities in vaccine distribution (Olufadewa et al. 2021).

Consider Intersections of Virus Dynamics with Other Contexts

As noted above, the impacts of HIV have been closely connected with impacts of other contexts of disadvantage and vulnerability, whose intersections must be recognized when designing policy and program interventions. For example, the impacts of AIDS worsened preexisting gender imbalances, so service providers have learned to take into account the role of gender-based violence, relative autonomy in health-seeking behaviors, and mental health in women's ability to access healthcare services, including HIV testing and care.

Like HIV, the negative impacts of COVID-19 were particularly acute among groups rendered vulnerable by overlapping characteristics of race, ethnicity, and disability, exposing intersectional disadvantages among groups already marginalized (Gerada 2021). Just as with HIV, these socioeconomic burdens fell particularly harshly upon women, who are more likely to be caregivers (facing higher risk of infection) and who may have been exposed to particular hardship associated with gender-based violence during lockdown (Olufadewa et al. 2021). For example, one study showed high prevalence of specific health concerns (including skipping meals, depression, and fear) related to COVID-19 among young women in Kenya (Population Council 2020). Effects of impact mitigation measures (e.g., movement restrictions) may also have exacerbated inequities, with disproportionately negative effects among the most vulnerable people, including people who live in informal settlements, rely on daily wages, or are dependent on the sex trade. Experiences learned from HIV include ensuring representation from among marginalized groups in the design and implementation of impact mitigation initiatives (Olufadewa et al. 2021).

Focus on Key Behaviors Associated with Transmission Risk

Acknowledging that HIV risk transmission is strongly associated with behaviors that may be hidden, stigmatized, or forced (e.g., sex work, injecting drugs, MSM), research has highlighted the importance of understanding the complex realities of human behaviors (Haseltine 2020). Harm reduction interventions can be employed to identify and reduce behavioral risks by creating enabling environments to support behavior change, rather than by cracking down on already stigmatized behaviors and driving them further underground, where they may become more risky (Hargreaves et al. 2020). Risk mitigation strategies must account for individuals assessing their own level of risk and risk tolerance and developing personal strategies for risk management. Such strategies include providing clean needles to people who inject drugs (PWIDs), rather than shaming them for their drug use, and promoting condom use during transactional sex rather than trying to eliminate sex work altogether (Wondergem et al. 2015; Lyss et al. 2020).[4] In Brazil, needle exchange programs became a key component of a national HIV prevention strategy emphasizing human rights and involvement of marginalized populations, contributing to a paradigm shift in responding to drug use as a question of public rather than criminal justice (Berkman et al. 2005).

Like HIV, in responding to COVID-19 in the absence of (or prior to) pharmaceutical solutions, nonpharmaceutical interventions sought to shift human behavior to reduce risk exposures by acknowledging the strengths and limitations of human decision-making (Hargreaves et al. 2020). Interventions aiming to change COVID-19 risk behaviors sought to address deeply embedded and personal behavioral norms, including social interactions and economic motivations (Haseltine 2020). People living in poverty may have faced specific barriers to adopting behaviors that protected against virus transmission, including limited access to clean running water, living in crowded locations, inability to comply with guidance for social distancing or movement restrictions, and inadequate supplies of PPE. A harm reduction approach to mitigating COVID-19 addresses the reasons why people might feel unable to comply with health guidance (e.g., if they were compelled to leave home to work in order to maintain their family's economic survival) and seeks to provide a pragmatic response to risk management under suboptimal circumstances. Messaging should address the realities of daily life in communities facing hardship in their response to COVID-19 (including older people, people with comorbidities, people who are already marginalized, people with limited access to health services, and families with young children) and should acknowledge that an "abstinence-only" approach to social interactions by staying at home and strictly maintaining physical distancing may not always be possible and may present or exacerbate other health risks (e.g., mental health) (Kutscher and Greene 2020; Carrasco et al. 2021). By acknowledging a spectrum of risk, supporting policies that reduce if not eliminate harm, and encouraging individuals to make informed choices, policy-makers can create an enabling environment in which to lower risk exposure and avoid stigma (Carrasco et al. 2021).

Evaluate Social and Structural Factors as Exogenous Drivers of Risk

Mitigating HIV transmission requires acknowledging the key roles of underlying socioeconomic and structural drivers[5] in determining health-seeking and risk-taking behaviors and underscores the potential for structural interventions (including community mobilization) to address these root causes (Strathdee et al. 2021). Factors driving HIV transmission risk and undermining prevention and treatment efforts include many socioeconomic and structural factors grounded in the intersection of HIV infection, racism, homophobia, and sexism.[6]

Like HIV, structural and social drivers contributed to adverse SARS-CoV-2 risk and outcomes, manifesting through multiple pathways, including social exclusion, unequal access to healthcare, physical environment, and living arrangements. In the United States, systemic racism affected virus transmission and prevention through deeply rooted structural mechanisms (Strathdee et al. 2021). For example, racial and ethnic minorities may have been overrepresented among essential workers exposed to elevated risks of virus transmission and with limited workplace protections (Strathdee et al. 2021). In many countries, access to health services is impeded by poverty, user fees, long distances to health facilities, and sociocultural practices. Opportunities to conduct structural interventions that address the root causes of these health-seeking and risk-taking behaviors include advocating for long-term, far-reaching policy change (including community mobilization for access to healthcare and paid sick leave), promoting testing and prevention strategies, and seeking housing for homeless people (Strathdee et al. 2021).

5. Intervention Strategies: Impacts and Responses

Employ Multiple Intervention Strategies Concurrently

Contextualizing HIV response strategies recognizes the need to implement multiple interventions concurrently, including nonpharmaceutical strategies (e.g., behavior change communications, partner reduction) alongside pharmaceutical strategies (HIV testing and treatment, PrEP/PEP [pre- and post-exposure prophylaxis]). Interventions can be tailored to context by selecting from a range of layered intervention options spanning community mobilization, social protection, and healthcare delivery across HIV prevention, testing, care, and treatment (Hargreaves et al. 2020). For example, the DREAMS Partnership implemented among young women in ten sub-Saharan African countries sought to reduce HIV incidence through a "combination HIV prevention" package layering evidence-based behavioral, biological, and structural interventions tailored to population need (Dehne et al. 2016; Abdool Karim, Baxter, and Birx 2017; Saul et al. 2018).

Like HIV, responding efficiently and effectively to SARS-CoV-2 requires policy-makers and program implementers to employ multiple strategies simultaneously for virus prevention and mitigation. Nonpharmaceutical interventions such as behavior change communication strategies, ventilation and filtration, wearing masks, and social distancing should be employed alongside pharmaceutical interventions including promoting testing and vaccination (Carrasco et al. 2021). The "Swiss cheese model," originally developed to minimize the role of human error in advancing technologies, was adapted to represent the concurrent layering of COVID-19 interventions, accepting that no single intervention offers a watertight guarantee against virus spread (Reason 1990; Mackay 2020; Roberts 2020).

Focus on the Most Relevant Interventions for the Most Vulnerable People

Intervention strategies aiming to address the most private and deeply rooted norms of sexual behavior have historically been difficult to implement, particularly among people who are marginalized through gender inequalities and stigma (including MSM, sex workers, and women living in fear of gender-based violence), who are least empowered to change their risk exposures though their own behaviors (Haseltine 2020). Evidence supports the introduction of behavior change interventions that recognize the roles of community participation and social capital in shaping social norms in order to address risk exposure and create enabling environments (Carrasco et al. 2021; Hargreaves et al. 2020). A central principle of the UNAIDS pandemic response is "know your local epidemic,"[7] underscoring the critical importance of recognizing and responding to the specific populations and sociocultural settings most affected by HIV and AIDS within their local contexts (UNAIDS 2014). One size does not fit all: there is no single HIV prevention strategy that is universally appropriate, acceptable, and effective among all people in all settings (Halperin 2020; Carrasco et al. 2021). The most efficient and effective HIV response strategies are those that acknowledge the diversity of populations infected and affected and target specific population groups with particular characteristics. Such strategies recognize the holistic context of vulnerabilities and assets found among various population groups and select the most fitting health education messages based on the range of biomedical and behavioral interventions[8] on offer, such as partner reduction, condom use, VMMC, PrEP, etc. (Anderson et al. 2014; Lin et al. 2016; Cordie et al. 2021; Carrasco et al. 2021).

Like HIV, intervention opportunities to prevent and mitigate the spread of SARS-CoV-2 should be targeted to prioritize resource allocation based on need, addressing specific contextual challenges while utilizing messages, language, and imagery appropriate for the intended audience (Carrasco et al. 2021). Services and commodities (e.g., diagnostic testing, PPE, tailored health messages) should be targeted to communities in most need, recognizing the realities and complexities of living circumstances (Olufadewa et al. 2021). For example, low-wage workers without financial safety nets are less likely to be able to abide by restrictions on movement due to losing income, so interventions might offer food and financial support alternatives; residents of crowded or informal settlements and multigenerational households are less likely to be able to comply with physical distancing recommendations, so interventions might offer guidance for masking in indoor or outdoor interactions.

Engage with Community Groups in a Coordinated Multisectoral Response

Experiences responding to HIV have illustrated the importance of active community engagement in developing and implementing prevention and mitigation strategies. Tailoring interventions to meet specific local needs requires partnership and participation with members of key affected population groups, community-based groups, and community health workers to build community engagement, knowledge, and trust as a vital component of a multisectoral response. Collaborations between government-led initiatives and community-based programs have been crucial to the design and implementation of appropriate, relevant interventions that genuinely address lived experiences, by employing trusted and effective strategies adapted to local needs (Carrasco et al. 2021; Berkman et al. 2005). Cooperation with civil society groups[9] has been key to fostering community engagement, improving community knowledge and communication, and developing trust in relationships. For example, community groups have been recruited to play key roles in encouraging treatment uptake by using local networks to engage those most at risk, disseminating evidence-based information, and addressing misinformation and harmful community norms (Cordie et al. 2021; Carrasco et al. 2021). Community and civil society groups have an especially valuable contribution to make toward developing relationships with marginalized groups (e.g., sex workers, PWIDs, MSM, LGBTQ+, PLHIV), building credibility, and improving communications and operations of interventions (Berkman et al. 2005). Another way in which communities have contributed to the implementation of HIV interventions is by active involvement in recruitment and training for key staffing roles, where community members serve as a link between key populations and intervention delivery (Berkman et al. 2005). Local community members engaged in peer education and other fieldwork roles have used their intimate community knowledge to enhance service outreach and quality. Further possibilities of "up-skilling"[10] may improve the uptake and effectiveness of HIV programmatic responses (Uwimana et al. 2012; Guilamo-Ramos et al. 2021). Extending the multisectoral response to also include international agencies and public-private partnerships can provide further opportunities for leveraging the comparative advantage of each sector to foster innovation and efficiency. This is especially relevant when considering the distribution of pharmaceutical commodities, which requires a strong and coordinated approach (Eisinger, Lerner, and Fauci 2021).

Like HIV, interventions to reduce transmission of SARS-CoV-2 will be enhanced by the implementation of a multisectoral response through innovative program design, implementation, and evaluation (Hargreaves et al. 2020). Across the range of possible interventions, encompassing pharmaceutical and nonpharmaceutical approaches, urgent multisectoral efforts are required to promote uptake (Carrasco et al. 2021). Responding appropriately to COVID-19 with effective and culturally sensitive interventions requires the input of community members in the design of outreach tools and messaging aimed at vulnerable population groups (Carrasco et al. 2021; Cordie et al. 2021).

Rise above Stigma and Fear to Avoid Driving Risk Behaviors Underground

Since the earliest days of the HIV pandemic, stigma has served as a significant barrier to reaching the people most at risk of infection with services to address prevention, care, and treatment (Piot et al. 2009). Fear and stigma have continued to spread in parallel with the virus, with discriminating actions manifest in homes, communities, healthcare facilities, and workplaces, exacerbating stigma experienced among at-risk communities already marginalized due to behaviors or social status (Kutscher and Greene 2020; Nyblade et al. 2020; Pulerwitz et al. 2010). Characterizing the struggle against stigma as central to the HIV response has been vital to supporting approaches that address the social consequences of HIV and avoiding the spread of prejudices and irrational fears, including through partnerships with civil society and community groups (Halperin 2020; Berkman et al. 2005; Hargreaves et al. 2020). Interventions to address stigma and discrimination have sought to develop community-sensitive solutions through mass sensitization and awareness-raising, in order to avoid driving stigmatized behaviors underground where risks may be elevated (Cordie et al. 2021).

Like HIV, it was critical to address the barriers presented by stigma when considering the fears associated with SARS-CoV-2. Initial stigmatizing behaviors presented as prejudices against people who looked Chinese, fueled by racist statements from political leaders speculating on the origins of the virus. The unintended consequences of stigmatizing a COVID-19 diagnosis include the possibility that people will avoid complying with guidance for quarantine, isolation, and even treatment, thus exacerbating conditions favoring virus transmission (Halperin 2020; Hargreaves et al. 2020).

Consider Direct and Indirect Impacts on Families

The direct impacts of HIV fell initially on adults, especially those who could be described as members of high-risk groups, including MSM, PWIDs, and sex workers. However, it soon became clear that indirect impacts of the epidemic were manifesting as serious adverse effects on members of their families and households. Across high HIV-prevalence countries of sub-Saharan Africa, orphans and vulnerable children were dropping out of school due to poverty and taking increased responsibilities for caregiving and earning income, while entire households were facing elevated food insecurity, exacerbated within a preexisting context of pressure from climate change, conflict, and economic instability (Olufadewa et al. 2021; Esu-Williams et al. 2006). Interventions targeted at members of at-risk households (not just the person living with HIV) have proven effective at mitigating the indirect impacts of HIV, including addressing impaired educational, health, and psychosocial outcomes among children in AIDS-affected households (Olufadewa et al. 2021; Brown et al. 2009; Schenk 2009; Schenk et al. 2010).

Like HIV, COVID-related deaths among adults have created a new generation of children exposed to the social, emotional, and economic vulnerabilities associated with orphanhood (Hillis et al. 2021; Kidman 2021). Experiences of parental mortality and morbidity globally have illustrated the long-term impacts on families and communities, and also the potential for support interventions to address children's well-being (Barenbaum and Smith 2016; Bergman, Axberg, and Hanson 2017). Furthermore, as the effects of COVID-19 led to school closures aimed at curtailing virus transmission, children worldwide faced prolonged interruptions to their education, especially those without access to reliable power and internet connections for online school. Even in areas where online schooling was available, children enrolled in remote learning lacked opportunities for psychosocial interactions and community support provided by in-person schooling. Emerging data demonstrated adverse mental health outcomes related to COVID-19 for learners in different settings (Population Council 2020). The impacts of COVID-19 also affected food security, due to reduced household incomes and obstacles to trade when borders closed, and have been associated with rising malnutrition (Olufadewa et al. 2021; International Committee of the Red Cross 2020). Communications about the impacts of COVID-19 frequently focus on a general population message while failing to address the situations of families with children aged under 12, who were not yet eligible for vaccination (Schenk and Stuart 2021).

Prioritize the Role of Data in Driving Evidence-Based Policies and Programs

The use of epidemiological data to describe and explore the underlying drivers of the spread of disease remains a key tool for understanding how to prevent and mitigate it. During the HIV pandemic, increasingly rigorous methods of data collection and modeling have become established as important tools to inform the development of policies and programs and to evaluate their impacts. Collecting and triangulating quantitative and qualitative data has enabled scientists to build a comprehensive picture of trends, including tracking the spread of the virus, characterizing its natural history, identifying risk and protective factors, and evaluating interventions to prevent, mitigate, and treat (Strathdee et al. 2021; Ellenberg and Morris 2021). The development of evidence-based, data-driven policies and programs has become a fundamental principle in moving the field away from the influence of politics and ideology and learning from reliable scientific methodologies and observations.

Like HIV, experiences with SARS-CoV-2 had already begun to benefit from sound methodologies for data collection and analysis to develop policies and programs driven by the available evidence rather than political leanings. Scientists conducting research into SARS-CoV-2 were able to leverage research networks and laboratory platforms originally developed for the creation of clinical trials for HIV treatment (Dean 2021). However, even in the wealthiest of countries, efforts to record and collate reliable data were hampered by an out-of-date public health system that lacked modern data capabilities (Schenk 2021). Furthermore, incorporating messages that reflect data-driven findings and policies into popular media and public engagement tools remains an ongoing challenge (Dean 2021).

Support Individuals to Assess Risk and Implement Realistic Protective Behaviors

Experiences developing interventions and public health messaging for HIV have demonstrated the value of communicating science-based information, educating about risk, and encouraging individuals to make informed decisions about risk tolerance and implement realistic risk-reduction strategies accordingly. For example, providing young people with information about HIV risk and encouraging them to know their partners' status and use condoms has proven to be a more effective strategy than an abstinence-only approach (Haseltine 2020). Risk assessment and reduction strategies can help people who are HIV-positive to access treatment and learn how to avoid transmitting HIV to other people. Harm reduction interventions (see above) promote education that helps individuals distinguish between situations that pose high or low levels of risk and support realistic decision-making (Halperin 2020).

Like HIV, SARS-CoV-2 presented the opportunity to provide education about behaviors and assessing virus transmission risk. Young people who assumed that they were unlikely to become severely ill may have underestimated the possibility of long-term consequences and contributed to viral spread and the emergence of mutations (Haseltine 2020). Learning to distinguish between virus transmission risks indoors and outdoors, the role of social distancing, and other background information for preventive measures may permit individuals and communities to find their own norms, allowing the development of evidence-based risk behaviors that reflect social and economic realities (Halperin 2020; Kutscher and Greene 2020).

Build and Strengthen Reliable Supply Chains for Necessary Commodities

Practical lessons from HIV have demonstrated the value of building reliable supply chains for the commodities necessary for building and sustaining critical interventions, including the supply of pharmaceutical treatments for HIV, HIV tests and lab supplies, and PPE. A global movement to address the challenges of supply chain logistics has drawn attention and funding to streamlining infrastructure and staffing demands for transport and storage, resulting in improvements to procurement, security, data, and efficiency (Pastakia et al. 2018)

Like HIV, the commodity needs for interventions to address SARS-CoV-2 can be addressed through acting on the transferable lessons learned for efficient and cost-effective supply chains. Specific commodity and transport needs must be recognized, including cold chain storage requirements for vaccines and the supply needs to transform vaccines into vaccinations, including gloves, syringes, etc. In addition, an effective supply chain to deliver shots into arms requires the availability of skilled staff to organize clinics and administer vaccine doses.

SUMMARY AND LESSONS LEARNED

Context Is Everything

In this chapter, we have described our observations of similarities and differences between the characteristics of the HIV and COVID-19 pandemics and their strategic responses. Many diverse experiences from the global response to HIV provide instructive lessons for decision-making in the emergency response to COVID-19. However, HIV has taught us the need to contextualize: there exists no single homogeneous experience or prepackaged approach to responding to a pandemic of infectious disease. In every location, response will be shaped by a unique history that encompasses the full diversity of culture, institutions, resources, social forces, and civil society (Berkman et al. 2005). We argue that the common thread underlying intervention strategies for the prevention and mitigation of COVID-19 (like other communicable diseases) must surely be the use of evidence-based approaches based explicitly upon scientific data, encompassing clinical and community-based research studies, epidemiological modeling, and real-world operational research, in order to inform policy and programs. The guiding principles of knowing your local epidemic and knowing your local community learned from HIV remain crucial to the design of appropriate interventions addressing COVID-19.

Global Responsibility to Address Health Inequities

Experiences with HIV have encouraged the global community to focus on clearly stated goals and coalesce behind them in united action to stop transmission, reduce deaths, prevent future outbreaks, and support affected communities (Hargreaves et al. 2020). A focus on the equivalent goals for a COVID-19 resurgence or for future pandemics requires the global community to mobilize scientific resources and political capital to improve our understanding of the virus and how to combat it, and to avert the worsening challenge in the poorest of countries (Ellenberg and Morris 2021; El-Sadr and Justman 2020). We seek coordination between global, regional, and country responses to confront the devastating effects of COVID-19 in managing emergency and long-term responses to the virus, including allocating scarce resources where they are most needed. We seek strong, unequivocal leadership from the WHO (e.g., through the WHO-led ACT-Accelerator partnership) and collaboration with partners in government and industry to ensure that key priorities for pandemic response are aligned, responsive, and nimble. We look to these experts and institutions for robust leadership on coordinating global surveillance, epidemiology, modeling, diagnostics, clinical care, and other ways to manage the virus and limit transmission. We seek guidance and tools for clear public health messaging that can be tailored locally to the needs of specific and diverse audiences. In particular, we seek moral leadership and commitment to urgently address and avert the predictable inequities emerging between resource-rich and resource-poor countries in accessing vaccines. We see clear practical and moral imperatives for leveraging resources to increase global access to vaccination.

Impacts of COVID on HIV

Both HIV and SARS-CoV-2 viruses have brutally exposed weaknesses within healthcare systems throughout the globe, especially in countries with highly inequitable access to a wide range of development resources and funding (Carrasco et al. 2021; Schenk 2021). Recognizing healthcare as a fundamental human right requires increased attention to the role of strengthening health systems and prioritizing public health as a central aspect of governmental responsibility to promote efficiency and innovation in the pandemic response (Berkman et al. 2005; Olufadewa et al. 2021). We strive to ensure that the impact of COVID-19 or future pandemics on health systems globally does not derail the progress that has been made in recent years in addressing service delivery for HIV prevention and treatment and for other common health conditions associated with poverty, including the communicable diseases of childhood (Stegling 2020). Having witnessed the detrimental impacts of COVID-19 reversing precious gains in health indicators globally, we must seek to improve flexibility and adapt health services to maintain their resilience in the face of significant challenges to infrastructure and environment (Vrazo et al. 2020; Sarwer et al. 2020; Venter 2020). We urge providers of HIV services to adapt and maintain service delivery for HIV testing, treatment, and care even as a pandemic might divert attention from the cause, in order to avoid further mortality and morbidity indirectly attributable to the pandemic (UNAIDS 2020; Olufadewa et al. 2021).

We also seek further evidence of how to respond to the juxtaposition of the HIV and COVID-19 pandemics and their associated comorbidities (e.g., HIV and TB in sub-Saharan Africa, SARS-CoV-2 and obesity in the United States). Are people who are HIV-positive particularly vulnerable to COVID-19 and its complications (including long term) due to respiratory symptoms, or vice versa? What are the specific clinical and public health needs that relate to coinfection with HIV and SARS-CoV-2 simultaneously? These and related questions are important areas for continuing research and application in public health policy and practices (Eisinger, Lerner, and Fauci 2021; Anjorin et al. 2021; Cooper et al. 2020).

Lessons from COVID to HIV

As we offer lessons learned from past experiences of HIV and their applicability to COVID-19, we also suggest that lessons might also be taken from our recent experiences of COVID-19 and applied in the future to HIV and other communicable diseases (Rebeiro et al. 2020; Millett 2020; CBC 2021). Recent experiences developing innovative technologies to deliver and enhance health services and information have leveraged robust use of digital technologies and mobile interventions to monitor and track patient data, some of which might next be leveraged for HIV service reporting and for health systems use more widely (WHO 2016; Balhara and Anwar 2019; Maharana et al. 2020). Promoting a transition to robust health data and information systems will be of enormous benefit in countries where public health information systems are either effectively lacking or significantly limited in capacity and reach (Cordie et al. 2021; Schenk 2021). In particular, the experiences of developing COVID-19 vaccine research, approvals, and distribution at unprecedented speeds point the way toward future opportunities for accelerating vaccine development and distribution for other pathogens (including HIV, TB, and malaria) from both scientific and regulatory perspectives. We emphasize, however, that transferring learnings from prior epidemics to future epidemics only remains a viable strategy for as long as funding exists *between* outbreaks, stressing the importance of maintaining funding for public health preparedness and response even when not in outbreak emergency mode (Haseltine 2020).

CONCLUSION

Throughout our work on the front lines of the COVID-19 emergency response, we repeatedly heard the equivalent of "We're building the plane while flying it" as an explanation for obstacles to services delivery and suboptimal outcomes. However, we argue that even from the early days of the emergence of the global COVID-19 pandemic, the experiences of prior outbreaks of infectious disease, especially HIV, have already provided us with model "planes" that can teach us how to fly.

CLASS EXERCISE

Draw a table that illustrates lessons learned from experiences with a prior epidemic of infectious disease and how the same principle might be transferred to experiences with SARS-CoV-2.

E.G.:

Lesson learned	Example from HIV (or H1N1 or MERS or . . .)	SARS-CoV-2 example

NOTES

1. It took four years from initial reports of AIDS to development of the first antibody test for HIV, and a further year until availability of the first viral detection assay (Alexander 2016). Prior to availability of laboratory testing, health providers diagnosed HIV by assessing patient symptoms, using a clinical case definition including weight loss, cancer, tuberculosis, and pneumonia

to assess stage of disease (Keou et al. 1992; WHO 2005). Early testing efforts were designed to reach a limited at-risk population readily described by specific behavioral and biomedical exposures (Ellenberg and Morris 2021). Even after laboratory tests for HIV became widely available, processing could take weeks, and positive results required confirmatory testing—all of which added delays to diagnosis and subsequent contact tracing, especially at a frightening time when cooperation with tracing was frequently difficult to obtain (Slotten 2020).

2. At a time when discussions invoking sexual behaviors and other risky exposures to HIV were taboo, reluctance of international political leaders to discuss HIV resulted in a lack of action, favoring widespread rumors and conspiracy theories about the origins of HIV that slowed the response. Although CDC officials were well aware of AIDS from 1981, it was not until 1985 that US president Ronald Reagan mentioned it publicly. President Reagan avoided mentioning AIDS (and condoms) and funding AIDS research until it was unavoidable, and further contributed to misinformation and discrimination by calling into question the safety of sending his child to school with children who were HIV-positive (Olufadewa et al. 2021; Strathdee et al. 2021; Haseltine 2020; Reagan 1985). Even in South Africa, where the impacts of HIV were soon being felt on a widespread population basis, President Nelson Mandela did not mention AIDS publicly until 1997 and his successor, President Thabo Mbeki, came under the influence of dissident scientists questioning the origins and implications of the virus (Macinnis 1997; Fassin 2013).

3. For example, in the United States, initial communications from health authorities discouraged the public from using facemasks, aiming to preserve supplies of PPE for health workers. When new evidence emerged supporting the benefit of masks in preventing asymptomatic transmission in a context of widespread community spread, guidance was updated to recommend mask use in public. The resulting mixed messages were portrayed by populist media as a confusing U-turn when they actually reflected a growing knowledge base (Stankevitz et al. 2019; Carrasco et al. 2021). Scientists in the United Kingdom and United States also struggled to communicate the complexities of herd immunity in an accessible way to people with varying levels of scientific education (Halperin 2020).

4. Similar approaches have also underpinned interventions to address teenage pregnancy (Kutscher and Greene 2020; Arnold 2021).

5. Within the HIV discourse, the term *structural drivers* is used to describe a range of factors that shape and influence patterns of risk behavior by facilitating or impeding ability to access services or adhere to treatment. Macro-level structural drivers may influence a range of other community-level factors (e.g., harmful gender and social norms, stigma and discrimination, violence against women and girls, and alcohol use), which may then act as mediators to influence the more proximal determinants of HIV risk (e.g., sexual behavior, prevalence of STI symptoms, ability to access health services) (STRIVE Research Consortium 2019).

6. For example, healthcare providers who initially blamed and abused MSM for transmitting the "gay plague."
7. Formerly "know your epidemic."
8. Targeted behavioral intervention strategies to address HIV prevention and treatment focus on key populations who are at high risk of HIV due to exposures associated with their behaviors (e.g., injecting drugs, sex work) or social or structural factors (e.g., criminalization, access to healthcare, socioeconomic inequalities), and offer specific supports that recognize those vulnerabilities (e.g., condom distribution among sex workers, clean needles among PWIDs) (Iversen et al. 2020; Carrasco et al. 2021; Olufadewa et al. 2021). Strategies recognizing the vulnerabilities of key at-risk population groups also include leveraging community engagement and social structures to promote access to services among, for instance, people living in regions of conflict and people living with disabilities, and have also been included in national HIV strategies (Olufadewa, Adesina, and Ayorinde 2020; Olufadewa et al. 2021).
9. Including community-based organizations, religious groups, youth groups, and nongovernmental organizations.
10. Also known as "task-shifting."

REFERENCES

Abdool Karim, Quarraisha, Cheryl Baxter, and Deborah Birx. 2017. "Prevention of HIV in Adolescent Girls and Young Women: Key to an AIDS-Free Generation." *JAIDS Journal of Acquired Immune Deficiency Syndrome* 75, no. S1 (May): S17–S26. https://doi.org/10.1097/QAI.0000000000001316.

Alexander, Thomas S. 2016. "Human Immunodeficiency Virus Diagnostic Testing: 30 Years of Evolution." *Clinical and Vaccine Immunology* 23, no. 4 (April): 249–53. https://doi.org/10.1128/CVI.00053-16.

Anderson, Sarah-Jane, Peter Cherutich, Nduku Kilonzo, Ide Cremin, Daniela Fecht, Davies Kimanga, Malayah Harper, et al. 2014. "Maximising the Effect of Combination HIV Prevention through Prioritisation of the People and Places in Greatest Need: A Modelling Study." *Lancet* 384, no. 9939 (July): 249–56. https://doi.org/10.1016/S0140-6736(14)61053-9.

Anjorin, A. A., A. I. Abioye, O. E. Asowata, A. Soipe, M. I. Kazeem, I. O. Adesanya, M. A. Raji, et al. 2021. "Comorbidities and the COVID-19 Pandemic Dynamics in Africa." *Tropical Medicine & International Health* 26, no. 1 (January): 2–13. https://doi.org/10.1111/tmi.13504.

Arnold, Carrie. 2021. "Covid-19: How the Lessons of HIV Can Help End the Pandemic." *BMJ* 372:n216. https://doi.org/10.1136/bmj.n216.

Arons, Melissa M., Kelly M. Hatfield, Sujan C. Reddy, Anne Kimball, Allison James, Jesica R. Jacobs, Joanne Taylor, et al. 2020. "Presymptomatic SARS-CoV-2 Infections and Transmission in a Skilled Nursing Facility." *New England Journal of Medicine* 382, no. 22: 2081–90. https://doi.org/10.1056/NEJMoa2008457.

Atkins, Kaitlyn, Ping Teresa Yeh, Caitlin E. Kennedy, Virginia A. Fonner, Michael D. Sweat, Kevin R. O'Reilly, Rachel Baggaley, George W. Rutherford, and Julia

Samuelson. 2020. "Service Delivery Interventions to Increase Uptake of Voluntary Medical Male Circumcision for HIV Prevention: A Systematic Review." *PLOS ONE* 15, no. 1: e0227755. https://doi.org/10.1371/journal.pone.0227755.

Babiker, Ahmed, Charlie W. Myers, Charles E. Hill, and Jeannette Guarner. 2020. "SARS-CoV-2 Testing: Trials and Tribulations." *American Journal of Clinical Pathology* 153, no. 6 (June): 706–8. https://doi.org/10.1093/ajcp/aqaa052.

Bacchetti, Peter, and Andrew R. Moss. 1989. "Incubation Period of AIDS in San Francisco." *Nature* 338, no. 6212: 251–53. https://www.nature.com/articles/338251a0.

Balhara, Yatan Pal Singh, and Nazneen Anwar. 2019. "BehavioR: A Digital Platform for Prevention and Management of Behavioural Addictions." *WHO South-East Asia Journal of Public Health* 8, no. 2 (September): 101–3. https://www.who.int/southeastasia/publications/who-south-east-asia-journal-of-public-health/whoseajphv8n2.

Barenbaum, Edna, and Tamarah Smith. 2016. "Social Support as a Protective Factor for Children Impacted by HIV/AIDS across Varying Living Environments in Southern Africa." *AIDS Care* 28, Supp. 2 (July): 92–99. https://doi.org/10.1080/09540121.2016.1176683.

Bergman, Ann-Sofie, Ulf Axberg, and Elizabeth Hanson. 2017. "When a Parent Dies: A Systematic Review of the Effects of Support Programs for Parentally Bereaved Children and Their Caregivers." *BMC Palliative Care* 16, art. no. 39: 1–15. https://doi.org/10.1186/s12904-017-0223-y.

Berkman, Alan, Jonathan Garcia, Miguel Muñoz-Laboy, Vera Paiva, and Richard Parker. 2005. "A Critical Analysis of the Brazilian Response to HIV/AIDS: Lessons Learned for Controlling and Mitigating the Epidemic in Developing Countries." *American Journal of Public Health* 95, no. 7 (July): 1162–72. https://doi.org/10.2105/AJPH.2004.054593.

Boobalan, J., T. R. Dinesha, S. Gomathi, E. Elakkiya, A. Pradeep, D. Chitra, K. G. Murugavel, et al. 2019. "Pooled Nucleic Acid Testing Strategy for Monitoring HIV-1 Treatment in Resource Limited Settings." *Journal of Clinical Virology* 117:56–60. https://doi.org/10.1016/j.jcv.2019.05.012.

Brown, Lisanne, Tonya R. Thurman, Janet Rice, Neil W. Boris, Joseph Ntaganira, Laetitia Nyirazinyoye, Jean De Dieu, and Leslie Snider. 2009. "Impact of a Mentoring Program on Psychosocial Wellbeing of Youth in Rwanda: Results of a Quasi-Experimental Study." *Vulnerable Children and Youth Studies* 4, no. 4: 288–99. https://doi.org/10.1080/17450120903193915.

Carrasco, Maria A., Kaitlyn Atkins, Ruth Young, Joseph G. Rosen, Suzanne M. Grieb, Vincent J. Wong, and Paul J. Fleming. 2021. "The HIV Pandemic Prevention Efforts Can Inform the COVID-19 Pandemic Response in the United States." *American Journal of Public Health* 111, no. 4 (April): 564–67. https://doi.org/10.2105/ajph.2021.306158.

CBC (Canadian Broadcasting Corporation). "Could COVID Technology Offer New Hope in the Fight against HIV." 2021. *The National,* CBC Television, June 16, 2021. http://www.proquest.com/docview/2541671974/citation/55C7B6A345D04C72PQ/1.

Chou, Roger, Tracy Dana, Sara Grusing, and Christina Bougatsos. 2019. "Screening for HIV Infection in Asymptomatic, Nonpregnant Adolescents and Adults: Updated Evidence Report and Systematic Review for the US Preventive Services Task Force." *JAMA* 321, no. 23: 2337–48. https://doi.org/10.1001/jama.2019 .2592.

Cooper, T. J., B. L. Woodward, S. Alom, and A. Harky. 2020. "Coronavirus Disease 2019 (COVID-19) Outcomes in HIV/AIDS Patients: A Systematic Review." *HIV Medicine* 21, no. 9 (October): 567–77. https://doi.org/10.1111/hiv.12911.

Cordie, A., M. AbdAllah, A. Vergori, B. Kharono, M. Karkouri, and G. Esmat. 2021. "Human Immunodeficiency Virus (HIV) and Coronavirus Disease 2019: Impact on Vulnerable Populations and Harnessing Lessons Learned from HIV Programmes." *New Microbes and New Infections* 41:100857. https://doi.org /10.1016/j.nmni.2021.100857.

Davtyan, Mariam, Brandon Brown, and Morenike Oluwatoyin Folayan. 2014. "Addressing Ebola-Related Stigma: Lessons Learned from HIV/AIDS." *Global Health Action* 7, no. 1: 26058. https://doi.org/10.3402/gha.v7.26058.

Dean, Natalie. 2021. "Statistical Successes and Failures during the COVID-19 Pandemic: Comments on Ellenberg and Morris." *Statistics in Medicine* 40, no. 11: 2515–17. https://doi.org/10.1002/sim.8934.

Dehne, Karl L., Gina Dallabetta, David Wilson, Geoff P. Garnett, Marie Laga, Elizabeth Benomar, Ade Fakoya, Rachel C. Baggaley, Lisa J. Nelson, and Susan Kasedde. 2016. "HIV Prevention 2020: A Framework for Delivery and a Call for Action." *Lancet HIV* 3, no. 7 (July): e323–32. https://doi.org/10.1016/s2352 -3018(16)30035-2.

Drain, Paul K. 2015. "Ebola: Lessons Learned from HIV and Tuberculosis Epidemics." *Lancet Infectious Diseases* 15, no. 2 (February): 146–47. https://doi.org /10.1016/S1473-3099(14)71079-5.

Eisinger, Robert W., Andrea M. Lerner, and Anthony S. Fauci. 2021. "Human Immunodeficiency Virus/AIDS in the Era of Coronavirus Disease 2019: A Juxtaposition of 2 Pandemics." *Journal of Infectious Diseases* 224, no. 9 (November): 1455–61. https://doi.org/10.1093/infdis/jiab114.

Ellenberg, Susan S., and Jeffrey S. Morris. 2021. "AIDS and COVID: A Tale of Two Pandemics and the Role of Statisticians." *Statistics in Medicine* 40, no. 11: 2499–510. https://doi.org/10.1002/sim.8936.

El-Sadr, Wafaa M., and Jessica Justman. 2020. "Africa in the Path of Covid-19." *New England Journal of Medicine* 383, no. 3: e11. https://doi.org/10.1056 /NEJMp2008193.

Esu-Williams, E., K. D. Schenk, S. Geibel, J. Motsepe, A. Zulu, P. Bweupe, and E. Weiss. 2006. "'We Are No Longer Called Club Members but Caregivers': Involving Youth in HIV and AIDS Caregiving in Rural Zambia." *AIDS Care* 18, no. 8 (November): 888–94. https://doi.org/10.1080/09540120500308170.

Farquharson, Wilfred H., and Carmen J. Thornton. 2020. "Debate: Exposing the Most Serious Infirmity—Racism's Impact on Health in the Era of COVID-19." *Child and Adolescent Mental Health* 25, no. 3 (September): 182–83. https://doi .org/10.1111/camh.12407.

Fassin, Didier. 2013. "A Case for Critical Ethnography: Rethinking the Early Years of the AIDS Epidemic in South Africa." *Social Science & Medicine* 99:119–26. https://doi.org/10.1016/j.socscimed.2013.04.034.

Fauci, Anthony S. 2021. "The Story behind COVID-19 Vaccines." *Science* 372, no. 6538: 109. https://doi.org/10.1126/science.abi8397.

Gandhi, Monica, Deborah S. Yokoe, and Diane V. Havlir. 2020. "Asymptomatic Transmission, the Achilles' Heel of Current Strategies to Control Covid-19." *New England Journal of Medicine* 382, no. 22: 2158–60. https://doi.org/10.1056/NEJMe2009758.

Gerada, Clare. 2021. "Tackling Intersectionality Must Be Our Post-Covid Legacy." *BMJ* 372:n766. https://doi.org/10.1136/bmj.n766.

Guan, Wei-jie, Zheng-yi Ni, Yu Hu, Wen-hua Liang, Chun-quan Ou, Jian-xing He, Lei Liu, et al. 2020. "Clinical Characteristics of Coronavirus Disease 2019 in China." *New England Journal of Medicine* 382, no. 18: 1708–20. https://doi.org/10.1056/NEJMoa2002032.

Guilamo-Ramos, Vincent, Marco Thimm-Kaiser, Adam Benzekri, Andrew Hidalgo, Yzette Lanier, Sheila Tlou, María de Lourdes Rosas López, Asha B. Soletti, and Holly Hagan. 2021. "Nurses at the Frontline of Public Health Emergency Preparedness and Response: Lessons Learned from the HIV/AIDS Pandemic and Emerging Infectious Disease Outbreaks." *Lancet Infectious Diseases* 21, no. 10 (October): e326–33. https://doi.org/10.1016/S1473-3099(20)30983-X.

Hahn, Beatrice H., George M. Shaw, Kevin M. De Cock, and Paul M. Sharp. 2000. "AIDS as a Zoonosis: Scientific and Public Health Implications." *Science* 287, no. 5453: 607–14. https://doi.org/10.1126/science.287.5453.607.

Halperin, Daniel T. 2020. "Coping With COVID-19: Learning From Past Pandemics to Avoid Pitfalls and Panic." *Global Health: Science and Practice* 8, no. 2: 155–65. https://doi.org/10.9745/GHSP-D-20-00189.

Hargreaves, James, Calum Davey, Judith Auerbach, Jamie Blanchard, Virginia Bond, Chris Bonell, Rochelle Burgess, Joanna Busza, Tim Colbourn, and Frances Cowan. 2020. "Three Lessons for the COVID-19 Response from Pandemic HIV." *Lancet HIV* 7, no. 5 (May): e309–11. https://doi.org/10.1016/S2352-3018(20)30110-7.

Haseltine, William A. 2020. "Lessons from AIDS for the COVID-19 Pandemic." *Scientific American,* October 1, 2020. https://doi.org/10.1038/scientificamerican1020-35.

He, Xi, Eric H. Y. Lau, Peng Wu, Xilong Deng, Jian Wang, Xinxin Hao, Yiu Chung Lau, et al. 2020. "Temporal Dynamics in Viral Shedding and Transmissibility of COVID-19." *Nature Medicine* 26:672–75. https://doi.org/10.1038/s41591-020-0869-5.

HealthGap Global Access Project. 2020. "Uganda's COVID-19 Response Is Terrorizing Women with Arbitrary Detention, Blackmail, and Violence." HealthGap Global Access Project, April 30, 2020. https://healthgap.org/press/ugandas-covid19-response-is-terrorizing-women-with-arbitrary-detention-blackmail-and-violence/.

Hillis, Susan D., Alexandra Blenkinsop, Andrés Villaveces, Francis B. Annor, Leandris Liburd, Greta M. Massetti, Zewditu Demissie, et al. 2021. "COVID-19-Associated Orphanhood and Caregiver Death in the United States." *Pediatrics* 148, no. 6: e2021053760. https://doi.org/10.1542/peds.2021-053760.

Ibitoye, Mobolaji, Timothy Frasca, Rebecca Giguere, and Alex Carballo-Diéguez. 2014. "Home Testing Past, Present and Future: Lessons Learned and Implications for HIV Home Tests." *AIDS and Behavior* 18:933–49. https://doi.org/10.1007/s10461-013-0668-9.

International Committee of the Red Cross. 2020. "Nigeria: Sharp Increase in Food Prices Caused by COVID-19 Raises Fear of Hunger." International Committee of the Red Cross, October 16, 2020. https://www.icrc.org/en/document/nigeria-sharp-increase-food-prices-caused-covid-19-raises-fear-hunger.

Iversen, Jenny, Keith Sabin, Judy Chang, Ruth Morgan Thomas, Garrett Prestage, Steffanie A. Strathdee, and Lisa Maher. 2020. "COVID-19, HIV and Key Populations: Cross-Cutting Issues and the Need for Population-Specific Responses." *Journal of the International AIDS Society* 23, no. 10 (October): e25632. https://doi.org/10.1002/jia2.25632.

Jürgens, Ralf, Jonathan Cohen, Edwin Cameron, Scott Burris, Michaela Clayton, Richard Elliott, Richard Pearshouse, Anne Gathumbi, and Delme Cupido. 2009. "Ten Reasons to Oppose the Criminalization of HIV Exposure or Transmission." *Reproductive Health Matters* 17, no. 34 (November): 163–72. https://doi.org/10.1016/S0968-8080(09)34462-6.

Kalbarczyk, Anna, Wendy Davis, Sam Kalibala, Scott Geibel, Aisha Yansaneh, Nina A. Martin, Ellen Weiss, Deanna Kerrigan, and Yukari C. Manabe. 2019. "Research Capacity Strengthening in Sub-Saharan Africa: Recognizing the Importance of Local Partnerships in Designing and Disseminating HIV Implementation Science to Reach the 90-90-90 Goals." *AIDS and Behavior* 23, no. S2: 206–13. https://doi.org/10.1007/s10461-019-02538-0.

Keou, F. X., L. Bélec, P. M. Esunge, N. Cancre, and G. Gresenguet. 1992. "World Health Organization Clinical Case Definition for AIDS in Africa: An Analysis of Evaluations." *East African Medical Journal* 69, no. 10 (October): 550–53.

Kidman, Rachel. 2021. "Use HIV's Lessons to Help Children Orphaned by COVID-19." *Nature* 596, no. 7871 (August): 185–88. https://doi.org/10.1038/d41586-021-02155-9.

Kim, Young Soo. 2015. "World Health Organization and Early Global Response to HIV/AIDS: Emergence and Development of International Norms." *Journal of International and Area Studies* 22, no. 1 (June): 19–40.

Knight, Lindsay. 2008. *UNAIDS: The First Ten Years, 1996–2006*. Geneva, Switzerland: UNAIDS.

Kutscher, Eric, and Richard E. Greene. 2020. "A Harm-Reduction Approach to Coronavirus Disease 2019 (COVID-19)—Safer Socializing." *JAMA Health Forum* 1, no. 6: e200656. https://doi.org/10.1001/jamahealthforum.2020.0656.

Larson, Heidi J. 2020. *Stuck: How Vaccine Rumors Start—and Why They Don't Go Away*. New York: Oxford University Press.

Lerner, Andrea M., Robert W. Eisinger, and Anthony S. Fauci. 2020. "Comorbidities in Persons with HIV: The Lingering Challenge." *JAMA* 323, no. 1: 19–20. https://doi.org/10.1001/jama.2019.19775.

Lin, Feng, Paul G. Farnham, Ram K. Shrestha, Jonathan Mermin, and Stephanie L. Sansom. 2016. "Cost Effectiveness of HIV Prevention Interventions in the U.S." *American Journal of Preventive Medicine* 50, no. 6: 699–708. https://doi.org/10.1016/j.amepre.2016.01.011.

Logie, Carmen H. 2020. "Lessons Learned from HIV Can Inform Our Approach to COVID-19 Stigma." *Journal of the International AIDS Society* 23, no. 5 (May): e25504. https://doi.org/10.1002/jia2.25504.

Lyss, Sheryl B., Kate Buchacz, R. Paul McClung, Alice Asher, and Alexandra M. Oster. 2020. "Responding to Outbreaks of Human Immunodeficiency Virus among Persons Who Inject Drugs—United States, 2016–2019: Perspectives on Recent Experience and Lessons Learned." *Journal of Infectious Diseases* 222, no. S5: S239–49. https://doi.org/10.1093/infdis/jiaa112.

Macinnis, R. 1997. "Mandela Calls for Greater Commitment and Leadership in Fighting AIDS: The World Economic Forum—Policy and Business in a World of HIV/AIDS." *AIDSlink: Eastern, Central & Southern Africa* 43:1–3.

Mackay, Ian M. 2020. "The Swiss Cheese Infographic That Went Viral." *Virology Down Under,* December 26, 2020. https://virologydownunder.com/the-swiss-cheese-infographic-that-went-viral/.

Maharana, Adyasha, Morine Amutorine, Moinina David Sengeh, and Elaine O. Nsoesie. 2020. "Use of Technology and Innovations in the COVID-19 Pandemic Response in Africa." *ArXiv Preprint* 2012.07741. https://doi.org/10.48550/arXiv.2012.07741.

Mann, J. M. 1987. "The World Health Organization's Global Strategy for the Prevention and Control of AIDS." *Western Journal of Medicine* 147, no. 6 (December): 732–34.

Mateo-Urdiales, Alberto, Samuel Johnson, Rhodine Smith, Jean B. Nachega, and Ingrid Eshun-Wilson. 2019. "Rapid Initiation of Antiretroviral Therapy for People Living with HIV." *Cochrane Database of Systematic Reviews* 6, no. 6: CD012962. https://doi.org/10.1002/14651858.CD012962.pub2.

Millett, Gregorio A. 2020. "New Pathogen, Same Disparities: Why COVID-19 and HIV Remain Prevalent in U.S. Communities of Colour and Implications for Ending the HIV Epidemic." *Journal of the International AIDS Society* 23, no. 11: e25639. https://doi.org/10.1002/jia2.25639.

Moynihan, Donald, and Gregory Porumbescu. 2020. "Trump's 'Chinese Virus' Slur Makes Some People Blame Chinese Americans. But Others Blame Trump." *Washington Post,* September 16, 2020. https://www.washingtonpost.com/politics/2020/09/16/trumps-chinese-virus-slur-makes-some-people-blame-chinese-americans-others-blame-trump/.

National Public Radio. 2018. "Long before Facebook, The KGB Spread Fake News about AIDS." *National Public Radio,* August 22, 2018. https://www.npr.org/2018/08/22/640883503/long-before-facebook-the-kgb-spread-fake-news-about-aids.

Nyblade, Laura, Rebecca J. Mbuya-Brown, Mangi J. Ezekiel, Nii A. Addo, Amon N. Sabasaba, Kyeremeh Atuahene, Pfiraeli Kiwia, et al. 2020. "A Total Facility Approach to Reducing HIV Stigma in Health Facilities: Implementation Process and Lessons Learned." *AIDS (London)* 34, no. S1: S93–102. https://doi.org /10.1097/QAD.0000000000002585.

Oduor, Michael. 2021. "President Magufuli Warns Tanzanians against Covid-19 Vaccines." *Africanews,* January 27, 2021. https://www.africanews.com/2021/01 /27/president-magufuli-warns-tanzanians-against-covid-19-vaccines/.

Olufadewa, Isaac Iyinoluwa, Miracle Ayomikun Adesina, and Toluwase Ayorinde. 2020. "From Africa to the World: Reimagining Africa's Research Capacity and Culture in the Global Knowledge Economy." *Journal of Global Health* 10, no. 1 (June): 010321. https://doi.org/10.7189/jogh.10.010321.

Olufadewa, Isaac Iyinoluwa, Ifeoluwa Oduguwa, Miracle Adesina, Koton Ibiang, Nnenne Eke, Blessing Adewumi, Inimfon Ebong, Funmilayo Abudu, and Nancy Adeyelu. 2021. "COVID-19: Learning from the HIV/AIDS Pandemic Response in Africa." *International Journal of Health Planning and Management* 36, no. 3 (May): 610–17. https://doi.org/10.1002/hpm.3133.

Park, Mirae, Ryan S. Thwaites, and Peter J. M. Openshaw. 2020. "COVID-19: Lessons from SARS and MERS." *European Journal of Immunology* 50, no. 3: 308–11. https://doi.org/10.1002/eji.202070035.

Parmet, Wendy E., and Jeremy Paul. 2020. "COVID-19: The First Posttruth Pandemic." *American Journal of Public Health* 110, no. 7 (July): 945–46. https://doi .org/10.2105/AJPH.2020.305721.

Pastakia, Sonak D., Dan N. Tran, Imran Manji, Cassia Wells, Kyle Kinderknecht, and Robert Ferris. 2018. "Building Reliable Supply Chains for Noncommunicable Disease Commodities: Lessons Learned from HIV and Evidence Needs." *AIDS (London)* 32, no. S1: S55–61. https://doi.org/10.1097/QAD .0000000000001878.

Piot, Peter, Richard G. A. Feachem, Jong-Wook Lee, and James D. Wolfensohn. 2004. "A Global Response to AIDS: Lessons Learned, Next Steps." *Science* 304, no. 5679: 1909–10. https://doi.org/10.1126/science.1101137.

Piot, Peter, Michel Kazatchkine, Mark Dybul, and Julian Lob-Levyt. 2009. "AIDS: Lessons Learnt and Myths Dispelled." *Lancet* 374, no. 9685: 260–63. https://doi .org/10.1016/S0140-6736(09)60321-4.

Population Council. 2020. *Social, Health, Education and Economic Effects of COVID-19 on Adolescent Girls in Kenya: Results from Adolescent Surveys in Kilifi, Nairobi, Wajir, and Kisumu.* COVID-19 Research and Evaluations Brief. Nairobi: Population Council.

Pulerwitz, Julie, Annie Michaelis, Ellen Weiss, Lisanne Brown, and Vaishali Mahendra. 2010. "Reducing HIV-Related Stigma: Lessons Learned from Horizons Research and Programs." *Public Health Reports* 125, no. 2 (March–April): 272–81. https://doi.org/10.1177/003335491012500218.

Reagan, Ronald. 1985. "The President's News Conference." Ronald Reagan Presidential Library and Museum, September 17, 1985. https://www.reaganlibrary .gov/archives/speech/presidents-news-conference-16.

Reason, James T. 1990. *Human Error*. Cambridge: Cambridge University Press.

Rebeiro, Peter F., Stephany N. Duda, Kara K. Wools-Kaloustian, Denis Nash, and Keri N. Althoff. 2020. "Implications of COVID-19 for HIV Research: Data Sources, Indicators and Longitudinal Analyses." *Journal of the International AIDS Society* 23, no. 10: e25627. https://doi.org/10.1002/jia2.25627.

Reed, Jason B., Rupa R. Patel, and Rachel Baggaley. 2018. "Lessons from a Decade of Voluntary Medical Male Circumcision Implementation and Their Application to HIV Pre-exposure Prophylaxis Scale Up." *International Journal of STD & AIDS* 29, no. 14 (December): 1432–43. https://doi.org/10.1177/0956462418787896.

Roberts, Siobhan. 2020. "The Swiss Cheese Model of Pandemic Defense." *New York Times,* December 5, 2020. https://www.nytimes.com/2020/12/05/health/coronavirus-swiss-cheese-infection-mackay.html.

Sarwer, Abdullah, Bilal Javed, Erik B. Soto, and Zia-ur-Rehman Mashwani. 2020. "Impact of the COVID-19 Pandemic on Maternal Health Services in Pakistan." *International Journal of Health Planning and Management* 35, no. 6 (November): 1306–10. https://doi.org/10.1002/hpm.3048.

Saul, Janet, Gretchen Bachman, Shannon Allen, Nora F. Toiv, Caroline Cooney, and Ta'Adhmeeka Beamon. 2018. "The DREAMS Core Package of Interventions: A Comprehensive Approach to Preventing HIV among Adolescent Girls and Young Women." *PLOS ONE* 13, no. 12: e0208167. https://doi.org/10.1371/journal.pone.0208167.

Schenk, Katie D. 2009. "Community Interventions Providing Care and Support to Orphans and Vulnerable Children: A Review of Evaluation Evidence." *AIDS Care* 21, no. 7 (July): 918–42. https://doi.org/10.1080/09540120802537831.

———. 2021. "Biden's COVID Plan Is Just a Beginning." *Scientific American,* February 25, 2021. https://www.scientificamerican.com/article/bidens-covid-plan-is-just-a-beginning/.

Schenk, Katie D., Annie Michaelis, Tobey Nelson Sapiano, Lisanne Brown, and Ellen Weiss. 2010. "Improving the Lives of Vulnerable Children: Implications of Horizons Research among Orphans and Other Children Affected by AIDS." *Public Health Reports* 125, no. 2 (March–April): 325–36. https://doi.org/10.1177/003335491012500223.

Schenk, Katie D., and Elizabeth A. Stuart. 2021. "Don't Let Children under 12 Slip through the Cracks in the Fight against Covid." *STAT,* August 10, 2021. https://www.statnews.com/2021/08/10/dont-let-children-under-12-slip-through-the-cracks-in-the-fight-against-covid/.

Schenk, Katie D., Waimar Tun, Meredith Sheehy, Jerry Okal, Emmanuel Kuffour, Grimond Moono, Felix Mutale, et al. 2018. "'Even the Fowl Has Feelings': Access to HIV Information and Services among Persons with Disabilities in Ghana, Uganda, and Zambia." *Disability and Rehabilitation* 42, no. 3 (February): 335–48. https://doi.org/10.1080/09638288.2018.1498138.

Sherlock, Christopher H., Steffanie A. Strathdee, Tom Le, Don Sutherland, Michael V. O'Shaughnessy, and Martin T. Schechter. 1995. "Use of Pooling and Outpatient Laboratory Specimens in an Anonymous Seroprevalence Survey of HIV Infection in British Columbia, Canada." *AIDS (London)* 9, no. 8 (August): 945–50. https://doi.org/10.1097/00002030-199508000-00017.

Slotten, Ross A. 2020. *Plague Years: A Doctor's Journey through the AIDS Crisis.* Chicago: University of Chicago Press.

Stankevitz, Kayla, Katie Schwartz, Theresa Hoke, Yixuan Li, Michele Lanham, Imelda Mahaka, and Saiqa Mullick. 2019. "Reaching At-Risk Women for PrEP Delivery: What Can We Learn from Clinical Trials in Sub-Saharan Africa?" *PLOS ONE* 14, no. 6: e0218556. https://doi.org/10.1371/journal.pone.0218556.

Stegling, Christine. 2020. "Opinion: We Must Not Let Covid Undo a Decade of Progress in HIV Prevention." *Independent,* December 1, 2020. https://www.independent.co.uk/voices/coronavirus-hiv-world-aids-day-b1764388.html.

Strathdee, Steffanie A., Natasha K. Martin, Eileen V. Pitpitan, Jamila K. Stockman, and Davey M. Smith. 2021. "What the HIV Pandemic Experience Can Teach the United States about the COVID-19 Response." *Journal of Acquired Immune Deficiency Syndrome* 86, no. 1: 1–10. https://doi.org/10.1097/QAI.0000000000002520.

STRIVE Research Consortium. 2019. *Addressing the Structural Drivers of HIV: A STRIVE Synthesis.* London: London School of Hygiene & Tropical Medicine.

UNAIDS. 2014. *The Gap Report.* Geneva, Switzerland: UNAIDS. https://www.unaids.org/en/resources/campaigns/2014/2014gapreport/gapreport.

———. 2020. "Modelling the Extreme—COVID-19 and AIDS-Related Deaths." *UNAIDS,* May 25. https://www.unaids.org/en/resources/presscentre/featurestories/2020/may/20200525_modelling-the-extreme.

Uwimana, J., C. Zarowsky, H. Hausler, and D. Jackson. 2012. "Training Community Care Workers to Provide Comprehensive TB/HIV/PMTCT Integrated Care in KwaZulu-Natal: Lessons Learnt." *Tropical Medicine & International Health* 17, no. 4 (April): 488–96. https://doi.org/10.1111/j.1365-3156.2011.02951.x.

Venter, Francois. 2020. "How the Covid Fight Has Crippled Efforts to Fight HIV and TB." *Daily Maverick,* September 29, 2020. http://www.proquest.com/docview/2447098315/citation/A66AAC98237B488DPQ/1.

Vrazo, Alexandra C., Rachel Golin, Nimasha B. Fernando, Wm P. Killam, Sheena Sharifi, B. Ryan Phelps, Megan M. Gleason, et al. 2020. "Adapting HIV Services for Pregnant and Breastfeeding Women, Infants, Children, Adolescents and Families in Resource-Constrained Settings during the COVID-19 Pandemic." *Journal of the International AIDS Society* 23, no. 9 (September): e25622. https://doi.org/10.1002/jia2.25622.

WHO (World Health Organization). 2005. "Interim WHO Clinical Staging of HIV/AIDS and HIV/AIDS Case Definitions for Surveillance: African Region." Report WHO/HIV/2005.02. Geneva, Switzerland: World Health Organization. https://apps.who.int/iris/handle/10665/69058/WHO_HIV_2005.02.pdf.

———. 2016. *Global Diffusion of eHealth: Making Universal Health Coverage Achievable: Report of the Third Global Survey on eHealth.* Geneva, Switzerland: World Health Organization.

———. 2020a. "COVAX." World Health Organization. https://www.who.int/initiatives/act-accelerator/covax.

————. 2020b. *Report of the WHO-China Joint Mission on Coronavirus Disease 2019 (COVID-19)*. Geneva, Switzerland: World Health Organization. https://www.who.int/publications/i/item/report-of-the-who-china-joint-mission-on-coronavirus-disease-2019-(covid-19).

Wondergem, Peter, Kimberly Green, Samuel Wambugu, Comfort Asamoah-Adu, Nana Fosua Clement, Richard Amenyah, Kyeremeh Atuahene, and Michael Szpir. 2015. "A Short History of HIV Prevention Programs for Female Sex Workers in Ghana: Lessons Learned over 3 Decades." *Journal of Acquired Immune Deficiency Syndrome* 68, no. S2: S138–45. https://doi.org/10.1097/QAI.0000000000000446.

Part 5

POLICY AND POLITICS

10

Policy and Politics of COVID-19 Response Mask Mandates

*The Conflict between Individual Autonomy and Public Health Mandates
in the United States*

ADAEZE AROH, RAFEEK A. YUSUF, UGONWA AROH, AND ZENAB I. YUSUF

Public health law, according to Lawrence Gostin, is "the study of the legal powers and duties of the state to ensure the conditions for people to be healthy . . . , and the limitations on the power of the state to constrain the autonomy, privacy, liberty, proprietary, or other legally protected interests of individuals for protection or promotion of community health." (Gostin 2000b). Gostin also specifies that the word *public* in "public health law" refers primarily to the democratically elected entity—the government (which can decide to partner with the private sector), legitimized by the political process to act in the interest of the citizens—exercising powers and duties meant for the protection, promotion, and preservation of the health of the citizens (Gostin 2000b; Bowser and Gostin 1998; Tobey 1927). In other words, public health laws at the federal, state, and local government levels, including statutes, regulations, ordinances, and mandates, provide governments at these different levels with powers and duties to safeguard the health of the population. These safeguards include ensuring injury and disease prevention and health promotion (Gostin 2000b; Parmet 1993). Public health laws at the population level make healthier choices easier to adopt by attempting to change behavior and providing regulatory oversight, ultimately resulting in healthier and safer lives (Silverman 2005; Christoffel and Gallagher 2006; Parmet 2009; Wing et al. 2007). Examples of public health laws to prevent injury and disease and promote population health include seatbelt (Giubilini and Savulescu 2019) and helmet laws, increased taxation on tobacco products (Wilson and Thomson 2005) and beverages sweetened with sugar (Allcott, Lockwood, and Taubinsky 2019), regulations requiring safer product designs and labeling, built-environment codes preventing injury and disease while promoting physical activities, regulations on environmental emissions, restrictions on advertising of hazardous products, and awareness campaigns to encourage healthy behaviors and discourage risky behaviors. Members of the communities whose well-being the government is required to protect, promote, and preserve are expected to subordinate themselves to the powers and duties of the government (Walzer 2008; Beauchamp 1988). As such, these individuals acknowledge that achieving public health and safety requires collective actions rather than individual pursuits.

Individual autonomy, on the other hand, is the right of individuals to liberty, self-determination, privacy, and property rights (Gostin 2000b). Individual autonomy as it relates to health and healthcare is predicated on the notion that individuals will take necessary and sufficient steps to safeguard their personal well-being (Gostin 2000b; Walzer 2008; Oliver 2006; Buchanan 2008; Beauchamp 1988; Coggon and Miola 2011). Importantly, even when exercising their autonomy, individuals cannot guarantee the protection, promotion, and preservation of the health of the communities in which they reside and the larger society (Entwistle et al. 2010; Gostin 2007a).

Overall, ensuring communal participation through public health laws and not individual self-determination will guarantee common goods such as prevention and control of infectious diseases, healthy nutrition and potable drinking water, clean air and reduced emissions, unpolluted surface waters, safe natural and built environments, environmental protection and sanitation, and others (Gostin 2000b).

In this chapter, we review the policy and politics of mask mandates in the United States' response to the COVID-19 pandemic. In addition, we explore how these mandates specifically highlight the conflict between individual autonomy and public health mandates. Furthermore, we provide theoretically grounded recommendations on how existing mask mandates can be improved and/or new mask mandates enacted to align with prevailing politics. This alignment between policy and politics is necessary in order to ensure that due consideration is given to both individual autonomy and public health mandates in the context of COVID-19 response.

It is our hope that this review and associated recommendations will stimulate constructive and prolific discussions aimed at reducing the conflict between individual autonomy and public health mandates related to current and future pandemics.

BACKGROUND

Coronavirus disease 2019 (COVID-19), caused by the severe acute respiratory syndrome–related coronavirus (SARS-CoV-2), initially affected humans in the city of Wuhan in China's Hubei Province in late December 2019. Thereafter, it spread rapidly worldwide, was declared a public health emergency of international concern on January 30, 2020, and subsequently gained official pandemic status on February 11, 2020 (WHO 2020).

As of the time of this review, there were 250,131,482 cases and 5,057,989 deaths worldwide attributed to COVID-19. In the United States, there were 47,287,033 cases and 774,726 deaths (Worldometer 2021). The first case of COVID-19 in the United States presented at a healthcare facility in Washington State on January 19, 2020, and was confirmed by real-time reverse-transcriptase–polymerase-chain-reaction (rRT-PCR) assay on January 20, 2020 (Holshue et al. 2020).

In the United States, public wearing of face masks to mitigate transmission of SARS-CoV-2 was first recommended on April 3, 2020, by the Centers for Disease Control and Prevention (CDC 2021d). New Jersey was the first state to enact and implement a statewide mask mandate on April 10, 2020 (Ballotpedia 2021). As of July 2020, thirty-one out of fifty states had orders mandating the wearing of facial coverings. These mandates ranged from directives to the general public to specific directives to businesses (covering employers, employees, or both), with some exemptions for individuals with medical conditions or disabilities that make wearing facial coverings more challenging (Gostin, Cohen, and Koplan 2020).

SCOPE OF THE PROBLEM

One of the most effective tools to mitigate the spread of COVID-19 is wearing face masks. Research has established the efficacy of face masks in decreasing respiratory transmission of SARS-CoV-2 within twenty days of local implementation of mask mandates (Guy et al. 2021; Fischer et al. 2020; Peeples 2020). Despite evidence in support of face masks, conflicts exist between individual autonomy and mandating of face masks in the interest of public health (Gostin, Cohen, and Koplan 2020; An et al. 2021). These conflicts arise because individuals perceive such public health mandates as usurping their individual rights and freedom of choice (WHO 2020; Network for Public Health Law 2021).

Over a year and half into the COVID-19 pandemic, with vaccination rates plateauing in the United States and other parts of the world and despite evidence supporting the efficacy of mask mandates, public health officials were still struggling to get many individuals to wear facial covering in public to slow the transmission of the virus. Those refusing to wear masks were arguing that the mandate violated their First Amendment rights, was intrusive, and restricted their personal liberty. The issue was politicized to such an extent that opponents of the mandates sued various state governments for violating their individual rights and liberties (Scurlock 2020). In such a situation, public health policy-makers and even practitioners were faced with the task of reconciling the conflicts that exist between individual autonomy and mandating of face masks for the common good.

To better understand the reasoning as to why government has the power to interfere in individual autonomy, it is necessary to evaluate mask mandates using legal and policy theories and constructs that are important but not in themselves determinative.

LEGAL AND POLICY THEORIES AND CONSTRUCTS RELATED TO MASK MANDATES

Legal Appropriateness of Mask Mandates

In a public health crisis, it is often theoretically assumed that, given adequate information by regulatory bodies or public health agencies, individuals will act in a rational manner to protect themselves and the general public from harm. However, this is not always the case in reality. Through their actions and inactions, individuals and institutions produce significant negative or positive effects known as externalities (Oliver 2006). Actions such as smoking, driving while intoxicated, harmful sexual practices, and vaccine hesitancy lead to negative health outcomes (Oliver 2006) and often require governments to intervene in the form of policies, laws, mandates, and ordinances to encourage healthy behavior (Gostin 2000a). To determine and justify when it is appropriate for government to infringe on individual liberty and to what extent, a legal question to ask would be, Does a mask mandate pass the *reasonableness test* in terms of coercion? From the perspective of the good of the public as a whole, a mask mandate is reasonable because it is cost-effective and less invasive than the vaccine or total lockdown (Gee and Gupta 2020). Furthermore, from the same perspective, because many individuals are more concerned about individual autonomy or liberty than broader public health, governments (federal, state, and local) *need* to mandate the use of facial masks, as it is much more socially and politically difficult to mandate COVID-19 vaccination or outright lockdown (Gostin 2000b).

Constitutionality of Mask Mandates

In order to understand the role of government or any other public entity in protecting public health, it is important to first understand the meaning of the *public* whose health is at stake. First, the government is a public entity which by virtue of the political process has the legitimacy to act on behalf of the people. So, when there is a public health crisis, a democratically elected government is constitutionally granted the right to exercise its powers or duties to protect and promote public health (Gostin 2000b). By this analysis, state governments thus have the constitutional right and authority to institute mask mandates or other laws to reduce or stop the spread of the COVID-19 virus.

The Tenth Amendment of the US Constitution expressly reserves for state governments what are known as "police powers," which are not granted to the federal government. These police powers are meant for states to use to promote the welfare of their citizens (Gostin 2000c). The police power of the state is defined as "the inherent authority of the state (and through delegation, local governments) to enact laws and promulgate regulations to protect, preserve, and promote the health, safety, morals, and general welfare of the people. To achieve these communal benefits, the state retains the power to restrict, within federal and state constitutional limits, personal interests in liberty, autonomy, privacy, and expression, as well as economic interests in freedom of contract and uses of property" (Gostin 2000c).

The police powers of the state authorize the states to legislate, regulate, and adjudicate in manners that may necessarily interfere with, limit, or even eliminate private interests, autonomy, privacy, or liberty within moral standards in order to keep communities safe (Gostin 2000c). Given the natural history of SARS-CoV-2 and the contagious nature of COVID-19, the state is well within its rights to require its citizens to wear facial coverings to reduce the spread of the virus through respiratory transmission.

A legal precedent supporting the legitimacy and application of police powers of the state is the 1905 landmark case of *Jacobson v. Massachusetts* (1905). Interestingly, the original case arose from a mandate by the City of Cambridge, based on a Massachusetts law, ordering compulsory vaccination during an outbreak of smallpox. The Supreme Court's ultimate decision articulated the view that the freedom of the individual must sometimes be subordinated to the common welfare and is subject to the police power of the state (Colgrove and Bayer 2005).

Risk to Others

Alongside the question of the common good, also at the core of most discussions about government intervention in public health issues, there is individual autonomy: the personal governance of the self, free from controlling interferences. It is assumed that an autonomous person is free to hold views and to make choices based on personal values. Advocates for the primacy of individual autonomy argue that neither government nor others should restrain competent adults in the absence of adequate justification (Gostin, Cohen, and Koplan 2020). Yet the natural history of the COVID-19 virus and the mode and the speed of its transmission pose serious harm to the public. This provides adequate justification for constraining individual autonomy. Referencing John Stuart Mill, one of the most important foundational thinkers in the development of our conception of modern democracy, Gostin argues that "persons should be free to think, speak, and behave as they wish, provided they do not interfere with a like expression of freedom by others" (Gostin 2008). That is, an individual's personal freedom stops at their intrusion on the health, safety, and other legitimate interests of others, including the general population. In the case of COVID-19, the need to respect individual autonomy is superseded by the need to protect the general population from the risks of contracting the virus (Gostin 2000d).

Magnitude of the Problem and Probability of Risk

COVID-19 imposed substantial negative impacts on economic, social, and environmental resources in the United States and globally (Kontis et al. 2020). We have already noted staggering statistics on cases and deaths in the United States and globally at the time of this writing. The International Monetary Fund, in its *World Economic Outlook* report of April 2021, estimated that the global economy had contracted by 3.5% due to the COVID-19 pandemic. As for resources, governmental expenditures triggered by the response to the pandemic were estimated at approximately $16 trillion, equivalent to roughly 15% of global gross domestic product (GDP) (Yeyati and Filippini 2021). In the United States, there are various ways to determine the viability of the economy, such as the ratio of employment to population, unemployment rate, percent of the population making unemployment insurance claims, consumer spending, and small business employment (Udalova 2021). When using the employment-to-population ratio, the economy is said to be on the decline if employment loss exceeds predictions based on the historical trend. During the early pandemic months, specifically in April 2020, the actual employment-to-population ratio was 51.5%, while the predicted employment-to-population ratio was 61.3%, showing a significant 9.8% shortfall in employment due to the pandemic (Amara et al. 2021). The Bureau of Economic Analysis estimated that the US GDP fell by $1.73 trillion, at an annualized rate of 31.7%, from the first quarter of 2020 to the second quarter of 2020. This negative impact was attributed primarily to a $1.35 trillion reduction in consumer spending during the peak of the pandemic (Wang et al. 2020; Chetty et al. 2020). The consumer spending makes up the largest part of the US GDP (Chetty et al. 2020). Seventy-four percent of small businesses were also not spared by the pandemic as they reported experiencing losses in revenues during the peak of the pandemic from April to May of 2020 (Wang et al. 2020). Given these negative socioeconomic impacts, it was logical for the government to want to protect and promote public health through mask mandates and other policies so as to bring the pandemic under control for return to economic and fiscal growth as soon as possible.

Paternalism

Paternalism in public health is defined as "interference with a person's liberty of action justified by the reason referring exclusively to the welfare of the person being coerced" or the common good (Buchanan 2008; Dworkin 1988). The major issue is deciding the extent to which government can interfere with an individual's autonomy to modify behaviors that affect or improve health outcomes. Childress (2020) defined the conditions that justify ethical interference in an individual's autonomy as (a) effectiveness, (b) proportionality, (c) necessity, (d) least infringement, and (e) public justification. Mask mandates meet the effectiveness, necessity, least infringement, and public justification criteria to warrant overriding individual autonomy. Paternalism is also based on the assumption that individuals are inadequately informed about their needs. To this end, mask mandates are reasonable based on the probable benefits or trade-offs between individual *autonomy and avoidance of harm* (Gostin 2007b, 2008). They can also be likened to seat belt and motorbike helmet laws, which are viewed as paternalistic. Individuals perceive these laws to be controlling given that the consequences of not using seat belts or not wearing helmets are self-imposed harms. Contrarily, these individual inactions are "deeply socially embedded and pervasively harmful to the public" (Gostin 2007b). Similarly, an individual who is infected with SARS-CoV-2 and asymptomatic (without symptoms) is still highly infectious and capable of spreading the disease to healthy individuals. It is the right of an individual not to wear a face mask, but it is also a moral responsibility not to expose others to the risk of contracting the virus. Therefore, mask mandates actually balance the common good with individual civil liberties. In the landmark US Supreme Court case of *Jacobson v. Massachusetts,* Justice Harlan found that "the whole people covenant with each citizen, and each citizen with the whole people, . . . all shall be governed by certain laws for the common good" (Gostin et al. 2002).

Equal Protection, Fairness in Public Health, and Distribution of Cost and Benefits

The goal of government and public health practitioners when initiating public health policies is to ensure fairness. Fairness in public health and public health policy is attained when the policy strives to achieve the common good by equitably distributing benefits, burdens, and costs among citizens (Gostin 2000d).

To what extent possible are mask mandates just? Do mandates provide necessary protection to those in need and place reasonable burdens and costs on those who endanger public health? SARS-CoV-2 is very pervasive and evasive (Bourne 2021), and thus everyone is at risk of contracting the virus if there are no interventions to reduce the spread. Mask mandates provide part of the necessary protection with very minimal burden on individuals. To mitigate the effects and uncertainties of the COVID-19 virus, it is reasonable that government impose a necessary action rather than just advising a voluntary response.

A mask mandate's fairness can also be analyzed through the lens of inclusiveness. A public health policy can be *underinclusive* or *overinclusive.* It is said to be underinclusive if government provides services to only a subgroup of those in need, or if it regulates only a subgroup of those who are dangerous. It is overinclusive if it extends to more people than necessary to achieve its purposes (unnecessarily benefits or penalizes a group of people) (Gostin 2000d).

For the reasons given above, mask mandates are equitably inclusive because they do not regulate only a subgroup of people nor protect a subgroup of people. Rather, they protect a wide set of individuals at a given period. In addition, they protect individuals with illnesses that prevent them from wearing masks to protect themselves against contracting the virus. Furthermore, if the SARS-CoV-2 was contained, there would be a reduction in lives lost due to the virus, businesses would be opened, and the economy would thrive.

Another contention raised against mask mandates was that they violate individuals' constitutional right to freedom of speech and equal protection under the law for people with disabilities. This assertion is not totally true, as the mask mandate recommendation by the Centers for Disease Control and Prevention (CDC) made exceptions for people who cannot wear masks, such as those with chronic obstructive pulmonary disease (Dorfman and Raz 2020). The CDC's recommendation made provision for people with disabilities to participate in the same activities as abled persons (Kaganovich 2021). Other instances of such accommodations are requiring businesses to make reasonable modifications to their mask policies to allow people with disabilities to wear a face shield instead of a face mask and allowing online orders and curbside pickup in restaurants (CDC 2021a; Kaganovich 2021). These accommodations ensure a balance between protecting the health and safety of employees, customers, and communities and still respecting individual liberty (Kaganovich 2021).

Another strong argument was that mask mandates violate an individual's "First Amendment right to the freedom of speech" (Kaganovich 2021). This argument was refuted by the United States District Court for the District of Maryland in *KOA v. Hogan* (2020). The plaintiffs alleged that wearing a mask was akin to a "sign of capture on the battlefield, and subservience to the captor," and was, as a result, compelled speech (Kaganovich 2021). However, the court rejected the claim that "the action of wearing a mask contained a subtextual message and explained that, in the face of the most severe health crisis in generations, wearing a face covering would be viewed as a means of preventing the spread of COVID-19, not as expressing any message" (Kaganovich 2021). Wearing a mask is neither an action that the government unduly compels, nor does it express a government-sanctioned message (Kaganovich 2021).

In the conflict between respecting individual autonomy and taking action in the face of a devastating public health emergency such as the COVID-19 pandemic, the states have found it necessary to exercise their police powers. According to the Arizona Supreme Court in 1909, "Necessity is the law of time and place, and the emergency calls into life the necessity . . . to exercise the power to protect the public health" (Dann, Lewis, and Dunseath 1909). Furthermore, when duly politically elected and accountable officials "undertake to act in areas fraught with medical and scientific uncertainties," their scope of action "must be especially broad." Where those broad limits are not exceeded, they should not be subject to second-guessing by an "unelected federal judiciary" which lacks the background, competence, and expertise to assess public health and is not accountable to the people (Price and Diaz 2020).

KINGDON'S THREE-STREAM FRAMEWORK AND RECOMMENDATIONS

Overview

Our recommendations concerning current and future mask mandates utilize John Kingdon's three-stream model, a policy framework for understanding how issues find their way into the political agenda. This framework will enable us to determine whether there is a window of opportunity for states to justify interference in individual autonomy to achieve the common good—in this case, mandating the wearing of face masks to reduce the spread of COVID-19 virus. The framework will also guide the understanding of the reasoning behind our recommendations to state policy-makers on how to strengthen existing or pass new mask mandates.

The three streams in Kingdon's model are *the problem, the politics,* and *the policy* streams. Each stream exists independently of the others, but the three must converge to form a window of opportunity before a policy can have a chance for action (Oliver 2006).

Kingdon's theoretical framework is critical when examining the politics of public health interventions. It provides an understanding of how certain issues work their way into the political agenda over others. The question here is, How did mask mandates become a politically controversial issue and how can they be leveraged in the battle against the COVID-19 virus and subsequent pandemics and/or any public health issues?

Kingdon (1984) defines the political agenda as "the list of subjects or problems which government officials, and people closely associated to those officials, are paying serious attention to at any given time." The window of opportunity is the time when a given policy option is most likely to be passed and acted upon. Policy windows rarely present themselves, and advocates must capitalize when they do, because another opportunity may not come (Atupem 2017; Kingdon 1984). During the pandemic the window closed for state governments to strengthen existing mask mandates or enact new ones. But the lessons learned from that experience can potentially provide the template for policies during future pandemics.

Problem stream: Kingdon posits that the problem stream marks the transition of an issue from a private problem to a public problem that the government should be involved in fixing. For instance, COVID-19 was initially endemic to Wuhan, China, and later became a worldwide pandemic as identified by WHO. In Kingdon's theory, a problem changes from private to public when an indicator shows a change in the state of a system; such an indicator can be the magnitude of a problem (Atupem 2017). In this current situation, the problem stream is well defined with the magnitude of the incidence, prevalence, mortality rates, and the socioeconomic burden due to COVID-19 in the United States and globally (Worldometer 2021; Kontis et al. 2020; Yeyati and Filippini 2021; Udalova 2021; Wang et al. 2020; Chetty et al. 2020). Even though these problems are well defined, individuals argue that the numbers are not compelling enough for government to interfere in their individual autonomy with a mask mandate. There is an argument that other interventions might be used instead to curb the spread of the virus, such as vaccination. Government can make a compelling argument that mask mandates are the cheapest and least invasive of all the other options, especially as there is still the issue of mid to low vaccine uptake. It is also important to stress the point that mask mandates will ensure full reopening of businesses and prevent further total lockdowns due to the spread of the virus.

Policy stream: This is the policy solution that is been proffered to potentially address the public health problem. The proof of concept of this policy solution would have been tested and established through scientific experiments (Fischer et al. 2020) and simulations before being recommended for implementation. Mask mandates are one of the strongest solutions that have been offered to curb the spread of the virus. Studies have shown that implementing mask mandates increase the percentage of people who wear masks by fifteen points and cuts the daily growth rate of confirmed cases by 0.6%–1.0% (Ruvo 2020). Mask mandates also prevent strict lockdowns, which have been shown to have negative impacts on consumer spending and national gross domestic product. The policy stream is important because for a problem to find its way onto the political agenda the idea must have viable policy alternatives.

Politics stream: The politics stream assesses the feasibility of an issue as well as the political climate surrounding it. The word *politics* refers to the art and tactics politicians use to convince members of the opposition to support their initiatives (Atupem 2017). In this case, it refers to the art and tactics they use to convince the public that it is necessary to interfere in individual autonomy for the common good by mandating the wearing of face masks. Scientific research continues to advance and improve our understanding of the natural history of SARS-CoV-2 (the virus that causes COVID-19) and COVID-19. Consequent upon this understanding is the identification and development of innovative, reliable, and validated solutions, including the wearing of face masks, to prevent transmission of SARS-CoV-2. For such a solution to have the desired meaningful outcome at the population level, it needs to become a policy legitimized by law. However, only the persistent and concerted political willingness of decision-makers and government in the face of challenges such as fiscal accountability and limitations, competing political interests, and pressure from interest groups can lead to adopting and implementing such policies. In spite of scientific proof of concept, these policies are usually implemented with caution, incrementally rather than comprehensively (Oliver 2006). This may be due in part to government awareness, particularly in the United States, that individuals—who tend to be more inclined to voluntary participation—are usually more wary of government policies and actions that attempt to control them by restricting their autonomy and freedom of expression than of policy reforms that benefit them individually (Rothman 1997; Shafer 1989, 1991; Tocqueville 1969; Hofstadter 2011; Lawrence 1996; Morone 1990). Additionally, while scientific research may provide findings that inform and provide impetus for the government to act to protect, promote, and preserve the population's health, it also provide ammunition for individuals, groups of individuals, and businesses not to subordinate to or comply with government policies or mandates perceived as controlling and usurping their individual autonomy (Weiss 1989; Stone 1997; Lindblom and Cohen 1979). To this end, science, though necessary, is usually not sufficient to cause the government to act; the perceived threat of the issues at hand to social well-being also needs to be considered and may play a more significant role in political decision-making and action by government and compliance by individuals (Oliver 2006; Kersh and Morone 2002; Nathanson 1999; Wallack et al. 1993). Thus the perennial conflict between individual autonomy and government policy and politics even in the presence of catastrophic public health problems such as the COVID-19 pandemic.

Furthermore, given the understanding of governments at all levels that benefits conferred and costs imposed largely determine the politics of an issue, governments may ultimately practice *entrepreneurial* or *client* politics. Entrepreneurial politics imposes costs on a concentrated segment of the population with the aim of ensuring that broad and unpredictable benefits accrue to a wider segment of the population. In client politics, identifiable segments of the population are offered concentrated benefits with the imposition of diffuse costs across a broader segment of the population (Oliver and Paul-Shaheen 1997; Oliver 2006). Thus, in responding to the COVID-19 pandemic, government may view public health mask mandates as a type of entrepreneurial politics and individual autonomy related to mask mandates as client politics. As a result, while governments at all levels may have initially perceived mask mandates as entrepreneurial politics, as the pandemic became protracted, and faced with challenges such as fiscal accountability and limitations, competing political interests, and pressure from interest groups, some may have chosen to adopt client politics so as to facilitate concentrated benefits by way of large, direct, and immediate assistance for an identifiable segment of the population while at the same time imposing only diffuse costs across the rest of the population within their jurisdictions. This may have influenced their unwillingness to justify using paternalistic interventions in the interest of public health to override individual autonomy and instead to revoke mask mandates entirely, implement them incrementally, or implement them on an as-needed basis. This assertion of the effects of politics on mask mandates can be further demonstrated by comparing state-level mask mandates at two different time periods during the COVID-19 pandemic—July 2020 and August 2021.

As of July 2020 in the United States, thirty-one of fifty states plus the District of Columbia had mask mandates, compared to eleven with mask mandates in August 2021 (Gostin, Cohen, and Koplan 2020; Fischer et al. 2021; Hubbard 2021). In July 2020, before the development, approval, and use of vaccines, the number of COVID-19 cases and COVID-19 related mortality were mixed, with both low and high numbers of cases and low and high mortality, regardless of whether mask mandates were comprehensive, partial, or nonexistent. Comprehensive mask mandates required wearing of masks by all citizens, while partial mask mandates excluded certain portions of the population from wearing masks, such as children as well as people with disabilities and other ailments for whom complications might arise if they wore face masks (Fischer et al. 2021; Hubbard 2021). The lowest number of COVID-19 cases (40,424 cases per 1 million population) and lowest mortality due to COVID-19 (399 deaths per 1 million population) were in the only state (Hawai'i) with a comprehensive mask mandate. Conversely, the states with no mask mandates recorded the highest number of COVID-19 cases (151,568 cases per 1 million population in Rhode Island) and COVID-19 related mortality (3,014 deaths per 1 million population in New Jersey) (Fischer et al. 2021; Hubbard 2021; Peeples 2020). However, it is important to note that this correlation may not be due wholly to mask mandates but also to the combined effects of all nonpharmacologic preventive and control measures to curb the spread of COVID-19. Furthermore, as explained above, sustained challenges faced by state governments during the pandemic may have caused some state governments to shift from entrepreneurial to client politics, thus revoking earlier mask mandates instituted by executive orders—as was the case with New Jersey. Additionally, the discovery, emergency use authorization (EUA) approval, and subsequent administration following clinical trials of the vaccine against COVID-19 in the United States starting on

December 14, 2020 (Guarino et al. 2020), may also have contributed to the decision to revoke mask mandates by some state governments.

Notwithstanding the introduction of vaccines, by August 2021 the wearing of face masks to help with preventing the transmission of SARS-CoV-2 was still relevant and significant, albeit controversial, as 41% of the US population was still not fully vaccinated (CDC 2021b). In addition, it had been empirically established that individuals vaccinated against COVID-19 were still susceptible to and capable of transmitting SARS-CoV-2 (Peeples 2020; Boyarsky et al. 2021; CDC 2021c).

RECOMMENDATIONS

Following are our recommendations to strengthen mask mandates and to enact new mask mandates for the future or reemergent COVID-19 cases.

Policy Language

An important requirement of policy adoption and effectiveness is the crafting and framing of the policy language. The wording and language of the policies must be strong, compelling, and clear (free of ambiguities) to prevent inconsistencies in adoption downstream. For instance, the first mask mandate for the state of Hawai'i, issued on April 25, 2020, was not clear in its language, resulting in inconsistencies in implementation because it allowed for each of the four counties to choose its own exemptions. However, a revised proclamation on November 17, 2020, added clarity to the language so it clearly stated that the mask mandate was mandatory for all persons without exemption (Office of the Governor, State of Hawai'i 2020a, 2020b).

Policy Legislation

State governors should continue to use appropriate executive orders during the emergency phase of a pandemic as necessary. Concomitantly, during the state of emergency, legislative mechanisms should be set in motion to transform the executive orders into laws.

Public-Private Partnerships

In areas where government might not be able to enforce total control of the mandates, government can partner with private organizations to implement mask mandates to ensure total compliance. An instance of private business enforcing mask mandates is the case of Walmart's masking rules, which are independent of government regulations. Government can provide incentives in the form of additional tax breaks and small business loans to encourage adoption and enforcement of mask mandates within an organization to ensure that there is no loss of revenue while protecting members of staff of the organization and the public (Gee and Gupta 2020).

Enforcement Initiatives

Applying enforcement strategies from similar past policies such as seat belt and helmet laws could improve compliance. For instance, when the State of New York made wearing seat belts a recommendation only, the results were minimal, but when seat belts became mandatory, road traffic mortalities decreased by 17% (Gee and Gupta 2020).

While the Constitution does not give the federal government the authority to make universal laws like a mask mandate, the government can, through the Centers for Disease Control and Prevention (CDC), collect data for monitoring and evaluating existing mandates to prove their effectiveness and provide adequate education and awareness to the public on their importance (Gee and Gupta 2020; Gostin, Cohen, and Koplan 2020).

Federal and state public health regulatory agencies can issue compliance orders with as specified duration to businesses found in violation of mask mandates.

During peaks in the pandemic, the federal government can declare a state of national emergency, issue an executive order to states to enact mandatory mask mandates, and provide financial support to the states that enact such mandates. Financial support can be continued after the state of emergency has been lifted, as long as the states continue mask mandates.

CONCLUSION

As of the writing of this chapter, in the United States the COVID-19 pandemic continued to pose significant disease, economic, and social burdens. In spite of scientifically proven mitigating interventions such as transmission prevention and control measures, including wearing of face masks and vaccination, conflicts persisted between compliance with government-enacted policies such as public health mask mandates instituted to curb transmission of the coronavirus and individuals who saw such policies as infringing on their autonomy. However, in other to protect, promote, and preserve the health and well-being of the population, the government has a duty to exercise its constitutional powers to protect the public from harm while still giving due consideration to individual autonomy within moral standards.

LESSONS LEARNED

What Worked?

- Clear policy language

- Concise public messaging

- Continuous awareness campaigns

What Did Not Work?

- Conflicting messages and guidelines

- Mask mandate enforcement through punitive measures such as fines

RECOMMENDATIONS FOR FUTURE PRACTICE

Uniformity and clarity of public health policy language and enforcement initiatives should be ensured to engender harmonious messaging and avoid inconsistent interpretation and implementation of public health policies.

States should endeavor not to pass preemptive mask mandates to avoid weakening local mandates that are already in place.

DISCUSSION QUESTIONS

- How might the fundamental legal theories related to public health practice and interventions be applied?

- What are the criteria for selecting government-based solutions to public health issues?

- How do public health problems, policies, and politics interact?

REFERENCES

Allcott, Hunt, Benjamin B. Lockwood, and Dmitry Taubinsky. 2019. "Should We Tax Sugar-Sweetened Beverages? An Overview of Theory and Evidence." *Journal of Economic Perspectives* 33, no. 3: 202–27. https://doi.org/10.1257/jep.33.3 .202.

Amara, Sara A., Estefany D. Diaz, Lakshmi K. Menon, Priyanka Singh, Liudmila Rozanova, and Antoine Flahault. 2021. "COVID-19 Outbreak Management and Vaccination Strategy in the United States of America." *Epidemiologia (Basel)* 2, no. 3: 426–53. https://doi.org/10.3390/epidemiologia2030031.

An, Brian Y., Simon Porcher, Shui-Yan Tang, and Eunji Emily Kim. 2021. "Policy Design for COVID-19: Worldwide Evidence on the Efficacies of Early Mask Mandates and Other Policy Interventions." *Public Administration Review* 81, no. 6 (November/December): 1157–82. https://doi.org/10.1111/puar.13426.

Atupem, George. 2017. "Applying John Kingdon's Three Stream Model to the Policy Idea of Universal Preschool." Honors thesis, Bridgewater State University. https://vc.bridgew.edu/honors_proj/245.

Ballotpedia. 2021. "State-Level Mask Requirements in Response to the Coronavirus (COVID-19) Pandemic, 2020–2021." Ballotpedia. Last modified August 19, 2021. https://ballotpedia.org/State-level_mask_requirements_in_response_to_the_coronavirus_(COVID-19)_pandemic,_2020-2021.

Beauchamp, Dan E. 1988. *The Health of the Republic: Epidemics, Medicine, and Moralism as Challenges to Democracy.* Philadelphia: Temple University Press.

Bourne, Ryan. 2021. "The Economic Case against New Mask Mandates." Cato Institute. Last modified August 4, 2021. https://www.cato.org/commentary/economic-case-against-new-mask-mandates.

Bowser, Rene, and Lawrence O. Gostin. 1998. "Managed Care and the Health of a Nation." *Southern California Law Review* 72, no. 5 (July): 1209–95.

Boyarsky, Brian J., William A. Werbel, Robin K. Avery, Aaron A. R. Tobian, Allan B. Massie, Dorry L. Segev, and Jacqueline M. Garonzik-Wang. 2021. "Antibody Response to 2-Dose SARS-CoV-2 mRNA Vaccine Series in Solid Organ Transplant Recipients." *JAMA* 325, no. 21 (February): 2204–6. https://doi.org/10.1001/jama.2021.7489.

Buchanan, David R. 2008. "Autonomy, Paternalism, and Justice: Ethical Priorities in Public Health." *American Journal of Public Health* 98, no. 1 (January): 15–21. https://doi.org/10.2105/AJPH.2007.110361.

CDC (Centers for Disease Control and Prevention). 2021a. "Considerations for Restaurant and Bar Operators." Centers for Disease Control and Prevention. Last modified June 14, 2021. https://www.cdc.gov/coronavirus/2019-ncov/community/organizations/business-employers/bars-restaurants.html (page discontinued).

———. 2021b. "COVID-19 Vaccinations in the United States." Centers for Disease Control and Prevention. Accessed November 21, 2021. https://covid.cdc.gov/covid-data-tracker/#vaccinations_vacc-total-admin-rate-total.

———. 2021c. "Frequently Asked Questions about COVID-19 Vaccination." Centers for Disease Control and Prevention. Last modified November 5, 2021. https://www.cdc.gov/coronavirus/2019-ncov/vaccines/faq.html.

———. 2021d. "Your Guide to Masks." Centers for Disease Control and Prevention. Last modified August 13, 2021. https://www.cdc.gov/coronavirus/2019-ncov/prevent-getting-sick/about-face-coverings.html.

Chetty, Raj, John N. Friedman, Nathaniel Hendren, Michael Stepner, and Opportunity Insights Team. 2020. *How Did COVID-19 and Stabilization Policies Affect Spending and Employment? A New Real-Time Economic Tracker*

Based on Private Sector Data. Cambridge, MA: National Bureau of Economic Research.

Childress, James F. 2020. "Paternalism in Healthcare and Health Policy." In *Public Bioethics: Principles and Problems,* 38–52. Oxford: Oxford University Press.

Christoffel, Tom, and Susan Scavo Gallagher. 2006. *Injury Prevention and Public Health: Practical Knowledge, Skills, and Strategies.* 2nd ed. Burlington, MA: Jones & Bartlett Learning.

Coggon, John, and José Miola. 2011. "Autonomy, Liberty, and Medical Decision-Making." *Cambridge Law Journal* 70, no. 3 (November): 523–47. https://doi.org /10.1017/S0008197311000845.

Colgrove, James, and Ronald Bayer. 2005. "Manifold Restraints: Liberty, Public Health, and the Legacy of *Jacobson v Massachusetts.*" *American Journal of Public Health* 95, no. 4 (April): 571–76. https://doi.org/10.2105/AJPH.2004.055145.

Dann, F. P., Ernest William Lewis, and James R. Dunseath. 1909. *Reports of Cases Argued and Determined in the Supreme Court of the Territory of Arizona.* Vol. 10. San Francisco: Bancroft-Whitney.

Dorfman, Doron, and Mical Raz. 2020. "Mask Exemptions during the COVID-19 Pandemic—A New Frontier for Clinicians." *JAMA Health Forum* 1, no. 7: e200810. https://doi.org/10.1001/jamahealthforum.2020.0810.

Dworkin, Gerald. 1988. *The Theory and Practice of Autonomy.* Cambridge: Cambridge University Press.

Entwistle, Vikki A., Stacy M. Carter, Alan Cribb, and Kirsten McCaffery. 2010. "Supporting Patient Autonomy: The Importance of Clinician-Patient Relationships." *Journal of General Internal Medicine* 25, no. 7 (July): 741–45. https:// doi.org/10.1007/s11606-010-1292-2.

Fischer, Charlie B., Nedghie Adrien, Jeremiah J. Silguero, Julianne J. Hopper, Abir I. Chowdhury, and Martha M. Werler. 2021. "Mask Adherence and Rate of COVID-19 across the United States." *PLOS ONE* 16, no. 4: e0249891. https:// doi.org/10.1371/journal.pone.0249891.

Fischer, Emma P., Martin C. Fischer, David Grass, Isaac Henrion, Warren S. Warren, and Eric Westman. 2020. "Low-Cost Measurement of Face Mask Efficacy for Filtering Expelled Droplets during Speech." *Science Advances* 6, no. 36: eabd3083. https://doi.org/10.1126/sciadv.abd3083.

Gee, Rebekah E., and Vin Gupta. 2020. "Mask Mandates: A Public Health Framework for Enforcement." Health Affairs Forefront, October 5, 2020. https:// www.healthaffairs.org/do/10.1377/hblog20201002.655610/full/.

Giubilini, Alberto, and Julian Savulescu. 2019. "Vaccination, Risks, and Freedom: The Seat Belt Analogy." *Public Health Ethics* 12, no. 3 (November): 237–49. https://doi.org/10.1093/phe/phz014.

Gostin, Lawrence O. 2000a. "Legal and Public Policy Interventions to Advance the Population's Health." In *Promoting Health: Intervention Strategies from Social and Behavioral Research,* edited by Brian D. Smedley and S. Leonard Syme, 390–416. Washington, DC: National Academy Press.

———. 2000b. "Public Health Law in a New Century: Part I: Law as a Tool to Advance the Community's Health." *JAMA* 283, no. 21: 2837–41. https://doi.org/10 .1001/jama.283.21.2837.

————. 2000c. "Public Health Law in a New Century: Part II: Public Health Powers and Limits." *JAMA* 283, no. 22: 2979–84. https://doi.org/10.1001/jama.283.22.2979.

————. 2000d. "Public Health Law in a New Century: Part III: Public Health Regulation: A Systematic Evaluation." *JAMA* 283, no. 23: 3118–22. https://doi.org/10.1001/jama.283.23.3118.

————. 2007a. "General Justifications for Public Health Regulation." *Public Health* 121, no. 11 (November): 829–34. https://doi.org/10.1016/j.puhe.2007.07.013.

————. 2007b. "Law as a Tool to Facilitate Healthier Lifestyles and Prevent Obesity." *JAMA* 297, no. 1: 87–90. https://doi.org/10.1001/jama.297.1.87.

————. 2008. "A Theory and Definition of Public Health Law." In *Public Health Law: Power, Duty, Restraint*, 3–41. Rev. and exp. 2nd ed. Berkeley: University of California Press / Milbank Memorial Fund.

Gostin, Lawrence O., I. Glenn Cohen, and Jeffrey P. Koplan. 2020. "Universal Masking in the United States: The Role of Mandates, Health Education, and the CDC." *JAMA* 324, no. 9: 837–38. https://doi.org/10.1001/jama.2020.15271.

Gostin, Lawrence, Jason Sapsin, Stephen Teret, Scott Burris, Julie Mair, James G. Hodge Jr., and Jon Vernick. 2002. "The Model State Emergency Health Powers Act: Planning for and Response to Bioterrorism and Naturally Occurring Infectious Diseases." *JAMA* 288, no. 5: 622–28. https://doi.org/10.1001/jama.288.5.622.

Guarino, Ben, Ariana Eunjung Cha, Josh Wood, and Griff Witte. 2020. "'The Weapon That Will End the War': First Coronavirus Vaccine Shots Given Outside Trials in U.S." *Washington Post*, December 14, 2020. https://www.washingtonpost.com/nation/2020/12/14/first-covid-vaccines-new-york/.

Guy, Gery P., Jr., Florence C. Lee, Gregory Sunshine, Russell McCord, Mara Howard-Williams, Lyudmyla Kompaniyets, Christopher Dunphy, et al. 2021. "Association of State-Issued Mask Mandates and Allowing On-Premises Restaurant Dining with County-Level COVID-19 Case and Death Growth Rates—United States, March 1–December 31, 2020." *Morbidity and Mortality Weekly Report (MMWR)* 70, no. 10 (March 12): 350–54. https://www.cdc.gov/mmwr/volumes/70/wr/mm7010e3.htm.

Hofstadter, Richard. 2011. *The American Political Tradition and the Men Who Made It*. New York: Random House.

Holshue, Michelle L., Chas DeBolt, Scott Lindquist, Kathy H. Lofy, John Wiesman, Hollianne Bruce, Christopher Spitters, et al. 2020. "First Case of 2019 Novel Coronavirus in the United States." *New England Journal of Medicine* 382, no. 10: 929–36. https://doi.org/10.1056/nejmoa2001191.

Hubbard, Kaia. 2021. "These States Have COVID-19 Mask Mandates." *US News and World Report*. Last modified October 27, 2021. https://www.usnews.com/news/best-states/articles/these-are-the-states-with-mask-mandates.

Kaganovich, Katerina. 2021. "Mask Mandates Are Constitutional. Here Is Why." *Columbia Political Review*, January 4, 2021. http://www.cpreview.org/blog/2021/1/mask-mandates-are-constitutional-here-is-why.

Kersh, Rogan, and James Morone. 2002. "The Politics of Obesity: Seven Steps to Government Action." *Health Affairs* 21, no. 6 (November–December): 142–53. https://doi.org/10.1377/hlthaff.21.6.142.

Kingdon, John W. 1984. *Agendas, Alternatives, and Public Policies.* Boston: Little, Brown.

Kontis, Vasilis, James E. Bennett, Theo Rashid, Robbie M. Parks, Jonathan Pearson-Stuttard, Michel Guillot, Perviz Asaria, et al. 2020. "Magnitude, Demographics and Dynamics of the Effect of the First Wave of the COVID-19 Pandemic on All-Cause Mortality in 21 Industrialized Countries." *Nature Medicine* 26, no. 12 (December):1919–28. https://doi.org/10.1038/s41591-020-1112-0.

Lawrence, Christopher. 1996. Review of *The Health of Nations: Public Opinion and the Making of American and British Health Policy,* by Lawrence R. Jacobs. *English Historical Review* 111, no. 441 (April): 540–42.

Lindblom, Charles Edward, and David K. Cohen. 1979. *Usable Knowledge: Social Science and Social Problem Solving.* New Haven, CT: Yale University Press.

Morone, James A. 1990. "American Political Culture and the Search for Lessons from Abroad." *Journal of Health Politics, Policy and Law* 15, no. 1: 129–43. https://doi.org/10.1215/03616878-15-1-129.

Nathanson, Constance A. 1999. "Social Movements as Catalysts for Policy Change: The Case of Smoking and Guns." *Journal of Health Politics, Policy and Law* 24, no. 3 (June): 421–88. https://doi.org/10.1215/03616878-24-3-421.

Network for Public Health Law. 2021. "Individual Rights and the Public's Health: Constitutional, Ethical, and Political Aspects of COVID-19 Measures and Their Enforcement." Network for Public Health Law, February 24, 2021. https://www.networkforphl.org/news-insights/individual-rights-and-the-publics-health-constitutional-ethical-and-political-aspects-of-covid-19-measures-and-their-enforcement/.

Office of the Governor, State of Hawai'i. 2020a. "Fifteenth Proclamation Related to the Covid-19 Emergency." Office of the Governor, State of Hawai'i. November 16.

———. 2020b. "Sixth Supplementary Proclamation Amending and Restating Prior Proclamations and Executive Orders Related to the Covid-19 Emergency." Office of the Governor, State of Hawai'i, April 7, 2020. https://dod.hawaii.gov/hiema/sixth-supplementary-proclamation/.

Oliver, Thomas R. 2006. "The Politics of Public Health Policy." *Annual Review of Public Health* 27:195–233. https://doi.org/10.1146/annurev.publhealth.25.101802.123126.

Oliver, Thomas R., and Pamela Paul-Shaheen. 1997. "Translating Ideas into Actions: Entrepreneurial Leadership in State Health Care Reforms." *Journal of Health Politics, Policy and Law* 22, no. 3 (June): 721–89. https://doi.org/10.1215/03616878-22-3-721.

Parmet, Wendy E. 1993. "Health Care and the Constitution: Public Health and the Role of the State in the Framing Era." *Hastings Constitutional Law Quarterly* 20, no. 2: 267–335.

———. 2009. *Populations, Public Health, and the Law.* Washington, DC: Georgetown University Press.

Peeples, Lynne. 2020. "Face Masks: What the Data Say." *Nature* 586, no. 7828: 186–89. https://doi.org/10.1038/d41586-020-02801-8.

Price, Polly J., and Patrick C. Diaz. 2020. "Face-Covering Requirements and the Constitution." Expert Forum: Law and Policy Analysis. American Constitution Society, June 3, 2020. https://www.acslaw.org/expertforum/face-covering -requirements-and-the-constitution/.

Rothman, David J. 1997. *Beginnings Count: The Technological Imperative in American Health Care.* Oxford: Oxford University Press.

Ruvo, Christopher. 2020. "Study: Mask Mandate Would Benefit US Economy." Advertising Specialty Institute, July 1, 2020. https://www.asicentral.com/news /newsletters/promogram/june-2020/study-mask-mandate-would-benefit-us -economy/.

Scurlock, Stephanie. 2020. "Lawsuits against Mask Ordinances Filed across the Country." WREG Memphis, July 2, 2020. https://www.wreg.com/news/lawsuits -against-mask-ordinances-filed-across-the-country/.

Shafer, Byron E. 1989. "'Exceptionalism' in American Politics?" *PS: Political Science & Politics* 22, no. 3: 588–94. https://doi.org/10.2307/419626.

———. 1991. *Is America Different? A New Look at American Exceptionalism.* Oxford: Oxford University Press.

Silverman, Ross D. 2005. Review of *The Public Health Law Manual,* 3rd ed., by Frank P. Grad. *Journal of Legal Medicine* 26, no. 2: 293–301. https://doi.org/10 .1080/01947640590953332.

Stone, Deborah A. 1997. *Policy Paradox: The Art of Political Decision Making.* New York: W. W. Norton.

Tobey, James A. 1927. "Public Health and the Police Power." *New York University Law Review* 4:126.

Tocqueville, Alexis de. 1969. *Democracy in America.* Edited by J. P. Mayer. Translated by George Lawrence. New York: Doubleday. First published 1835–40.

Udalova, Victoria. 2021. "Pandemic Impact on Mortality and Economy Varies across Age Groups and Geographies." United States Census Bureau, March 8, 2021. https://www.census.gov/library/stories/2021/03/initial-impact-covid-19 -on-united-states-economy-more-widespread-than-on-mortality.html.

Wallack, Lawrence, Lori Dorfman, David Jernigan, and Makani Themba. 1993. *Media Advocacy and Public Health: Power for Prevention.* Thousand Oaks, CA: Sage.

Walzer, Michael. 2008. *Spheres of Justice: A Defense of Pluralism and Equality.* New York: Basic Books.

Wang, Jialan, Jeyul Yang, Benjamin Charles Iverson, and Raymond Kluender. 2020. "Bankruptcy and the COVID-19 Crisis." Working Paper 21–041. Harvard Business School. https://doi.org/10.2139/ssrn.3690398.

Weiss, Carol H. 1989. "Congressional Committees as Users of Analysis." *Journal of Policy Analysis and Management* 8, no. 3 (Summer): 411–31. https://doi.org/10 .2307/3324932.

WHO (World Health Organization). 2020. "Rolling Updates on Coronavirus Disease (COVID-19)." World Health Organization. Last modified July 31, 2020. https://www.who.int/emergencies/diseases/novel-coronavirus-2019/events-as -they-happen.

Wilson, Nick, and George Thomson. 2005. "Tobacco Taxation and Public Health: Ethical Problems, Policy Responses." *Social Science & Medicine* 61, no. 3 (August): 649–59. https://doi.org/10.1016/j.socscimed.2004.11.070.

Wing, Kenneth R., Wendy K. Mariner, George J. Annas, and Daniel S. Strouse. 2007. *Public Health Law.* New York: LexisNexis.

Worldometer. 2021. "Coronavirus Cases." Worldometer.com. Last modified August 21, 2021. https://www.worldometers.info/coronavirus/.

Yeyati, Eduardo Levy, and Federico Filippini. 2021. *Social and Economic Impact of COVID-19.* Background Paper 13. May 2021. N.p.: Secretariat for the Independent Panel for Pandemic Preparedness and Response. https://ycsg.yale.edu/sites/default/files/files/Social%20and%20Economic-impact%20of%20covid%2019.pdf.

11

COVID-19 and the American Overdose Crisis

EMMA T. BIEGACKI, KENNETH L. MORFORD, AND ROBERT HEIMER

People use substances for many reasons—for pleasure; to enhance social experiences; to cope with pain, illness, trauma, difficult emotions, and hardship; to gain functionality (e.g., to stay awake, have more energy, or feel more focused); and more (Duff 2008; Fraser, Moore, and Keane 2014). Most people who use psychoactive drugs (PWUD) do not develop a substance use disorder (SUD). An individual's likelihood of developing a SUD and experiencing adverse outcomes is mediated by myriad risk factors and protective factors that operate at personal, relational, community, and cultural levels, as well as by access to, options for, and quality of prevention, treatment, and support services (Krieger 2001; Rhodes 2009; Collins et al. 2019). That is to say, SUD can affect anyone but does not occur in a vacuum. Inequities in life course exposures produce disparities in SUD risk and adverse outcomes. People of color, particularly Black Americans, are disproportionately affected (Goedel et al. 2020; Parlier-Ahmad, Pugh, and Martin 2021). These disparities reflect the far-reaching health effects of structural racism in American society, which is embedded in the preconceptions, policies, and practices that conceptualize and shape responses to substance use (Smedley, Stith, and Nelson 2003; Paradies et al. 2015; James and Jordan 2018; ASAM 2021). The COVID-19 pandemic, in its numerous, multilevel impacts on PWUD and those with a SUD, intensified preexisting disparities and illuminated critical deficits in the care we provide for this population.

A widely reported consequence of the pandemic was an increase in drug overdose fatalities. From 1999 to 2022, drug overdoses claimed the lives of nearly 841,000 people in the United States, likely more when accounting for unreported and mislabeled deaths (CDC 2022a). Amidst the pandemic, overdose deaths topped 100,000 over a twelve-month period for the first time in US history, a 28.5% increase from the year prior (Ahmad, Rossen, and Sutton 2021). Overdose mortality increased despite the existence of effective SUD treatments and supports, including evidence-based medications, behavioral health interventions, harm reduction strategies, and other services. Existence of treatments and supports does not, unfortunately, guarantee access.

Even prior to the pandemic, a major challenge in addressing overdose and treating SUD more broadly has been a vast and persistent treatment gap. In a given year, only 10%–12% of the more than 20 million people with a SUD in the United States receive any form of treatment (SAMHSA 2020a). Numerous barriers contribute to the treatment gap, including accessibility, cost, stigma, and the effects of systemic racism and drug criminalization. Consequently, many PWUD and those with a SUD contend every day with heightened risk for preventable harms like overdose and transmission of infectious diseases such as HIV, hepatitis C, and bacterial infections. The COVID-19 pandemic added additional barriers to care, exacerbating the treatment gap and the ongoing overdose crisis.

This chapter reviews foundational concepts for understanding SUDs, with a focus on opioid use disorder (OUD). We discuss the historical and political contexts of illicit drug use in the United States, the addiction treatment landscape, and the American overdose crisis leading up to the onset of the COVID-19 pandemic. We then discuss the multilevel impacts of the pandemic on PWUD and SUD treatment systems. We conclude with lessons learned and implications for future policy and practice.

FOUNDATIONAL CONCEPTS FOR UNDERSTANDING SUBSTANCE USE, SUDs, AND RELATED RISKS

What Is a Substance Use Disorder?

A substance use disorder is broadly defined as a preventable and treatable chronic medical disease characterized by compulsive substance use and related behaviors despite harmful consequences. SUDs involve complex interactions among brain circuits, genetics, structural and environmental factors, as well as social determinants of health (ASAM, n.d.-b). Table 11.1 summarizes the diagnostic criteria for SUD. The number of criteria met correspond to SUD severity: Mild = 2–3, Moderate = 4–5, and Severe = 6 or more (APA 2013; APF 2020). Severe SUD is commonly referred to as addiction (NIDA 2020b).

TABLE 11.1. SUMMARY DSM-5 CRITERIA FOR SUBSTANCE USE DISORDER

Symptom type	Criteria
Impaired control	Substance is often taken in larger amounts and/or over longer periods than intended.
	Persistent attempts or one or more unsuccessful efforts made to cut down or control substance use.
	Craving, strong desire, or urge to use the substance.
Social challenges	A great deal of time is spent on activities necessary to obtain the substance, use the substance, or recover from effects.
	Recurrent substance use resulting in a failure to fulfill major obligations at work, school, or home.
	Continued substance use despite having persistent or recurrent social or interpersonal problems caused or exacerbated by the effects of the substance.
	Important social, occupational, or recreational activities given up or reduced because of substance use.
Risky use	Recurrent substance use in physically hazardous situations.
	Substance use is continued despite knowledge of having a persistent or recurring physical or psychological problem likely to have been caused or exacerbated by the substance.
Physical dependence	Tolerance, as defined by any of the following: • Markedly increased amounts of the substance in order to achieve intoxication or desired effect • Markedly diminished effect with continued use of the same amount
	Withdrawal, as manifested by either of the following: • The characteristic withdrawal syndrome for the substance • The same (or a closely related) substance is taken to relieve or avoid withdrawal symptoms.

Source: APA (2013).

What Is an Overdose?

An overdose occurs when someone takes a toxic amount of one or more substances. Among psychoactive substances, opioids carry the greatest risk for overdose and were involved in over 70% of fatal poisonings in 2019 (CDC 2020a). Opioids decrease breathing functionality through their action on the brain's respiratory control center, the locus coeruleus. In the case of an opioid overdose, breathing stops, resulting in cardiac arrest, which prevents the circulation of blood to the brain and other organs and can lead to death. Respiratory depression, pinpoint (constricted) pupils, loss of consciousness, insensitivity to pain, clamminess, vomiting or gurgling, and cyanosis (blue- or purple-tinged fingernail beds or lips) characterize opioid overdoses (WHO 2021; Schiller, Goyal, and Mechanic 2020). The risk of a fatal opioid overdose increases when opioids are used concomitantly with other sedating substances such as benzodiazepines or alcohol (Tori, Larochelle, and Naimi 2020). Recent data show that overdoses involving stimulants and synthetic cannabinoids are on the rise. Stimulant overdoses produced by cocaine or methamphetamine-type stimulants may involve tremors, overactive reflexes, rapid breathing, chest pain, confusion, aggression, hallucinations, panic, fever, and convulsions (Vasan and Olango 2021). Symptoms of synthetic cannabinoid-involved poisonings include headache, severe anxiety, insomnia, nausea and vomiting, loss of appetite, and diaphoresis in less severe cases and catalepsy and loss of consciousness in more severe cases (Hermanns-Clausen, Szabo, and Auwäter 2012; Cooper 2016). Overdose risk is heightened when resuming substance use after a period of abstinence, which has lowered the body's tolerance for the substance. Additional factors contributing to risk of overdose and death include but are not limited to route of administration (most notably by injection) and using alone without another party present to respond if an overdose occurs.

What Tools and Services Are Available to Care for PWUD and Those with a SUD?

The current standard for addiction treatment in the United States includes a view of care as a stepped continuum progressing from early intervention via outpatient services up to intensive inpatient care (ASAM, n.d.-a). Available treatments generally fall into four categories: Medications, Behavioral Health Interventions, Harm Reduction, and Wrap-Around Services.

Medications

Medication-based treatments (MBTs) approved by the US Food and Drug Administration (FDA) are available to treat opioid, alcohol, and tobacco use disorders. Other medications are used to treat substance-related withdrawal syndromes, which occur when an individual abruptly stops using a substance to which they have developed a physical dependence. MBTs work in different ways to reduce cravings and/or withdrawal symptoms, enabling the recipient to cease or reduce their substance use sustainably. Studies have shown that receiving MBTs reduces mortality and related complications of opioid, alcohol, and tobacco use (Mattick et al. 2004;

Wakeman et al. 2020; D. E. Jones et al. 2014; Allan, Ivers, and Els 2011). Improvements in health and quality of life among those receiving MBTs vary with disease severity, medication choice, and the quality of the program delivering the medication. FDA-approved medications for opioid use disorder (MOUD), the type of SUD most associated with fatal and nonfatal overdose, include opioid agonists buprenorphine and methadone, as well as the opioid antagonist naltrexone. Opioid agonists bind to and activate opioid receptors in the brain, allowing for reduction of opioid craving and withdrawal symptoms. Opioid antagonists, on the other hand, act as blockers preventing opioids from attaching to and activating opioid receptors, which reduces overdose risk but does not directly treat craving or withdrawal symptoms. Several medications are under investigation to treat stimulant, benzodiazepine, cannabis, and other SUDs; none are currently approved by the FDA.

Behavioral Health Interventions

Behavioral health interventions represent first-line treatment for SUDs lacking effective medication treatments. Evidence-based behavioral health interventions, such as cognitive behavioral therapy, contingency management, motivational interviewing, and peer recovery support, offer different approaches to address underlying drivers of substance use; teach skills to recognize, avoid, and cope with circumstances that trigger use; and provide supportive relationships and communities as individuals pursue their treatment goals. Behavioral health interventions are often offered in combination with MBTs.

Harm Reduction

Harm reduction is at once a set of principles, a collection of strategies, and a political movement that centers PWUD and prioritizes their rights, autonomy, safety, and well-being (Collins et al. 2012; NHRC 2020). Harm reduction strategies are designed to meet PWUD wherever they are along the continuum of substance use and reduce risk of harm. Select strategies are summarized in table 11.2. When each of these approaches has been studied, the benefits consistently outweigh prospective detriments (Marlatt and Witkiewitz 2010; Hopwood and Treolar 2013; Abdul-Quader et al. 2013; Potier et al. 2014; Isvins et al. 2020). A key element in harm reduction for people using opioids is the distribution of naloxone, an FDA-approved medication that can reverse an opioid overdose and prevent an overdose fatality (NIDA 2022).

TABLE 11.2. SELECTED HARM REDUCTION STRATEGIES

Sterile equipment distribution	Distribution of sterile syringes and other drug-consumption equipment to PWUD (e.g., cookers, tourniquets, pipes, etc.), and collection of used syringes and equipment, to reduce transmission of infections associated with sharing and reusing these items or other unsanitary practices
Overdose education and naloxone distribution	Provision of naloxone and overdose response training to PWUD, their friends, and family members
Safer use education	Education of PWUD on safer and alternative ways to use their substance(s) of choice (e.g., safer injecting practices)
Drug checking	Provision of services and supplies allowing PWUD to check the drug they plan to use for the presence of fentanyl (e.g., fentanyl test strips) or other contaminants
Good Samaritan laws	Laws protecting individuals who call 911 in the setting of an overdose from legal penalties or other consequences for involvement in or proximity to illicit substance use
Supervised consumption	Operation of sites permitting consumption of illicit substances under the supervision of peers, healthcare workers, or others able to respond in the event of an overdose and connect those interested to treatment, supportive services, and other resources
Safe supply	Regulated provision of psychoactive substances to PWUD to eliminate exposure to potentially harmful adulterants in the illicit market

Source: Drug Policy Alliance (n.d.); NIDA (2022); Isvins et al. (2020).

Wrap-Around Services

For individuals with a SUD, other problems may present a more immediate challenge than the SUD itself. SUD treatment programs improve their effectiveness when they provide services supporting basic needs, including housing, education, employment, food security, and medical and psychiatric care for co-occurring illnesses (Pringle et al. 2002).

A BRIEF HISTORY OF US DRUG POLICY AND THE AMERICAN OVERDOSE CRISIS

To understand the impact of the COVID-19 pandemic on PWUD and those with a SUD, and the effects and implications of key response efforts, it is critical to consider the conditions of illicit substance use and addiction treatment in the United States leading up to the pandemic and to reflect on the troubled history that established those conditions.

Early efforts by the US government to control and regulate psychoactive substances may be characterized by three key pieces of federal legislation (Musto 1999; Courtwright 2015):

- The Pure Food and Drug Act of 1906 identified ten psychoactive substances, including cannabis, cocaine, opium, and other opiates, as addictive and dangerous and instituted the first regulations on the distribution, marketing, and sale of products containing these substances.

- The Opium Exclusion Act of 1909 banned possession, importation, and use of opium for nonmedicinal purposes.

- The Harrison Act of 1914 (a) established a system to tax and regulate production, importation, distribution, and sales of opium, coca leaves, and derivates, and (b) limited physicians' ability to prescribe opiates, particularly to individuals considered "dope fiends," effectively restricting what could be considered early forms of MOUD and codifying SUD as a moral and behavioral flaw, not a medical illness in need of treatment.

Around the same time the Harrison Act was passed, the unviability of an abstinence-based approach to treat OUD was becoming apparent. By 1920, medical reports concluded that upwards of 90% of people with problematic morphine or heroin use returned to use within six months of beginning an abstinence-based regimen (Bishop 1919). In the century since then, little if any evidence of improvement in rates of return to use for abstinence-based regimens has been presented. Nonetheless, with subsequent legislation and public policy, the US government embraced a program of criminalization and promotion of abstinence to combat substance use and address SUD (Courtwright 1992).

The movement toward criminalization of substance use and PWUD occurred gradually but is perhaps best encapsulated by the passage of the Comprehensive Drug Abuse Prevention and Control Act in 1970 and subsequent declaration by President Richard Nixon of a War on Drugs. Ostensibly launched to reduce illicit substance use and addiction, the War on Drugs had an underlying racist agenda, plainly articulated by John Ehrlichman, then assistant to the president for domestic affairs:

> The Nixon campaign in 1968, and the Nixon White House after that, had two enemies: the antiwar left and black people. You understand what I'm saying? We knew we couldn't make it illegal to be either against the war or black, but by getting the public to associate the hippies with marijuana and blacks with heroin, and then criminalizing both heavily, we could disrupt those communities. We could arrest their leaders, raid their homes, break up their meetings, and vilify them night after night on the evening news. Did we know we were lying about the drugs? Of course we did. (Quoted in Baum 2016)

Racism in American drug policy was, at this point, hardly novel. Restrictions on opium production, use, and sales in the early 1900s bore the influence of anti-Chinese sentiments of the time (Ahmad 2007). Proponents of the temperance movement that ultimately begat Prohibition frequently associated the perceived evils of alcohol consumption, including moral corruption, disorder, idleness, and poverty, with urban-dwelling, poor Black and immigrant populations (Hopkins 1925). The Marijuana Tax Act of 1937, which placed a hefty tax on cannabis and hemp products, was conceived amidst rising concerns about Mexican immigration to the United States and helped promote fears of dangerous foreign substances being trafficked into the country that persist well into the present (Hudak 2020).

In the 1970s and 1980s, robust antidrug campaigns popularized conceptions of PWUD as socially corrupt and violent. Black Americans, in particular, were disproportionately portrayed in these stigmatizing narratives and directly targeted in the enforcement of drug criminalization laws (Netherland and Hansen 2016). During the Reagan administration, the Comprehensive Crime Control Act of 1984 and the Anti-Drug Abuse Act of 1988 were passed, increasing mandatory minimum sentences for drug-related offenses and coming down particularly hard on possession and sales of "crack" cocaine, which, due to access, affordability, and other structural factors, was more popular among Black PWUD at the time (Mustard 2001; Palamar et al. 2015). Although crack and powder cocaine are pharmacologically identical, from 1986 to 2010 crack possession and distribution were penalized unequally: crack distribution carried a mandatory minimum sentence of five years for five grams, while powder cocaine carried the same sentence for five hundred grams (Vagins and McCurdy 2006). The War on Drugs and its local implementation precipitated the mass incarceration that exists in the United States today, described by Michelle Alexander as the "New Jim Crow." While rates of illicit substance use do not differ significantly by race or ethnicity in the United States, Black Americans are far more likely to be arrested and incarcerated for a drug-related offense. In fact, despite comprising just 13% of the US population, Black Americans account for over 40% of people incarcerated for drug-related offenses (Alexander 2010; Sentencing Project 2018; Sawyer and Wagner 2020). Two in three people in prison have a SUD, as do almost 60% of those held in jails (NIDA 2020a; Chamberlain et al. 2019). Likewise, individuals under community supervision, such as those on probation or parole, have rates of illicit opioid use four times higher (14.9%) than among the general public (3.6%) (SAMHSA 2019).

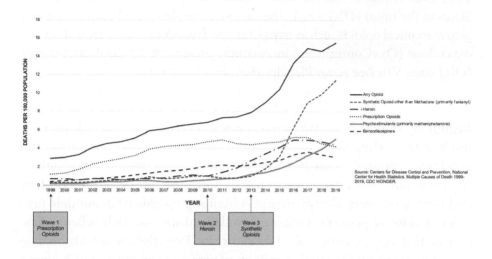

FIGURE 11.1. Trends in American overdose deaths from 1999 to 2019, including recent increases in stimulant- and benzodiazepine-involved deaths. Original figure created by the authors using publicly available data from the Centers of Disease Control and Prevention.

Conditions established by criminalization and the War on Drugs led to the American overdose crisis, commonly understood to have unfolded in three primary waves involving prescription opioids, followed by heroin and now high-potency synthetic opioids such as fentanyl (figure 11.1) (CDC 2022b).

Wave 1: Prescription Opioids

In the early 1980s, strict laws regulating prescription opioids effectively limited their use to treating pain related to terminal illness or surgical procedures. Concern that patients with pain who fell outside these two categories were not receiving appropriate pain management led to the development of a comprehensive national plan introducing new methods for assessing and treating pain. Importantly, this plan relaxed opioid-prescribing guidelines to include chronic, nonterminal pain (especially musculoskeletal pain) where benefits were unproven. Despite their addictive potential, opioid medications were marketed and prescribed as safe to use in large quantities for long-term, daily dosing. The medications were easily obtained from family members, friends, and others and diverted into the illicit market, where many individuals became physically dependent and sought a continuous supply to prevent withdrawal symptoms. By 2002, the number of people using illegally obtained pharmaceutical opioids was similar to that using cocaine (which, aside from cannabis, was the most common drug used illicitly in the United States at the time) (OIG 2019). The national overdose rate began to rise and pharmaceutical opioids such as oxycodone, hydrocodone, and extended-release oxycodone (OxyContin) were increasingly present in the illicit drug supply (OIG 2019; Van Zee 2009; Planalp, Hest, and Lahr 2019).

Wave 2: Heroin

Beginning around 2008, two approaches to curtail opioid overdoses were implemented. Guidelines were modified to reduce dosage, duration, and conditions appropriate for prescribing opioids. Prescription drug monitoring programs were established to track controlled substance prescriptions and help prescribers identify patients obtaining opioids from multiple providers and being prescribed other controlled substances, such as benzodiazepines, that may increase opioid-related risks. Prescription opioids became harder to acquire as the number and size of prescriptions fell by 40% between 2012 and 2018 (Pezalla et al. 2017; IQVIA 2020). Scarcity drove up the cost of pharmaceutical opioids on the illicit market. This reduction in access was not accompanied by an increase in access to alternative pain treatments nor treatments for OUD. Many individuals transitioned to using heroin, a more obtainable, affordable, and comparably potent alternative. Whereas the contents of prescribed substances are certifiable and the dosage consistent, the contents of substances produced on the illicit market are not. They may contain dangerous adulterants that increase overdose risk. Furthermore, because illicit substance use is a criminalized activity in the United States, and more heavily stigmatized than misuse of prescription medications, individuals may be more likely to use alone, in an unsafe environment, or in a rushed manner, and less likely to seek help or support. In 2010, Purdue Pharma replaced OxyContin with a new formulation difficult to crush, and demand for heroin increased even more (Ciccarone 2019). By 2017 the rate of heroin-involved overdose fatalities had risen to meet those involving prescription opioids.

Wave 3: Synthetic Opioids

A growing demand for heroin, coinciding with intensified domestic regulations to address illicit drug trafficking into the United States, produced a supply-side demand for a highly potent, transportable, and disguisable opioid that could be cheaply and easily made. Beginning in 2013, the prevalence of illicitly manufactured fentanyl, a synthetic opioid with sixty times the potency of heroin, increased substantially. By 2019, overdoses involving fentanyl and its analogs had risen by 1,040% from 1.0 to 11.4 per 100,000 (age-adjusted) (Mattson et al. 2021). The risk of encountering fentanyl is no longer limited to those seeking illicit opioids. Fentanyl and its analogs have been found in substances purchased as cocaine, methamphetamine, and benzodiazepines. This adulteration has contributed to increased stimulant- and benzodiazepine-involved overdoses (Fleming et al. 2020). In the twelve months leading up to May 2020, as COVID-19 spread across the United States, thirty-seven of thirty-eight US jurisdictions with available synthetic opioid data reported increases in synthetic opioid-involved overdose deaths, and eighteen of these jurisdictions reported increases exceeding 50% (CDC 2020b). At the onset of the COVID-19 pandemic, fentanyl was a primary driver of overdose deaths and remained so as the fatality rate continued to climb (Ciccarone 2021).

IMPACTS OF COVID-19 ON PEOPLE WHO USE DRUGS AND INDIVIDUALS WITH A SUD

The COVID-19 pandemic had multilevel impacts on the health and well-being of PWUD. Exposures in the course of obtaining or using substances placed PWUD at heightened risk for contracting SARS-CoV-2 (Wang et al. 2020; Walters et al. 2020; Volkow 2020b). Once they are infected, the poor health of many with severe SUDs and the broader risk environments they inhabit worsen outcomes, whether they are immunocompromised, unhoused, living in a congregate setting, engaged in sex work, or otherwise unable to isolate from others. Respiratory distress caused by COVID-19 compounds the breathing problems produced by opioid, alcohol, and benzodiazepine intoxication, by smoking, and by opioid withdrawal syndrome. Some clinical features of withdrawal from opioids and other drugs mimic COVID-19 symptoms, leading to false diagnosis, unnecessary isolation protocols, and delayed treatment of withdrawal symptoms.

As cases of COVID-19 proliferated in the United States in the spring and summer of 2020, the overdose crisis was expected to worsen (Becker and Fiellin 2020; Alexander et al. 2020; Volkow 2020a; Akiyama, Spaulding, and Rich 2020; Salisbury-Afshar, Rich, and Adashi 2020). The challenges of job loss, school closures, childcare interruptions, social isolation, and other stressors increased substance use through initiation, escalation, or resumption of use as people struggled to cope (Cziesler et al. 2020; Rogers et al. 2020). Efforts to practice social distancing led more individuals to use alone, and without others on hand to respond, overdoses turned fatal. Social distancing requirements and other COVID-19 precautions forced the closure or reduced operational capacity of many treatment, harm reduction, and basic needs programs. Overdose-prevention materials, such as naloxone and fentanyl test strips, and other harm reduction supplies became harder to obtain. Conversely, the effects of the pandemic on the illicit drug supply to the United States appeared relatively minimal (Vo et al. 2022). Anecdotal reports from PWUD, their providers, and organizations serving this population suggest relative continuity in access to and cost of illicit substances. Indeed, recent data from US Customs and Border Control show increased illicit drug seizures at US borders for fentanyl, cocaine, and methamphetamine (CBP 2021). Among the more than 93,000 accidental drug poisoning (including opioid overdose) deaths in the United States in 2020 alone, almost 75% involved opioids, 62% involved fentanyl or a fentanyl analogue, and 47% involved a stimulant such as cocaine or methamphetamine (Ahmad, Rossen, and Sutton 2021).

With the onset of the pandemic, many individuals engaged in or seeking SUD treatment experienced interruptions in their care or entry delays as treatment systems, which have historically heavily depended on in-person operations, struggled to implement alternative models of care. Lapsed access to SUD treatment can instigate return to or escalation of substance use (McQuaid, Jesseman, and Rush 2018). Particularly in the case of interruptions in MOUD, individuals may turn to illicit substances to manage symptoms of opioid withdrawal. Individuals returning to use following a disruption in abstinence-based treatments (e.g., discontinuation of Narcotics Anonymous meetings) face especially heightened risk of overdose, as periods of abstinence reduce opioid tolerance. In fact, overdose is a leading cause of death following cessation of abstinence-based treatment for OUD (Strang, Beswick, and Gossop 2003; Stein et al. 2017). In all cases, treatment cessation and subsequent return to illicit substance use during the pandemic occurred in a heightened risk environment rife with fentanyl and limited support structures.

The pandemic impacted initiation and management of MOUD. Two of the three medications available to treat OUD, buprenorphine and methadone, are opioid agonists, scheduled under the Controlled Substances Act and subject to special restrictions that limit access. Many people receiving buprenorphine for OUD are seen at least monthly by their provider. Prior to the pandemic, prescribers were required to complete eight to twenty-four hours of training to receive a special waiver, called an "X-waiver," from the US Drug Enforcement Agency (DEA) to prescribe buprenorphine. Even with an X-waiver, prescribers were restricted in the number of patients they may treat with buprenorphine. Most individuals receiving methadone must present daily to a specially licensed dispensing facility called an opioid treatment program (OTP) to receive their dose, which is taken under supervision. The pandemic limited in-person medical encounters, making methadone dispensing particularly difficult. To ensure continued treatment for their patients, providers were left to adapt policies and practices in MOUD management. Recently published studies suggest providers had more confidence maintaining established patients via telehealth than in starting new patients, and that patients delayed seeking treatment due to access challenges or concerns about COVID-19 exposure in a healthcare setting (Huskamp et al. 2020; Mark et al. 2021). MOUD access barriers have also appeared to vary by MOUD type, with patients receiving methadone experiencing more challenges than those receiving buprenorphine (Priest 2020; Peavy et al. 2020; Joudrey et al. 2021).

Many individuals unable to access care in the community, whether due to closures, reduced service capacity, inability to engage in telehealth services, or the broader impact of social disruptions, went without the care they needed, or presented to hospitals. SUD-related visits to US emergency departments (EDs), particularly for overdose, increased in early 2020 as compared to 2019, and remained high throughout the initial wave of the pandemic relative to visits unrelated to SUDs (Holland et al. 2021; Pines et al. 2021). Hospitals experienced a surge in admissions for SUDs and related complications (Komaromy et al. 2021; Harris et al. 2021). The increased need for hospital-based services challenged a general lack of infrastructure for addiction treatment in ED and inpatient settings and occurred alongside diversion of clinical resources to COVID-19 response efforts. Connecting patients with follow-up care in the community upon discharge from the hospital became especially challenging. With many shelter and respite facilities temporarily closed, operating at reduced capacity, or prioritizing COVID-19–positive patients, hospitalized individuals with a SUD who were homeless or unstably housed, particularly those who were also negative for COVID-19, frequently experienced extended hospital stays absent a viable discharge plan. In some cases, facilities otherwise open and available to receive people discharged from the hospital were inaccessible to those hospitalized with a SUD due to policies limiting their placement (e.g., restrictions on smoking or other substance use, possession of paraphernalia, and/or on MOUD).

Large-scale emergencies have a tendency to lay bare and intensify the harms of systemic inequity and structural oppression. Reflecting aforementioned racial and ethnic disparities involving SUDs, the pandemic posed unique risks and challenges disproportionately affecting PWUD of color (Friedman et al. 2021; Dorn, Cooney, and Sabin 2020; Essien and Venkataramani 2020). Black Americans who use drugs are at greater risk than White Americans for contracting COVID-19 and becoming seriously ill, as are Latinx and Native American PWUD (Wang et al. 2020; SAMHSA, n.d.; Khatri et al. 2021; Akee and Reber 2021). Delays and interruptions in OUD treatment due to challenges adapting methadone-dispensing practices disproportionately affected PWUD of color, reflecting a larger history of MOUD segregation, concentration of OTPs in communities of color, and restricted access to buprenorphine (Hansen et al. 2013; Lagisetty et al. 2019; Goedel et al. 2020). Since individuals who are incarcerated in the United States are disproportionately non-White, incarcerated individuals of color were most affected as COVID-19 transmission rates in prisons and jails ballooned during the spring and summer of 2020. Disparities among PWUD of color are foregrounded by racial and ethnic disparities in COVID-19 mortality more broadly, with one cross-sectional study finding that, had all racial and ethnic minorities experienced the COVID-19 mortality rates of college-educated non-Hispanic whites, racial and ethnic minorities would have seen 71% fewer deaths during 2020 (Feldman and Bassett 2021).

People exiting prisons and jails were among those most vulnerable as COVID-19 spread. In an effort to stem rampant virus transmission, some US prisons and jails released or transferred individuals near the end of their sentence or imprisoned for nonviolent offenses. Prior to the pandemic, overdose was the leading cause of death among those released from incarceration, and the risk was an order of magnitude higher in the first month following a period of incarceration (Seaman, Brettle, and Gore 1998; Binswanger et al. 2007; Merrall et al. 2010; Chang et al. 2015). The pandemic intensified this problem through a convergence of factors: lower opioid tolerance from imposed abstinence, lack of access to MOUD while incarcerated, COVID-imposed reductions to stabilizing resources upon release (housing, employment, public benefits, etc.), and the multiple stigmas associated with drug use and having a criminal record.

RESPONSE EFFORTS

Several key efforts were undertaken at the federal and state levels to address the needs of PWUD during the COVID-19 pandemic. These included rapid scale-up of telehealth services to provide virtual continuity of care in outpatient and inpatient settings; revisions in MOUD prescribing guidelines and practices; and expansion of curbside, mobile, and home delivery services.

Telehealth, having not been widely applied in addiction treatment prior to the pandemic, was adopted within months of the outset of the pandemic. Providing outpatient care continuity, it permitted patients to obtain buprenorphine prescriptions and engage in group and/or individual counseling amidst social distancing requirements. Healthcare systems across the United States worked speedily to transition patients to these platforms (Lee, Karsten, and Roberts 2020; Lin, Fernandez, and Bonar 2020). These efforts were facilitated by several key allowances enacted by federal and state government to reduce barriers:

- Coverage for telehealth services was expanded under Medicare, Medicaid, and the Children's Health Insurance Program (CHIP), and protections were put in place to ensure reimbursement parity (CMS 2020).

- Stipulations under the Health Insurance Portability and Accountability Act (HIPAA) and the Code of Federal Regulations 42, which govern patient privacy requirements, were relaxed to permit utilization of unconventional platforms such as Zoom, Skype, and FaceTime for patient care, and disclosure of identifying information in emergency situations (HHS 2021).

- Licensure requirements were relaxed to permit provision of care across state lines.

- An infusion of $200 million to the Federal Communication Commission to support nationwide telehealth services expansion was included in the Coronavirus Aid, Relief, and Economic Security (CARES) Act, passed by Congress in March 2020.

Virtual platforms were also adopted by peer-support groups, such as Alcoholics and Narcotics Anonymous, that were unable to convene in person.

These changes were coupled with significant revisions in guidelines for buprenorphine and methadone treatment. In March 2020, the DEA granted providers permission to prescribe buprenorphine and select other controlled substances using audio-visual telehealth without conducting a previously required in-person evaluation. This permission was later extended to include telehealth buprenorphine initiation (Prevoznik 2020). Research supports that these revisions played a critical role in retaining patients on buprenorphine during the pandemic and reducing overdose fatalities, as did relaxation of monitoring requirements such as regular urine toxicology screenings (ASAM 2020; C. M. Jones et al. 2023). Providers quickly adapted to telehealth bu-prenorphine treatment in high volume (Uscher-Pines et al. 2020; Cance and Doyle 2020; Nguyen et al. 2020). In May 2020, the US Department of Health and Human Services (HHS) reduced the requirements prescribers had to meet to obtain their X-waiver for buprenorphine prescribing. This was the first step toward eventual elimination of the X-waiver in 2022 (SAM-HSA 2023). Also in mid-March, the Substance Abuse and Mental Health Services Administration (SAMHSA) relaxed regulations governing metha-done dispensing. It issued guidance permitting OTPs to reduce or eliminate mandated counseling and drug-testing requirements and, most importantly, expanded the allowance of take-home methadone doses for up to twenty-eight days' supply for patients considered stable in their treatment, and up to fourteen days' supply for patients considered less stable (SAMHSA 2020b).

Extended take-home doses raised concerns among some providers that methadone would be diverted for nonmedical use and contribute to over-doses. Recent studies suggest these concerns were largely unfounded (Broth-ers, Viera, and Heimer 2021; Figgatt et al. 2021). Nonetheless, implementation of this guidance has been at the discretion of individual OTPs, and research examining how many US OTPs participated is ongoing. One study surveying OTP leaders from several US states ($n = 170$) found substantial variance in policies and practices for take-home methadone doses during the pandemic, with a majority but not all respondents endorsing adoption of revised dosing limits (Levander et al. 2022). In most cases, it has remained a requirement that patients pick up their take-home methadone in person. For patients quarantined or isolated due to suspected or confirmed COVID-19, SAMHSA permitted pickup by a surrogate family member or doorstep delivery. Imple-mentation of these distribution methods has varied substantially, particularly with respect to surrogate pickup. This option presents challenges for patients who do not have a trusted family member available to obtain their medica-tion or do not wish to disclose their SUD to others. Innovations in dose de-livery during the pandemic have included drive- or walk-up curbside systems and, more recently, mobile methadone dispensing (El-Sabawi et al. 2021).

Expansion of telehealth services and changes in MOUD prescribing guidelines also supported SUD care for individuals who were hospitalized. For example, rollout of e-consultations for patients who could not be seen at bedside due to COVID-19 precautions or high patient volume allowed hospi-tals equipped with addiction-consult services to provide SUD care, including MOUD, remotely. Still, many hospitals struggled to meet the needs of patients with a SUD, and particularly those whose treatment and discharge planning was complicated by a COVID-19 diagnosis (or in some cases, a lack thereof) and other factors such as housing instability. Hospital-based addiction-consult services that were well resourced prior to the pandemic were generally better able to scale, adapt, and sustain their services in a timely, responsive fashion. However, underresourced services scrambled to keep up with the volume and complexity of new admissions (Komaromy et al. 2021; Harris et al. 2021).

While the expansion of telehealth during the pandemic has generally helped initiate and retain individuals with a SUD in treatment, these adaptations have not worked well for everyone. Patients without regular access to technologies required for telehealth engagement (such as internet or a smartphone), who lack a private space to conduct telehealth visits, or who lack insurance with adequate telehealth coverage were left with limited options. To address the needs of individuals experiencing barriers to telehealth engagement, some organizations and health systems implemented new mobile treatment services, telephone hotline services, text-messaging outreach, and other interventions (Komaromy et al. 2021; Samuels et al. 2020). Telehealth also cannot completely replace the benefits of in-person services and supplies from harm reduction programs. At a time when the need for supplies was particularly high, distribution efforts remained hampered, notably by a national naloxone shortage and closure of several syringe-access facilities (Godvin 2021; Russell 2021; Tully 2021; Shelly 2021). Several states instituted policies to increase supply access, including elimination of one-to-one syringe-exchange requirements and expansion of infrastructure and permissions for delivery and mail-order supplies (Antezzo, Mette, and Manz 2020; French, Favaro, and Aronowitz 2021; Barnett et al. 2021). The American Rescue Plan Act, passed in March 2020, signaled renewed interest from the federal government in harm reduction as a vital tool to address substance use and SUDs, during and beyond the pandemic. Out of $4 billion intended for SUD and mental health services, $30 million was earmarked specifically to support evidence-based harm reduction programming (Newman 2021). However, the federal government has been slow to embrace the full spectrum of evidence-based harm reduction interventions, refusal to fund provision of safer smoking materials being one example (SAMHSA 2022).

A Connecticut Case Study

Federal efforts to address the dual crises of COVID-19 and overdose during the pandemic were coupled with local efforts that varied substantially given state-to-state differences in governance structures, resources, and attitudes toward substance use and PWUD. In a brief case study of Connecticut (CT), we dive further into pandemic outcomes and response efforts at the state and municipal levels.

As of November 2021, CT had seen nearly 382,173 laboratory-confirmed COVID-19 cases and 8,865 deaths (State of Connecticut 2021). In the twelve months following the start of the pandemic, the state recorded 1,444 opioid-involved fatalities, a 14.8% increase in overdose deaths from the previous year (CT-DPH 2021). Consistent with national trends, key challenges in the care of PWUD and those with a SUD during the pandemic included continuity of services and support for unhoused individuals, addressing the needs of the incarcerated and recently released, and preserving access to inpatient and outpatient SUD treatment services. Some of the localized actions to address these challenges are summarized below.

Continuity of Services for Unhoused PWUD

Amidst facility and service closures during the first surge of the pandemic, many experiencing housing insecurity in CT lost their places of refuge and access to basic needs, including sanitary facilities, in addition to reduced harm reduction and SUD treatment services.

KEY ACTIONS AND OUTCOMES

- Following the statewide shutdown in March 2020, efforts were undertaken to inform PWUD on steps they could take to protect themselves from COVID-19, overdose, and other harms within the heightened risk environment of the pandemic. This was achieved, in part, through partnerships between harm reduction advocates in CT municipalities and public health professionals in CT government and universities, to create compact, comprehensive information guides on risk of COVID-19 for PWUD and safer use practices. These materials were disseminated in English and Spanish (Heimer, McNeil, and Vlahov 2020).

- Programs that remained open to serve high-need populations such as the unhoused expanded services to account for reduced access elsewhere. In New Haven, CT, about one year into the pandemic, a new drop-in center was opened offering sanitary facilities and other services (Heimer, McNeil, and Vlahov 2020; Yu 2021).

- Advocacy efforts were undertaken to suspend policies prohibiting drugs and paraphernalia in shelters and ensure no one would be turned away because of substance use from facilities already operating at reduced capacity due to social distancing requirements.

- Efforts in several municipalities ensured that isolation spaces were available for unhoused individuals diagnosed with COVID-19 at local hotels and other converted spaces, and accepted PWUD and individuals receiving MOUD.

- In August 2021, the City of New Haven established a new Department of Community Resilience within the city's Community Service Administration. This department focuses on coordination and planning of mental health, public health, and social policy services in New Haven, and supports advancement of local efforts in SUD treatment and harm reduction (Breen 2021).

Addressing the Needs of the Incarcerated and Recently Released

Early in the pandemic, many correctional facilities across the country became hot spots for COVID-19 infections. But the CT unified correctional system was an exception. There were only sporadic introductions of COVID-19 by newly incarcerated individuals or corrections staff infected in the community, and one small-scale outbreak resulting from prisoner transfer between facilities. The first two cases of COVID-19 in a CT prison were reported in the last week of March 2020 and the first deaths shortly thereafter (Rondinone 2020; Krasselt 2020). In contrast to the large outbreaks that characterized correctional settings in many parts of the United States, resulting in more than 661,000 incarcerated people and staff infected and nearly 3,000 dead during the first year of the pandemic, CT experienced fewer than 3,000 cumulative cases and thirteen deaths among those in custody during the first year (Wallace 2020; *New York Times* 2023). The number of deaths in CT has since crept up to thirty (Connecticut Open Data, n.d.).

Formerly incarcerated individuals accounted for over 50% of fatal opioid overdoses in CT from 2016 to 2018, well before the pandemic introduced new risks and challenges (Lyons 2020). While it remains to be seen how many among those released during the pandemic period perished, preliminary unpublished analyses by Robert Heimer indicate that 47% of overdose deaths in 2020, and 53% in 2021, occurred among individuals with prior incarceration.

KEY ACTIONS AND OUTCOMES

- Advocates for criminal justice reform and the well-being of incarcerated people campaigned to hasten prison releases, improve conditions inside the CT correctional system, and ensure support for people upon their release, including linkage to SUD treatment and harm reduction services. These efforts included coordinated joint letter-writing to relevant state officials, opinion pieces in state media, and public demonstrations. CT reduced its census in prisons and jails by nearly 3,500 between March 2020 and April 2021, not through inmate releases but because court closures reduced those remanded to custody. In the meantime, the CT Department of Correction scaled up MOUD access in prisons and jails (Heimer, McNeil, and Vlahov 2020; Lyons and Pananjady 2021; CT-DOC 2021).

- A lawsuit filed by the CT American Civil Liberties Union prompted enhanced health and safety measures for individuals in CT prisons. The facility housing incarcerated people testing positive for COVID-19 was moved from the state's maximum-security prison to a lower-security environment. Systemwide changes required access to showers with running water, soap, cleaning supplies for common areas and cells, masks, and opt-in COVID-19 testing. Correctional staff were mandated to wear masks in 2020 and as of November 2021 were required to be vaccinated (ACLU-CT 2020).

Preserving Access to SUD Treatment Services

Delays and interruptions in both inpatient and outpatient SUD treatment affected PWUD in CT in several ways. Those experiencing housing instability or requiring linkage to a residential treatment facility or shelter were most adversely affected. In the late summer into early fall of 2020, several facilities and shelters that had reopened after initial closures either limited access for individuals coming from the hospital due to perceived risks of COVID-19 exposure, actively reserved space for patients testing positive for COVID-19 at the exclusion of those who were testing negative, or declined to receive patients on MOUD. Revisions to the OTP dispensing guidelines issued by SAMHSA proved highly beneficial. Where prior to the pandemic more than 55% of the state's 24,000 patients being treated with methadone were permitted to leave their OTP with just one or two days' worth of medication, the revised guidelines allowed CT OTPs to increase the number of take-home doses per patient, reducing crowding at dispensing stations and around program clinical sites. The revised guidelines also allowed certain intake assessments required by OTPs to be performed in the hospital, thus reducing barriers to continuing hospital-initiated methadone following discharge. Data from CT suggest that these changes occurred without increasing methadone-involved fatal overdose or decreasing the patient population treated with methadone (Brothers, Viera, and Heimer 2021).

KEY ACTIONS AND OUTCOMES

- Public health and healthcare professionals throughout the state worked to monitor and encourage timely and accurate local implementation of state and federal guidance around SUD treatment and support services.

- The revised methadone-prescribing guidelines were adopted in whole or in part by the majority of CT's eight OTPs (Brothers, Viera, and Heimer 2021).

- The percentage of patients with a methadone supply of two days or less fell to just 20% and the percentage with fourteen days and twenty-eight days increased to 26.8% and 16.8%, respectively (Brothers, Viera, and Heimer 2021).

- CT OTPs also sought to reduce the spread of COVID-19 by decreasing the mandated number of in-person counseling sessions and urine toxicology screenings.

- Telehealth counseling, nonexistent in OTPs prior to the pandemic, increased to account for 82.4% of all counseling visits by the summer of 2020. A significant shift was observed from group to individual counseling—from 57.5% to 84.5% of all counseling sessions in person or virtually, consistent with restrictions on group activities (Brothers, Viera, and Heimer 2021).

- Where some emergency shelters established for COVID-19–positive patients in New Haven, CT, initially declined access for individuals receiving MOUD, physician advocacy changed these policies and supported establishment of direct-to-shelter delivery of methadone doses.

Unanswered Questions

The impacts and outcomes of response efforts in CT are still being studied. Particularly difficult to evaluate is the impact of COVID-19-associated shutdowns, changes in the addiction treatment landscape, and related challenges for individuals seeking abstinence-based treatment options. For many engaged in traditionally abstinence-based programs like Alcoholics Anonymous and Narcotics Anonymous (AA/NA), closure of community meeting spaces and social distancing rapidly curtailed groups. Given the informal and autonomous nature of most of these groups, the national organizations of AA/NA left the establishment of virtual meetings up to individual groups (Pinney 2020). Lack of central coordination meant that it took time for these groups to identify mechanisms to begin virtual meetings. The extent to which lack of internet access to teleconferencing options or unwillingness to use mobile minutes or cellular data to connect by phone reduced participation and increased return to substance use has not yet been investigated.

LESSONS LEARNED

Lessons learned during the COVID-19 pandemic can inform improvements in the treatment and support of PWUD and those with a SUD as well as preparedness to meet the needs of this population in future crises. While substantial variance across the United States both in attitudes around substance use and addiction and in treatment access and quality makes cohesive planning challenging, the pandemic has shown that change on a national scale is possible.

The urgent need for solutions has opened the door to innovations and reforms long advocated by PWUD, advocates, and professionals in the fields of addiction treatment and harm reduction. Expansions in the use and coverage of telehealth services in addiction care are emergency provisions that should remain even after the pandemic is over. Similarly, relaxation in MOUD prescribing and monitoring practices for both methadone and buprenorphine was long overdue and should remain. With these changes, more PWUD will be able to access evidence-based treatment and supportive services and to engage in care from wherever they are. Initiation and management of MOUD is simpler for both providers and patients, and more options are available to care teams in structuring in-person and remote engagement in a manner that suits patients' needs. With these changes, MOUD now look and feel more like medication treatment for any other chronic disease. This has a destigmatizing effect (Frank et al. 2021). Early results indicate immense benefits and minimal if any detriments of these changes.

Pandemic-era changes that should be made permanent include the following:

- Expansion of insurance coverage for outpatient telehealth visits and inpatient consultations conducted via audio/video teleconferencing during implementation of isolation protocols.

- Key revisions under SAMHSA to MOUD prescribing guidelines, including:
    1. Ability to initiate and treat OUD with buprenorphine via tele-health, including audio only.
    2. Ability for OTPs to issue take-home doses of methadone in quantities up to twenty-eight days for stable patients and up to fourteen days for less stable patients, regardless of the amount of time they have been in treatment.

- Reductions in monitoring requirements for MOUD, including frequency of urine toxicology testing and counseling, neither of which is proven to improve care of stable patients (Khatri and Aronowitz 2021; Timko et al. 2016).

Decision-makers at the federal, state, and local levels should furthermore prioritize

- Supporting development of mobile methadone dosing and methadone dispensation at community pharmacies, to increase accessibility (El-Sabawi et al. 2021; Joudrey et al. 2020).

- Bringing all forms of evidence-based MOUD, naloxone, and comprehensive linkage-to-care programs to US prisons and jails to ensure individuals with OUD who are incarcerated can access treatment and reduce their risk of overdose death upon release.

- Pursuing approval of forms of MOUD currently unavailable or heavily restricted in the United States, such as injectable opioid agonist treatments and slow-release oral opiates (e.g., hydromorphone), that have been effectively implemented in other countries such as Canada, Switzerland, the Netherlands, and elsewhere (Uchtenhagen et al. 1997; Blanken et al. 2010; Ferri, Davoli, and Perucci 2011; Oviedo-Joekes et al. 2017; Fairbairn et al. 2019).

- Liberalizing policies governing dispensation and coverage of harm reduction supplies such as sterile syringes, safer smoking supplies, and naloxone through hospitals, to ensure PWUD for whom EDs and hospitals are a primary point of care have access to resources for safer use.

- Training inpatient and ED staff to recognize the unique and often complex needs of patients with a SUD and adjusting care delivery practices accordingly.

- Scaling evidence-based harm reduction strategies that have been successfully implemented abroad, including supervised consumption sites and safe supply programs.

- Expanding one-stop services that address overlapping SUD treatment, harm reduction, and basic needs such as food security, employment, and childcare.

- Enabling service providers to equip PWUD with basic material resources needed to stay engaged in care, such as phones and internet, for individuals lacking these.

Long-standing, persistent disparities in substance use, SUDs, and overdose, along lines of race, ethnicity, class, and other social determinants, have been starkly highlighted by the COVID-19 pandemic and ongoing overdose crisis. They indicate the urgent need for an equity lens in how we address these issues. Public health and healthcare systems must take up the work of upstream interventions to dismantle structural forms of oppression as fervently as they do interventions at the individual level such as MOUD provision and naloxone distribution. Drug criminalization, so thoroughly rooted in systemic racism, makes this foundational work difficult and has hindered efforts to respond to the overdose crisis and the COVID-19 pandemic every step of the way. Renewed investment in harm reduction services and evidence-based interventions presents an opportunity to move away from criminalizing policies around substance use, to implement the full arsenal of resources available to care for PWUD, to close the treatment gap for those with a SUD, and to strengthen our preparedness to meet the needs of this population in future emergencies. Some states, such as Oregon, Rhode Island, and New York, are already seizing this opportunity, advancing decriminalization and other critical interventions (State of Oregon 2020; RI-DH 2022; Mays and Newman 2021). These efforts will undoubtedly save lives that might otherwise be lost to overdose, other harms, or COVID-19.

DISCUSSION QUESTION

- What do you know about the impact of the COVID-19 pandemic on PWUD in the area where you live? How did your community respond? Have there been sustained changes as a result of these response efforts?

REFERENCES

Abdul-Quader, A. S., J. Feelemyer, S. Modi, E. S. Stein, A. Briceno, S. Semaan, T. Horvath, et al. 2013. "Effectiveness of Structural-Level Needle/Syringe Programs to Reduce HCV and HIV Infection among People Who Inject Drugs: A Systematic Review." *AIDS and Behavior* 17, no. 9 (November): 2878–92. https://pubmed.ncbi.nlm.nih.gov/23975473/.

ACLU-CT (American Civil Liberties Union—Connecticut). 2020. "Fight Continues to Protect Incarcerated People from COVID-19." American Civil Liberties Union—Connecticut, December 15, 2020. https://www.acluct.org/en/news/fight-continues-protect-incarcerated-people-covid-19.

Ahmad, D. L. 2007. *The Opium Debate and Chinese Exclusion Laws in the Nineteenth-Century American West.* Reno: University of Nevada Press.

Ahmad, F. B., L. M. Rossen, and P. Sutton. 2021. "Provisional Drug Overdose Death Counts." National Center for Health Statistics—Centers for Disease Control and Prevention. Last reviewed November 15, 2023. https://www.cdc.gov/nchs/nvss/vsrr/drug-overdose-data.htm.

Akee, R., and S. Reber. 2021. "American Indians and Alaska Natives Are Dying of COVID-19 at Shocking Rates." Brookings Institute. February 18, 2021. https://www.brookings.edu/research/american-indians-and-alaska-natives-are-dying-of-covid-19-at-shocking-rates/.

Akiyama, M. J., A. C. Spaulding, and J. D. Rich. 2020. "Flattening the Curve for Incarcerated Populations—COVID-19 in Jails and Prisons." *New England Journal of Medicine* 382:2075–77. https://www.nejm.org/doi/full/10.1056/NEJMp2005687.

Alexander, G. C., K. B. Stoller, R. L. Haffajee, and B. Saloner. 2020. "An Epidemic in the Midst of a Pandemic: Opioid Use Disorder and COVID-19." *Annals of Internal Medicine* 173, no. 1 (July): 57–58. https://www.acpjournals.org/doi/full/10.7326/M20-1141.

Alexander, Michelle. 2010. *The New Jim Crow: Mass Incarceration in the Age of Color Blindness.* New York: New Press.

Allan, G. M., N. Ivers, and C. Els. 2011. "Pharmacotherapy for Smoking." *Canadian Family Physician* 57, no. 1 (January): 47. https://cfp.ca/content/57/1/47.

Antezzo, M., E. Mette, and J. Manz. 2020. "Harm Reduction in the COVID-19 Era: States Respond with Innovations." National Academy for State Health Policy, October 19, 2020. https://www.nashp.org/harm-reduction-in-the-covid-19-era-states-respond-with-innovations/.

APA (American Psychiatric Association). 2013. *The Diagnostic and Statistical Manual of Mental Disorders.* 5th ed. Arlington, VA, 2013.

APF (Addiction Policy Forum). 2020. "DSM-5 Criteria for Addiction Simplified." Addiction Policy Forum, August 20, 2020. https://www.addictionpolicy.org/post/dsm-5-facts-and-figures.

ASAM (American Society of Addiction Medicine). 2020. "Adjusting Drug Testing Protocols." American Society of Addiction Medicine. https://www.asam.org/Quality-Science/covid-19-coronavirus/adjusting-drug-testing-protocols.

———. 2021. "Public Policy Statement on Advancing Racial Justice in Addiction Medicine." American Society of Addiction Medicine, February 25, 2021. https://www.asam.org/docs/default-source/public-policy-statements/asam -policy-statement-on-racial-justiced7a33a9472bc604ca5b7ff000030b21a.pdf ?sfvrsn=5a1f5ac2_2.

———. n.d.-a "ASAM Criteria." American Society of Addiction Medicine. Accessed December 1, 2022. https://www.asam.org/asam-criteria/about-the-asam -criteria.

———. n.d.-b "Definition of Addiction." American Society of Addiction Medicine. Accessed December 1, 2022. https://www.asam.org/Quality-Science/definition -of-addiction.

Barnett, B. S., S. E. Wakeman, C. S. Davis, J. Favaro, and J. D. Rich. 2021. "Expanding Mail-Based Distribution of Drug-Related Harm Reduction Supplies amid COVID-19 and Beyond." *American Journal of Public Health* 111, no. 6 (June): 1013–17. https://pubmed.ncbi.nlm.nih.gov/33950718/.

Baum, D. 2016. "Legalize It All." *Harper's Magazine,* April 2016. https://harpers.org /archive/2016/04/legalize-it-all/.

Becker, W., and D. A. Fiellin. 2020. "When Epidemics Collide: Coronavirus Disease 2019 (COVID-19) and the Opioid Crisis." *Annals of Internal Medicine* 173, no. 1: 59–60. https://pubmed.ncbi.nlm.nih.gov/32240291/.

Binswanger, I. A., M. F. Stern, R. A. Deyo, P. J. Heagerty, A. Cheadle, J. G. Elmore, and T. D. Koepsell. 2007. "Release from Prison—A High Risk of Death for Former Inmates." *New England Journal of Medicine* 356, no. 2: 157–65. https:// www.ncbi.nlm.nih.gov/pmc/articles/PMC2836121/.

Bishop, E. S. 1919. "Narcotic Drug Addiction: A Public Health Problem." *American Journal of Public Health* 9, no. 7 (July): 481–88. https://ajph.aphapublications .org/doi/pdf/10.2105/AJPH.9.7.481-a.

Blanken, P., V. Hendriks, J. M. van Ree, and W. van den Brink. 2010. "Outcome of Long-Term Heroin-Assisted Treatment Offered to Chronic, Treatment-Resistant Heroin Addicts in the Netherlands." *Addiction* 105, no. 2 (February): 300–308. https://doi.org/10.1111/j.1360-0443.2009.02754.x.

Breen, T. 2021. "New 'Resilience' Department Moves Ahead." *New Haven Independent,* August 10, 2021. https://www.newhavenindependent.org/index.php /archives/entry/community-resilience/.

Brothers, S., A. Viera, and R. Heimer. 2021. "Changes in Methadone Program Practices and Fatal Methadone Overdose Rates in Connecticut during COVID-19." *Journal of Substance Abuse Treatment* 131 (2021): 108449. https:// www.journalofsubstanceabusetreatment.com/article/S0740-5472(21)00175-6 /fulltext.

Cance, J. D., and E. Doyle. 2020. "Changes in Outpatient Buprenorphine Dispensing during the COVID-19 Pandemic." *JAMA* 324, no. 23: 2442–44. https://www .ncbi.nlm.nih.gov/pmc/articles/PMC7739121/.

CBP (US Customs and Border Protection). 2021. "Drug Seizure Statistics." US Customs and Border Protection. Accessed February 8, 2021. https://www.cbp.gov /newsroom/stats/drug-seizure-statistics.

CDC (Centers for Disease Control and Prevention). 2020a. "2019 Drug Overdose Death Rates." Centers for Disease Control and Prevention. Last reviewed March 22, 2021. https://www.cdc.gov/drugoverdose/deaths/2019.html.

———. 2020b. "Overdose Deaths Accelerating during COVID-19." Centers for Disease Control and Prevention. Last reviewed December 18, 2020. https://archive.cdc.gov/#/details?url=https://www.cdc.gov/media/releases/2020/p1218-overdose-deaths-covid-19.html.

———. 2022a. "Drug Overdose Deaths." Centers for Disease Control and Prevention. Last reviewed June 2, 2022. https://www.cdc.gov/drugoverdose/deaths/index.html.

———. 2022b. "Understanding the Epidemic." Centers for Disease Control and Prevention. Last reviewed June 1, 2022. https://www.cdc.gov/opioids/basics/epidemic.html.

Chamberlain, A., S. Nyamu, J. Aminawung, E. Wang, S. Shavit, and A. D. Fox. 2019. "Illicit Substance Use after Release from Prison among Formerly Incarcerated Primary Care Patients: A Cross-Sectional Study." *Addiction Science and Clinical Practice* 14, no. 1: 7. https://doi.org/10.1186/s13722-019-0136-6.

Chang, Z., P. Lichtenstein, H. Larsson, and S. Fazel. 2015. "Substance Use Disorders, Psychiatric Disorders, and Mortality after Release from Prison: A Nationwide Longitudinal Cohort Study." *Lancet Psychiatry* 2, no. 5 (May): 422–30. https://doi.org/10.1016/s2215-0366(15)00088-7.

Ciccarone, D. 2019. "The Triple Wave Epidemic: Supply and Demand Drivers of the US Opioid Overdose Crisis." *International Journal of Drug Policy* 71 (September): 183–88. https://www.ncbi.nlm.nih.gov/pmc/articles/PMC6675668/.

———. 2021. "The Rise of Illicit Fentanyls, Stimulants and the Fourth Wave of the Opioid Overdose Crisis." *Current Opinion in Psychiatry* 34, no. 4 (July): 344–50. https://journals.lww.com/co-psychiatry/fulltext/2021/07000/the_rise_of_illicit_fentanyls,_stimulants_and_the.4.aspx.

CMS (Centers for Medicare and Medicaid Services). 2020. "Medicare Telemedicine Health Care Provider Fact Sheet." Centers for Medicare and Medicaid Services, March 17, 2020. https://www.cms.gov/newsroom/fact-sheets/medicare-telemedicine-health-care-provider-fact-sheet.

Collins, A. B., J. Boyd, H. L. F. Cooper, and R. McNeil. 2019. "The Intersectional Risk Environment of People Who Use Drugs." *Social Science and Medicine* 234 (August): 112384. https://www.ncbi.nlm.nih.gov/pmc/articles/PMC6719791/.

Collins, S. E., S. L. Clifasefi, D. E. Logan, L. S. Samples, J. M. Somers, and G. A. Marlatt. 2012. "Current Status, Historical Highlights, and Basic Principles of Harm Reduction." In *Harm Reduction: Pragmatic Strategies for Managing High-Risk Behaviors,* edited by G. Alan Marlatt, Mary E. Larimer, and Katie Witkiewitz, 3–35. New York: Guilford.

Connecticut Open Data. n.d. "COVID-19 in Correctional Facilities." Accessed December 13, 2023. https://data.ct.gov/w/6t8i-du3u/wqz6-rhce?cur=_IVDjlsgYDD.

Cooper, Z. D. 2016. "Adverse Effects of Synthetic Cannabinoids: Management of Acute Toxicity and Withdrawal." *Current Psychiatry Reports* 18, no. 5 (May): 52. https://www.ncbi.nlm.nih.gov/pmc/articles/PMC4923337/.

Courtwright, D. T. 1992. "A Century of American Narcotic Policy." In *Treating Drug Problems*, vol. 2, *Commissioned Papers on Historical, Institutional, and Economic Contexts of Drug Treatment*, edited by D. R. Gerstein and H. J. Harwood, 1–62. Washington, DC: National Academies Press.

———. 2015. "Preventing and Treating Narcotic Addiction: A Century of Federal Drug Control." *New England Journal of Medicine* 373 (2015): 2095–97. https://www.nejm.org/doi/full/10.1056/NEJMp1508818.

CT-DOC (Connecticut Department of Correction). 2021. "Department of Correction Expands Medication for Opioid Use Disorder (MOUD) Programs." Connecticut Department of Correction, June 17, 2021. https://portal.ct.gov/-/media/DOC/Pdf/PressRelease/Press-Releases-2021/DOC-PRESS-RELEASE-re-DOC-Expands-MOUD-programs-061721.pdf.

CT-DPH (Connecticut Department of Health). 2021. "Fatal Unintentional and Undetermined Drug Overdose Report—2019–July 2021." Connecticut Department of Health. Accessed December 1, 2022. https://portal.ct.gov/-/media/DPH/Injury-Prevention/Opioid-Overdose-Data/Monthly-Reports/July-2021_2020-and-2019-Drug-Overdose-Deaths-Monthly-Report_CT_Updated_8-9-2021_Final.pdf (page discontinued).

Cziesler, M. É., R. I. Lane, E. Petrosky, J. R. Wiley, A. Christensen, R. Njai, M. D. Weaver, et al. 2020. "Mental Health, Substance Use, and Suicidal Ideation during the COVID-19 Pandemic—United States, June 24–30, 2020." *Morbidity and Mortality Weekly Report (MMWR)* 69, no. 32: 1049–57. https://www.cdc.gov/mmwr/volumes/69/wr/pdfs/mm6936-H.pdf.

Dorn, A. van, R. E. Cooney, and M. L. Sabin. 2020. "COVID-19 Exacerbating Inequalities in the US." *Lancet* 395, no. 10232: 1243–44. https://www.ncbi.nlm.nih.gov/pmc/articles/PMC7162639/.

Drug Policy Alliance. n.d. "Harm Reduction." Accessed December 12, 2022. https://www.drugpolicy.org/issues/harm-reduction.

Duff, C. 2008. "The Pleasure in Context." *International Journal of Drug Policy* 19, no. 5 (October): 384–92. https://pubmed.ncbi.nlm.nih.gov/17768037/.

El-Sabawi, T., M. Baney, S. L. Canzater, and S. R. Weizman. 2021. "The New Mobile Methadone Rules and What They Mean for Treatment Access." Health Affairs, August 4, 2021. https://www.healthaffairs.org/do/10.1377/hblog20210727.942168/full/.

Essien, U. R., and A. Venkataramani. 2020. "Data and Policy Solutions to Address Racial and Ethnic Disparities in the COVID-19 Pandemic." *JAMA Health Forum* 1, no. 4: e200535. https://jamanetwork.com/journals/jama-health-forum/fullarticle/2765498.

Fairbairn, N., J. Ross, M. Trew, K. Meador, J. Turnbull, S. MacDonald, E. Oviedo-Joekes, et al. 2019. "Injectable Opioid Agonist Treatment for Opioid Use Disorder: A National Clinical Guideline." *Canadian Medical Association Journal* 191, no. 38: e1049–56. https://doi.org/10.1503/cmaj.190344.

Feldman, J. M., and M. T. Bassett. 2021. "Variation in COVID-19 Mortality in the US by Race and Ethnicity and Educational Attainment." *JAMA Network Open* 4, no. 11: e135967. https://jamanetwork.com/journals/jamanetworkopen/fullarticle/2786466.

Ferri, M., M. Davoli, and C. A. Perucci. 2011. "Heroin Maintenance for Chronic Heroin-Dependent Individuals." *Cochrane Database Systematic Review* 2011, no. 12: CD003410. https://pubmed.ncbi.nlm.nih.gov/22161378/.

Figgatt, M. C., Z. Salazar, E. Day, L. Vincent, and N. Dasgupta. 2021. "Take-Home Dosing Experiences among Persons Receiving Methadone Maintenance Treatment during COVID-19." *Journal of Substance Abuse Treatment* 123 (April): 108276. https://www.journalofsubstanceabusetreatment.com/article/S0740-5472(21)0002-7/fulltext.

Fleming, T., A. Barker, A. Isvins, S. Vakharia, and R. McNeil. 2020. "Stimulant Safe Supply: A Potential Opportunity to Respond to the Overdose Epidemic." *Harm Reduction Journal* 17, no. 6. https://www.ncbi.nlm.nih.gov/pmc/articles/PMC6954588/.

Frank, D., P. Mateu-Gelabert, D. C. Perlman, S. M. Walter, L. Curran, and H. Guarino. 2021. "'It's Like Liquid Handcuffs': The Effects of Take-Home Dosing Policies on Methadone Maintenance Treatment (MMT) Patients' Lives." *Harm Reduction Journal* 18, no. 88. https://www.harmreductionjournal.biomedcentral.com/articles/10.1186/s12954-021-00535-y.

Fraser, S., D. Moore, and H. Keane. 2014. "Models of Addiction." In *Habits: Remaking Addiction,* 26–59. London: Palgrave Macmillan.

French, R., J. Favaro, and S. V. Aronowitz. 2021. "A Free Mailed Naloxone Program in Philadelphia amidst the COVID-19 Pandemic." *International Journal of Drug Policy* 94 (August): 1031199. https://www.sciencedirect.com/science/article/abs/pii/S0955395921000979?via%3Dihub.

Friedman, J., N. C. Mann, H. Hansen, P. Bourgois, J. Braslow, A. A. T. Biu, L. Beletsky, et al. 2021. "Racial/Ethnic, Social, and Geographic Trends in Overdose-Associated Cardiac Arrests Observed by US Emergency Medical Services during the COVID-19 Pandemic." *JAMA Psychiatry* 78, no. 8: 886–95. https://jamanetwork.com/journals/jamapsychiatry/fullarticle/2780427.

Godvin, M. 2021. "The US Faces a Naloxone Shortage at the Worst Possible Time." *Filter Magazine,* July 29, 2021. https://filtermag.org/us-naloxone-shortage/.

Goedel, W. C., A. Shapiro, M. Cerdá, J. W. Tsai, S. E. Hadland, and B. D. L. Marshall. 2020. "Association of Racial/Ethnic Segregation with Treatment Capacity for Opioid Use Disorder in Counties in the United States." *JAMA Network Open* 3, no. 4: e203711. https://jamanetwork.com/journals/jamanetworkopen/fullarticle/2764663.

Hansen, H. B., C. E. Siegal, B. G. Case, D. N. Bertollo, D. DiRocco, and M. Galanter. 2013. "Variation in Use of Buprenorphine and Methadone Treatment by Racial, Ethnic, and Income Characteristics of Residential Social Areas in New York City." *Journal of Behavioral Health Services Research* 40, no. 3 (July): 367–77. https://pubmed.ncbi.nlm.nih.gov/23702611/.

Harris, M. T. H., A. Peterkin, P. Back, H. Englander, E. Lapidus, T. Rolley, M. B. Weimer, and Z. M. Weinstein. 2021. "Adapting Inpatient Addiction Medicine Consult Services during the COVID-19 Pandemic." *Addiction Science and Clinical Practice* 16, no. 1: 13. https://pubmed.ncbi.nlm.nih.gov/33627183/.

Heimer, R., R. McNeil, and D. Vlahov. 2020. "A Community Responds to the COVID-19 Pandemic: A Case Study in Protecting the Health and Human

Rights of People Who Use Drugs." *Journal of Urban Health* 97:448–56. https://link.springer.com/article/10.1007/s11524-020-00465-3.

Hermanns-Clausen, M., B. Szabo, and V. Auwäter. 2012. "Acute Toxicity Due to the Confirmed Consumption of Synthetic Cannabinoids: Clinical and Laboratory Findings." *Addiction* 108, no. 3 (March): 534–44. https://pubmed.ncbi.nih.gov/22971158/.

HHS (US Department of Health and Human Services). 2021. "Notification of Enforcement Discretion for Telehealth Remote Communications during the COVID-19 Nationwide Public Health Emergency." US Department of Health and Human Services. Last reviewed January 20, 2021. https://www.hhs.gov/hipaa/for-professionals/special-topics/emergency-preparedness/notification-enforcement-discretion-telehealth/index.html.

Holland, K. M., C. Jones, A. M. Vivolo-Kantor, N. Idaikkader, M. Zwald, B. Hoots, E. Yard, et al. 2021. "Trends in US Emergency Department Visits for Mental Health, Overdose, and Violence Outcomes before and during the COVID-19 Pandemic." *JAMA Psychiatry* 78, no. 4: 372–79. https://jamanetwork.com/journals/jamapsychiatry/fullarticle/2775991.

Hopkins, R. J. 1925. "The Prohibition and Crime." *North American Review* 222, no. 828 (September–November): 40–44. https://www.jstor.org/stable/25113451?seq=1#metadata_info_tab_contents.

Hopwood, M., and C. Treolar. 2013. "International Policies to Reduce Illicit Drug-Related Harms and Illicit Drug Use." In *Interventions for Addiction: Comprehensive Addictive Behaviors and Disorders,* vol. 3, edited by Peter M. Miller, 735–43. San Diego: Academic Press.

Hudak, J. 2020. *Marijuana: A Short History.* Washington, DC: Brookings Institution Press.

Huskamp, H. A., A. B. Busch, L. Uscher-Pines, M. L. Barnett, L. Riedel, and A. Mehrotra. 2020. "Treatment of Opioid Use Disorder among Commercially Insured Patients in the Context of the COVID-19 Pandemic." *JAMA Network* 324, no. 23: 2440–42. https://jamanetwork.com/journals/jama/fullarticle/2774039.

IQVIA. 2020. "Prescription Opioid Trends in the United States: Measuring and Understanding Progress in the Opioid Crisis." IQVIA Institute, December 16, 2020. https://www.iqvia.com/insights/the-iqvia-institute/reports/prescription-opioid-trends-in-the-united-states.

Isvins, A., J. Boyd, L. Beletsky, and R. McNeil. 2020. "Tackling the Overdose Crisis: The Role of Safe Supply." *International Journal of Drug Policy* 80 (June): 102769. https://www.ncbi.nlm.nih.gov/pmc/articles/PMC7252037/.

James, K., and A. Jordan. 2018. "The Opioid Crisis in Black Communities." *Journal of Law, Medicine, and Ethics* 46, no. 2 (June): 404–21. https://pubmed.ncbi.nlm.nih.gov/30146996/.

Jones, D. E., H. R. Amick, C. Feltner, G. Bobashev, K. Thomas, R. Wines, M. M. Kim, et al. 2014. "Pharmacotherapy for Adults with Alcohol Use Disorders in Outpatient Settings: A Systematic Review and Meta-analysis." *JAMA* 311, no. 18: 1889–900. https://doi.org/10.1001/jama.2014.3628.

Jones, C. M., C. Shoff, C. Blanco, J. L. Losby, S. M. Ling, and W. M. Compton. 2023. "Association of Receipt of Opioid Use Disorder-Related Telehealth Services and Medications for Opioid Use Disorder with Fatal Drug Overdoses among Medicare Beneficiaries before and during the COVID-19 Pandemic." *JAMA Psychiatry* 80, no. 5: 508–14. https://doi.org/10.1001/jamapsychiatry.2023.0310.

Joudrey, P. J., Z. M. Adams, P. Bach, S. Buren, J. A. Chaiton, L. Ehrenfeld, M. E. Guerra, et al. 2021. "Methadone Access for Opioid Use Disorder during the COVID-19 Pandemic within the United States and Canada." *JAMA Network Open* 4, no. 7: e2118223. https://jamanetwork.com/journals/jamanetworkopen/fullarticle/2782211.

Joudrey, P. J., N. Chadi, P. Roy, K. Morford, P. Bach, S. Kimmel, E. A. Wang, et al. 2020. "Pharmacy-Based Methadone Dispensing and Drive Time to Methadone Treatment in Five States within the United States: A Cross-Sectional Study." *Drug and Alcohol Dependence* 211:107968. https://pubmed.ncbi.nlm.nih.gov/32268248/.

Khatri, Utsha G., and Shoshana V. Aronowitz. 2021. "Considering the Harms of Our Habits: The Reflexive Urine Drug Screen in Opioid Use Disorder Treatment." *Journal of Substance Use and Addiction Treatment* 123 (April): 108258. https://doi.org/10.1016/j.jsat.2020.108258.

Khatri, U. G., L. N. Pizzicato, K. Viner, E. Bobyock, M. Sun, Z. F. Meisel, and E. C. South. 2021. "Racial/Ethnic Disparities in Unintentional Fatal and Nonfatal Emergency Medical Services-Attended Opioid Overdoses during the COVID-19 Pandemic in Philadelphia." *JAMA Network Open* 4, no. 1: e2034878. https://jamanetwork.com/journals/jamanetworkopen/fullarticle/2775360.

Komaromy, M., M. Tomanovich, J. L. Taylor, G. Ruiz-Mercado, S. D. Kimmel, S. M. Bagley, K. M. Saia, et al. 2021. "Adaptation of a System of Treatment for Substance Use Disorders during the COVID-19 Pandemic." *Journal of Addiction Medicine* 15, no. 6 (November–December): 448–51. https://pubmed.ncbi.nlm.nih.gov/33298750/.

Krasselt, K. 2020. "CT Prison COVID Results: 'Either They Did Something Right or They Got Very Lucky.'" *Middletown Press,* July 1, 2020. https://www.middletownpress.com/news/coronavirus/article/CT-prison-COVID-results-Either-they-did-15380945.php.

Krieger, N. 2001. "Theories of Social Epidemiology in the 21st Century: An Ecosocial Perspective." *International Journal of Epidemiology* 30, no. 4 (August): 668–77. https://academic.oup.com/ije/article/30/4/668/705885.

Lagisetty, P. A., R. Ross, A. Bohnert, M. Clay, and D. T. Maust. 2019. "Buprenorphine Treatment Divide by Race/Ethnicity and Payment." *JAMA Psychiatry* 76, no. 9: 979–81. https://pubmed.ncbi.nlm.nih.gov/31066881/.

Lee, N. T., J. Karsten, and J. Roberts. 2020. "Removing Regulatory Barriers to Telehealth before and after COVID-19." Brookings Institute, May 6, 2020. https://www.brookings.edu/research/removing-regulatory-barriers-to-telehealth-before-and-after-covid-19/.

Levander, X. A., J. D. Pytell, K. B. Stoller, P. T. Korthuis, and G. Chander. 2022. "COVID-19-Related Policy Changes for Methadone Take-Home Dosing: A

Multisite Survey of Opioid Treatment Program Leadership." *Substance Abuse* 43, no. 1: 633–39. https://www.tandfonline.com/eprint/XET87VHR64V6EU93K9RK /full?target=10.1080/08897077.2021.1986768.

Lin, L., A. C. Fernandez, and E. E. Bonar. 2020. "Telehealth for Substance-Using Populations in the Age of Coronavirus Disease 2019." *JAMA Psychiatry* 77, no. 12: 1209–10. https://jamanetwork.com/journals/jamapsychiatry/fullarticle/2767300.

Lyons, K. 2020. "From Prison to the Grave: Former Inmates Now Account for More than Half of All Drug Overdose Deaths in Connecticut." *CT Mirror,* January 2, 2020. https://ctmirror.org/2020/01/02/from-prison-to-the-grave/.

Lyons, K., and K. Pananjady. 2021. "CT's Prison Population Shrunk During the Pandemic. Will It Last?" *CT Mirror,* April 13, 2021. https://ctmirror.org/2021/04 /13/cts-prison-population-shrunk-during-pandemic-will-it-last/.

Mark, T. L., B. Gibbons, A. Baronsky, H. Padwa, and V. Joshi. 2021. "Changes in Admissions to Specialty Addiction Treatment Facilities in California during the COVID-19 Pandemic." *JAMA Network Open* 4, no. 7: e2117029. https:// jamanetwork.com/journals/jamanetworkopen/fullarticle/2781940.

Marlatt, G. A., and K. Witkiewitz. 2010. "Update on Harm Reduction Policy and Intervention Research." *Annual Review of Clinical Psychology* 6:591–606. https://pubmed.ncbi.nlm.nih.gov/20192791/.

Mattick, R. P., J. Kimber, C. Breen, and M. Davoli. 2004. "Buprenorphine Maintenance versus Placebo or Methadone Maintenance for Opioid Dependence." *Cochrane Database of Systematic Reviews* 3: CD002207. https://pubmed.ncbi .nlm.nih.gov/15266465/.

Mattson, C. L., L. J. Tanz, K. Quinn, M. Kariisa, P. Patel, and N. L. David. 2021. "Trends and Geographic Patterns in Drug and Synthetic Opioid Overdose Deaths—United States 2013–2019." *Morbidity and Mortality Weekly Report (MMWR)* 70, no. 6: 202–7. https://www.cdc.gov/mmwr/volumes/70/wr /mm7006a4.htm.

Mays, J. C., and A. Newman. 2021. "Nation's First Supervised Drug-Injection Sites Open in New York." *New York Times,* November 30, 2021. https://www.nytimes .com/2021/nyregion/supervised-injection-sites-nyc.html.

McQuaid, R. J., R. Jesseman, and B. Rush. 2018. "Examining Barriers as Risk Factors for Relapse: A Focus on the Canadian Treatment and Recovery System of Care." *Canadian Journal of Addiction* 9, no. 3 (September): 5–12. https://www .ncbi.nlm.nih.gov/pmc/articles/PMC6110379/.

Merrall, E. L., A. Kariminia, I. A. Binswanger, M. S. Hobbs, M. Farrell, J. Marsden, S. J. Hutchinson, et al. 2010. "Meta-analysis of Drug-Related Deaths Soon after Release from Prison." *Addiction* 105, no. 9 (September): 1545–54. https:// pubmed.ncbi.nih.gov/20579009/.

Mustard, D. B. 2001. "Racial, Ethnic, and Gender Disparities in Sentencing: Evidence from the U.S. Federal Courts." *Journal of Law and Economics* 44, no. 1: 285–314. https://doi.org/10.1086/320276.

Musto, D. F. 1999. *The American Disease: Origins of Narcotic Control.* 3rd ed. New York: Oxford University Press.

Netherland, J., and H. B. Hansen. 2016. "The War on Drugs That Wasn't: Wasted Whiteness, 'Dirty Doctors,' and Race in Media Coverage on Prescription

Opioid Use." *Culture, Medicine, and Psychiatry* 40, no. 4 (December): 664–86. https://pubmed.ncbi.nlm.nih.gov/27272904/.

Newman, T. 2021. "Harm Reduction Receives Unprecedented $30 Million in Federal Funding through American Rescue Plan Act." Vital Strategies Press Room. March 12. https://www.vitalstrategies.org/harm-reduction-receives-unprecedented -30-million-in-federal-funding-through-american-rescue-plan-act/.

New York Times. 2023. "Coronavirus in the U.S.: Latest Map and Case Count." Last updated on March 23, 2023. Accessed December 13, 2023. https://www.nytimes .com/interactive/2021/us/covid-cases.html.

Nguyen, T. D., S. Gupta, E. Ziedan, S. I. Kosali, G. C. Alexander, B. Saloner, and B. D. Stein. 2020. "Assessment of Filled Buprenorphine Prescriptions for Opioid Use Disorder during the Coronavirus Disease 2019 Pandemic." *JAMA Internal Medicine* 181, no. 4: 562–65. https://jamanetwork.com/journals /jamainternalmedicine/fullarticle/2774272.

NHRC (National Harm Reduction Coalition). 2020. "Principles of Harm Reduction." National Harm Reduction Coalition. Revised 2020. https:// harmreduction.org/wp-content/uploads/2022/12/NHRC-PDF-Principles_Of_ Harm_Reduction.pdf.

NIDA (National Institutes of Drug Abuse). 2020a. "Criminal Justice DrugFacts." National Institutes of Drug Abuse. June 2020. https://www.drugabuse.gov /publications/drugfacts/criminal-justice.

———. 2020b. "Drug Misuse and Addiction." National Institutes of Drug Abuse. July 2020. https://www.drugabuse.gov/publications/drugs-brains-behavior -science-addiction/drug-misuse-addiction.

———. 2022. "Naloxone DrugFacts." National Institutes of Drug Abuse. January 2022. https://www.drugabuse.gov/publications/drugfacts/naloxone.

OIG (Office of the Inspector General). 2019. "Review of Drug Enforcement Administration's Regulatory and Enforcement Efforts to Control the Diversion of Opioids." US Department of Justice, Office of the Inspector General. Revised September 2019. https://oig.justice.gov/reports/2019/e1905.pdf.

Oviedo-Joekes, E., S. Brissette, S. MacDonald, D. Guh, K. Marchand, S. Harrison, A. Janmohamed, et al. 2017. "Safety Profile of Injectable Hydromorphone and Diacetylmorphine for Long-Term Severe Opioid Use Disorder." *Drug and Alcohol Dependence* 176:55–62. https://pubmed.ncbi.nlm.nih.gov/28521199/.

Palamar, J. J., S. Davies, D. C. Ompad, C. M. Cleland, and M. Weitzman. 2015. "Powder Cocaine and Crack Use in the United States: An Examination of Risk for Arrest and Socioeconomic Disparities in Use." *Drug and Alcohol Dependence* 149: 108–16. https://doi.org/10.1016/j.drugalcdep.2015.01.029.

Paradies, Y., J. Ben, N. Denson, A. Elias, N. Priest, A. Gupta, M. Kelaher, and G. Gee. 2015. "Racism as a Determinant of Health: A Systematic Review and Meta-Analysis." *PLOS ONE* 10, no. 9: e0138511. https://journals.plos.org/plosone /article?id=10.1371/journal.pone.0138511.

Parlier-Ahmad, A. B., M. Pugh Jr., and C. E. Martin. 2021. "Treatment Outcomes among Black Adults Receiving Medication for Opioid Use Disorder." *Journal of Racial and Ethnic Health Disparities* 9: 1557–67. https://link.springer.com /article/10.1007/s40615-021-01095-4.

Peavy, K. M., J. Darnton, P. Grekin, M. Russo, C. J. Banta Green, J. O. Merrill, C. Fotinos, et al. 2020. "Rapid Implementation of Service Delivery Changes to Mitigate COVID-19 and Maintain Access to Methadone among Persons with and at High-Risk for HIV in an Opioid Treatment Program." *AIDS and Behavior* 24, no. 9: 2469–72. https://www.ncbi.nlm.nih.gov/pmc/articles /PMC7186943/.

Pezalla, E. J., D. Rosen, J. G. Erensen, J. D. Haddox, and T. J. Mayne. 2017. "Secular Trends in Opioid Prescribing in the USA." *Journal of Pain Research* 10:383–87. https://pubmed.ncbi.nlm.nih.gov/28243142/.

Pines, J. M., M. S. Zocchi, B. S. Black, J. N. Carlson, P. Celedon, A. Moghtaderi, and A. Venkat. 2021. "How Emergency Department Visits for Substance Use Disorders Have Evolved during the Early COVID-19 Pandemic." *Journal of Substance Use Disorders* 129 (October): 108391. https://pubmed.ncbi.nih.gov/33994360/.

Pinney, J. 2020. "As 12-Step Meetings Halt in Person Due to the Coronavirus, Recovery Goes Online." Street Sense Media, April 16, 2020. https://www .streetsensemedia.org/article/12-step-meetings-coronavirus-recovery-online/# .YRWns5NKifV.

Planalp, C., R. Hest, and M. Lahr. 2019. "The Opioid Epidemic: National Trends in Opioid-Related Overdose Deaths from 2000–2017." State Health Access Data Assistance Center. June 2019. https://www.shadac.org/sites /default/files/publications/2019%20NATIONAL%20opioid%20brief%20FINAL %20VERSION.pdf.

Potier, C., V. Laprévote, F. Dubois-Arber, O. Cottencin, and B. Rolland. 2014. "Supervised Injection Services: What Has Been Demonstrated? A Systematic Literature Review." *Drug and Alcohol Dependence* 145 (December): 48–68. https:// www.sciencedirect.com/science/article/abs/pii/S0376871614018754.

Prevoznik, T. W. 2020. "DEA068—March 31, 2020." US Department of Justice Drug Enforcement Administration, March 31, 2020. https://www .deadiversion.usdoj.gov/GDP/(DEA-DC-022)(DEA068)%20DEA%20SAMHSA %20buprenorphine%20telemedicine%20%20(Final)%20+Esign.pdf.

Priest, K. 2020. "The COVID-19 Pandemic: Practice and Policy Considerations for Patients with Opioid Use Disorder." Health Affairs, April 3, 2020. https:// www.healthaffairs.org/do/10.1377/hblog20200331.557887/full/.

Pringle, J. L., L. A. Edmondston, C. L. Holland, K. Levent, N. P. Emptage, V. K. Balavage, W. E. Ford, et al. 2002. "The Role of Wrap Around Services in Retention and Outcome in Substance Abuse Treatment: Findings from the Wrap Around Services Impact Study." *Addictive Disorders and Their Treatment* 1, no. 4 (December): 109–18. https://journals.lww.com/addictiondisorders/Abstract/2002 /11000/The_Role_of_Wrap_Around_Services_in_Retention_and.1.aspx.

Rhodes, T. 2009. "Risk Environments and Drug Harms: A Social Science for Harm Reduction Approach." *International Journal of Drug Policy* 20, no. 3 (May): 193–201. https://pubmed.ncbi.nlm.nih.gov/19147339/.

RI-DH (State of Rhode Island Department of Health). 2022. "Harm Reduction Centers." State of Rhode Island Department of Health. Last updated July 21, 2022. https://health.ri.gov/addiction/about/harmreductioncenters/.

Rogers, A. H., J. M. Shepard, L. Garey, and M. J. Zvolensky. 2020. "Psychological Factors Associated with Substance Use Initiation during the COVID-19 Pandemic." *Psychiatry Research* 293 (November): 113407. https://www.ncbi.nlm.nih .gov/pmc/articles/PMC7434361/.

Rondinone, N. 2020. "COVID-19 Cases, Deaths Rise in Connecticut Prisons; DOC Brings on Additional Healthcare Workers, Increases Testing." *Hartford Courant,* December 25, 2020. https://www.courant.com/coronavirus /hc-news-coronavirus-covid-19-prisons-cases-deaths-rising-20201225 -pw4ymkakwvfancyig6hhfzexme-story.html.

Russell, J. 2021. "Scott County Officials Vote to Shut down Syringe Program 6 Years after HIV Outbreak." *Indianapolis Business Journal,* June 2, 2021. https://www .ibj.com/articles/scott-county-officials-vote-to-shut-down-syringe-exchange -program-six-years-after-hiv-outbreak.

Salisbury-Afshar, E. M., J. D. Rich, and E. Y. Adashi. 2020. "Vulnerable Populations: Weathering the Pandemic Storm." *American Journal of Preventive Medicine* 58, no. 6 (June): 892–94. https://www.ncbi.nlm.nih.gov/pmc/articles /PMC7174188.

SAMHSA (Substance Abuse and Mental Health Services Administration). 2019. "Key Substance Use and Mental Health Indicators in the United States: Results from the 2018 National Survey on Drug Use and Health." Substance Abuse and Mental Health Services Administration. Last updated August 2019. https://www.samhsa .gov/data/sites/default/files/cbhsq-reports/NSDUHNationalFindingsReport2018 /NSDUHNationalFindingsReport2018.pdf.

———. 2020a. "Key Substance Use and Mental Health Indicators in the United States: Results from the 2019 National Survey on Drug Use and Health." Substance Abuse and Mental Health Services Administration. Last updated September 2020. https://www.samhsa.gov/data/sites/default/files/reports/rpt29393 /2019NSDUHFFRPDFWHTML/2019NSDUHFFR1PDFW090120.pdf.

———. 2020b. "Opioid Treatment Program (OTP) Guidance." Substance Abuse and Mental Health Services Administration. Last updated March 19, 2020. https://www.samhsa.gov/sites/default/files/otp-guidance-20200316.pdf.

———. 2022. "Statement by HHS Secretary Xavier Becerra and ONDCP Director Rahul Gupta." Substance Abuse and Mental Health Services Administration, February 9, 2022. https://www.samhsa.gov/newsroom/statements/2022/hhs -secretary-ondcp-director.

———. 2023. "Waiver Elimination (MAT Act)." Substance Abuse and Mental Health Services Administration. Last updated October 10, 2023. https://www.samhsa .gov/medications-substance-use-disorders/waiver-elimination-mat-act.

———. n.d. "Double Jeopardy: COVID-19 and Behavioral Health Disparities for Black and Latino Communities in the U.S." Substance Abuse and Mental Health Services Administration. Accessed December 7, 2022. https://www .samhsa.gov/sites/default/files/covid19-behavioral-health-disparities-black -latino-communities.pdf.

Samuels, E. A., S. A. Clark, C. Wunch, L. A. Jordison Keeler, N. Reddy, R. Vanjani, and R. S. Wightman. 2020. "Innovation during COVID-19: Improving

Addiction Treatment Access." *Journal of Addiction Medicine* 14, no. 4 (July/August): e8–e9. https://pubmed.ncbi.nlm.nih.gov/32404652/.

Sawyer, W., and P. Wagner. 2020. "Mass Incarceration: The Whole Pie 2020." Prison Policy Initiative, March 24, 2020. https://www.prisonpolicy.org/reports/pie2020.html.

Schiller, Elizabeth Y., Amandeep Goyal, and Oren J. Mechanic. 2020. "Opioid Overdose." In *StatPearls [Internet]*, edited by Elizabeth Y. Schiller, Amandeep Goyal, and Oren J. Mechanic. Treasure Island, FL: StatPearls. https://www.ncbi.nlm.nih.gov/books/NBK470415/.

Seaman, S., R. Brettle, and S. M. Gore. 1998. "Mortality from Overdose among Injecting Drug Users Recently Released from Prison: Database Linkage Study." *BMJ* 316, no. 7129: 426–28. https://www.bmj.com/content/316/7129/426.

Shelly, M. 2021. "Murphy 'Disappointed' by Atlantic City Council Decision to Shut Down Needle Exchange." *Press of Atlantic City*, July 21, 2021. https://pressofatlanticcity.com/news/local/murphy-disappointed-by-atlantic-city-council-decision-to-shut-down-needle-exchange/article_c111de82-ea3f-11eb-aec8-5f4a5cc17f66.html.

Smedley, B. A., A. Y. Stith, and A. R. Nelson, eds. 2003. *Unequal Treatment: Confronting Racial and Ethnic Disparities in Health Care*. Washington, DC: National Academies Press.

State of Connecticut. 2021. "Connecticut COVID-19 Response." State of Connecticut. Accessed November 29, 2021. https://portal.ct.gov/coronavirus.

State of Oregon. 2020. *Measure 110: Drug Addiction Treatment and Recovery Act*. Oregon.gov. Last updated 2020. https://www.oregon.gov/oha/HSD/AMH/Pages/Measure110.aspx.

Stein, M. D., J. N. Flori, M. M. Risi, M. T. Conti, B. J. Anderson, and G. L. Bailey. 2017. "Overdose History Is Associated with Post-Detoxification Treatment Preference for Persons with Opioid Use Disorder." *Substance Abuse* 38, no. 4 (October–December): 389–93. https://www.ncbi.nlm.nih.gov/pmc/articles/PMC6077990/.

Strang, J., T. Beswick, and M. Gossop. 2003. "Loss of Tolerance and Overdose Mortality after Inpatient Opiate Detoxification: Follow Up Study." *Boston Medical Journal* 326, no. 7396: 959–60. https://www.ncbi.nlm.nih.gov/pmc/articles/PMC153851/.

The Sentencing Project. 2018. "Report to the United Nations on Racial Disparities in the U.S. Criminal Justice System." The Sentencing Project, April 19, 2018. https://www.sentencingproject.org/publications/un-report-on-racial-disparities/.

Timko, C., N. R. Schultz, M. A. Cucciare, L. Vittorio, and C. Garrison-Diehn. 2016. "Retention in Medication-Assisted Treatment for Opiate Dependence: A Systematic Review." *Journal of Addictive Diseases* 35, no. 1: 22–35. https://doi.org/10.1080/10550887.2016.1100960.

Tori, M. E., M. R. Larochelle, and T. S. Naimi. 2020. "Alcohol or Benzodiazepine Co-involvement with Opioid Overdose Deaths in the United States, 1999–2017." *JAMA Open Network* 3, no. 4: e202361. https://pubmed.ncbi.nlm.nih.gov/32271389/.

Tully, T. 2021. "As Overdoses Soar, This State's Largest Needle Exchange Is Being Evicted." *New York Times,* August 10, 2021. https://www.nytimes.com/2021/08/10/nyregion/nj-needle-exchange.html.

Uchtenhagen, A., F. Gutzwiller, A. D. Dobler-Mikola, and T. Steffen. 1997. "Programme for a Medical Prescription of Narcotics." *European Addiction Research* 3, no. 4: 160–63. https://www.karger.com/Article/Abstract/259173.

Uscher-Pines, L., J. Sousa, P. Raja, A. Mehrota, M. Barnett, and H. A. Huskamp. 2020. "Treatment of Opioid Use Disorder during COVID-19: Experiences of Clinicians Transitioning to Telemedicine." *Journal of Substance Abuse Treatment* 118 (November): 108–24. https://pubmed.ncbi.nlm.nih.gov/32893047/.

Vagins, D. J., and J. McCurdy. 2006. "Cracks in the System: Twenty Years of the Unjust Federal Crack Cocaine Law." American Civil Liberties Union, October 26, 2006. https://www.aclu.org/other/cracks-system-20-years-unjust-federal-crack-cocaine-law.

Van Zee, A. 2009. "The Promotion and Marketing of OxyContin: Commercial Triumph, Public Health Tragedy." *Health Policy and Ethics* 99, no. 2 (February): 221–27. https://www.ncbi.nlm.nih.gov/pmc/articles/PMC2622774/.

Vasan, S., and G. J. Olango. 2021. "Amphetamine Toxicity." In *StatPearls [Internet],* edited by Elizabeth Y. Schiller, Amandeep Goyal, and Oren J. Mechanic. Treasure Island, FL: StatPearls. https://www.ncbi.nlm.nih.gov/books/NBK470276/.

Vo, A. T., T. Patton, A. Peacock, S. Larney, and A. Borquez. 2022. "Illicit Substance Use and the COVID-19 Pandemic in the United States: A Scoping Review and Characterization of Research Evidence in Unprecedented Times." *International Journal of Environmental Research and Public Health* 19, no. 14 (July):8883. https://doi.org/10.3390/ijerph19148883.

Volkow, N. 2020a. "Collision of the COVID-19 and Addiction Epidemics." *Annals of Internal Medicine* 173, no. 1: 61–62. https://www.acpjournals.org/doi/full/10.7326/M20-1212.

———. 2020b. "New Evidence on Substance Use Disorders and COVID-19 Susceptibility." National Institute on Drug Abuse, October 5, 2020. https://www.drugabuse.gov/about-nida/noras-blog/2020/10/new-evidence-substance-use-disorders-covid-19-susceptibility.

Wakeman, S. E., M. R. Larochelle, O. Ameli, C. E. Chaisson, J. T. McPheeters, W. H. Crown, F. Azocar, et al. 2020. "Comparative Effectiveness of Different Treatment Pathways for Opioid Use Disorder." *JAMA Network Open* 3, no. 2: e1920622–e1920622. https://jamanetwork.com/journals/jamanetworkopen/fullarticle/2760032.

Wallace, M. 2020. "COVID-19 in Correctional and Detention Facilities—United States, February–April 2020." *Morbidity and Mortality Weekly Report (MMWR)* 69, no. 19: 587–90. https://www.cdc.gov/mmwr/volumes/69/wr/mm6919e1.htm.

Walters, S. M., D. W. Seal, T. J. Stopka, M. E. Murphy, and W. D. Jenkins. 2020. "COVID-19 and People Who Use Drugs: A Commentary." *Health Behavior Policy Review* 7, no. 5 (October): 489–97. https://doi.org/10.14485/hbpr.7.5.11.

Wang, Q. Q., D. C. Kaelber, R. Xu, and N. D. Volkow. 2020. "COVID-19 Risk and Outcomes in Patients with Substance Use Disorders: Analyses from Electronic

Health Records in the United States." *Molecular Psychiatry* 26, no. 1 (January): 30–39. https://doi.org/10.1038/s41380-020-00880-7.

WHO (World Health Organization). 2021. "Opioid Overdose." World Health Organization, August 4, 2021. https://www.who.int/news-room/fact-sheets/detail/opioid-overdose.

Yu, I. 2021. "Drop-In Center Opens for Homeless." *New Haven Independent,* June 11, 2021. https://www.newhavenindependent.org/index.php/archives/entry/desk_drop_incenter/.

Part 6

PUBLIC HEALTH PRACTICE

12

Lessons Learned from the COVID-19 Pandemic

Public Health Workforce, Data, and Information Systems Infrastructure Needs

CAROLYN NGANGA-GOOD AND ADANNA AGBO

BACKGROUND

COVID-19 Pandemic

On March 12, 2020, the World Health Organization (WHO) declared coronavirus 2 (SARS-CoV-2) a pandemic (Ciotti et al. 2020). SARS-CoV-2, commonly known as the 2019 coronavirus or COVID-19, is a betacoronavirus characterized by severe acute respiratory syndrome (Ciotti et al. 2020). The pandemic ravaged the world in 2020 and 2021, with death tolls and illness cases in the millions. It also destabilized economies, affected safety, and increased poverty (Ciotti et al. 2020). The pandemic put a strain on institutions and healthcare systems globally, and exposed flaws in the public health systems in the United States (US) and other parts of the world. Despite major advances in health, science, and technology in the twenty-first century, the COVID-19 pandemic showed that healthcare institutions, as structured, were not equipped to handle such a widespread outbreak. The pandemic also showed that healthcare workers, capacity, equipment, and planning were inadequate to address such a crisis. For example, Italy, despite having 3.2 hospital beds per 1,000 persons, still had difficulty meeting the needs of its population and providing care during the pandemic, due to the massive influx of patients into the health facilities and the short time frame in which they were arriving (Ciotti et al. 2020).

The US Public Health System

Public health is vital for the well-being of societies, and sound public health systems are key to responding to public health emergencies such as the COVID-19 pandemic. The issue is that public health systems were not equipped to address a global pandemic. To comprehend the state of the US public health system and its ability to adequately respond to the COVID-19 pandemic, it is imperative to reach back and understand its history and some of the policies that have affected it over time. The US public health system has been controlled by self-imposed restrictions over many decades (Fairchild et al. 2010). Historically, it has been involved in efforts to tackle issues like tobacco, lead poisoning, injuries, and the human immunodeficiency virus (HIV), among others. Current and growing public health challenges range from chronic diseases, climate change, disasters, and industrial pollution to bioterrorism and the lack of universal access to healthcare. These challenges pose a threat to the public's health and are further worsened by a weakened public health system. In the US, major deficits to the public health system infrastructure have been documented over time, especially to the workforce, information systems, and organizational capacity (Baker et al. 2005). This chapter will focus on the public health infrastructure, specifically the public health workforce and data/information systems. It will use the essentials of public health as the framework, with a focus on the public health's core function of assurance under the eighth and tenth essential functions—to build a diverse and skilled workforce and build and maintain a strong organizational infrastructure for public health (PHNCI and De Beaumont Foundation 2020).

Even though the public health system is strong in some areas, as evidenced by the efforts to curb tobacco use, vast areas of fragility still remain, caused by years of sapped infrastructure and budget cuts. Notable events in history such as the terrorist attacks of September 11, 2001 (9/11), and the COVID-19 pandemic harshly exposed the frailty of the public health system and highlighted the urgent need to reverse the course of continued inadequacy. The Institute of Medicine published two reports in 2003, *Future of the Public's Health in the 21st Century* and *Who Will Keep the Public Healthy?* (Institute of Medicine 2003), in which it assessed the public health system in the US and concluded that the system was in "disarray." The reports provided recommendations on how to repair the system in order to sufficiently support routine public health activities and respond adequately to emerging threats and emergencies. Federal funding has begun to prioritize public health through action such as the Public Health Improvement Act of 2000, aimed at ensuring the preparedness of every community in the nation by up-grading local and state infrastructure (Baker et al. 2005). Although there has been some federal traction in addressing public health infrastructure, more comprehensive and sustainable funding efforts and support are needed to achieve nationwide success. Without comprehensive national efforts, system gains made in one area of the nation may not materialize in others.

In addition to low prioritization at the federal level, state funding cuts for public health infrastructure and workforce endanger the public health gains that have been achieved and cast doubt on the ability to manage ongoing public health needs and the response to future threats (Baker et al. 2005). Even though cost-benefit analyses can show the economic impact of saving lives, the return on investment for public health efforts is not directly tied to larger economic returns (Butler and Diaz 2017; Stone 2016; Nganga-Good and McLaine 2017b). The US public health system yields its returns in lives improved and lives saved, and therefore is seen as a low priority by state and federal policy-makers. Cost-benefit analysis of Massachusetts Essential School Health Services showed a net benefit of $98.2 million to society and a $2.20 societal gain for every dollar invested in employing full-time school nurses (a subspecialty of public health nurses) (Butler and Diaz 2017). Funding reprogramming or reduction and cuts result in federal, state, and local levels of funding that are inadequate to support the infrastructure or routine core public health functions, or even carry out essential public health services.

Other challenges plaguing the US public health system include outdated policy foundation, decentralized governing authority, deficient organizational capacity, insufficient public health workforce, and limited technological capability (Baker et al. 2005). Ongoing budget cuts at the state level continue to substantially impact local public health departments. The National Association of County and City Health Officials (NACCHO) reported that in the first half of 2011 nearly half of local public health departments cut their staff and more than half cut programs in 2010 (Kuehn 2011). Fifty-five percent of local public health departments eliminated or decreased at least one of their public health programs in 2010 and 2011, while 11% completely eradicated their public health programs (Kuehn 2011). These types of funding cuts compounded losses to public health departments over the years, resulting in loss of funding for prevention efforts, which further hinder planned public health and prevention activities. Programs affected by cuts in public health budgets included health services for women and children, emergency preparedness efforts, and response to outbreaks (Kuehn 2011).

Public Health System Structure

The public health system in the US is not governed by one comprehensive authority, and the operations and oversight are not centralized through any one particular agency. Furthermore, in an effort to promote autonomy and creativity at the level of service provision, authority for the nation's health is divided among federal, state, and local agencies (Baker et al. 2005). The US Constitution was ratified to delegate authority over public health matters to the federal government (Baker et al. 2005). Additionally, Congress apportions public health duties and resources among federal executive agencies like the Centers for Disease Control and Prevention, Health Services and Resources Administration, and Food and Drug Agency through legislation, and also redelegates some responsibilities back to the states through spending programs (Baker et al. 2005). State authorities establish their own public health laws and delegate public health powers to the local authorities, such as cities, counties, and municipalities, as well as assign certain responsibilities to private-sector entities. In doing so, state authorities exercise their responsibility to protect the health of their citizens.

Even though this governing authority and policy foundation structure promotes autonomy and self-determination of public health, it has resulted in a decentralized, fragmented, and uneven public health system, susceptible to political and ideological influence at the state and local levels (Baker et al. 2005). During the COVID pandemic, this was evidenced by public health officials who expressed frustration when pressured not to impose shutdowns and mask mandates (Krisberg 2020; Narayan, Curran, and Foege 2021; DeSalvo et al. 2021). Self-determination and autonomy at the state level allow the ability to consider personal impact and private interests in public health matters, and also tend to enhance local control, appropriateness, and flexibility of programs and the entrusting of policies and programs to authorities at the local level to directly meet the needs of the local populations. The challenge is that policies, priorities, and preferences may differ from state to state, causing fragmentation and inequality in the supply, access, and quality of core public health functions and essential public health services carried out nationwide (Baker et al. 2005).

This funding and policy foundation also affects the infrastructure of the US public health system, creating deficits in organizational structure and capacity. Because the system is decentralized and states assume responsibility for their systems, there is variance in the infrastructure related to organizational structure, staffing, and types of services offered at the different state and local public health agencies (Baker et al. 2005). For example, in some local communities there may be no designated public health agency, leaving public health functions to be carried out by the state public health agencies or even relegated to private agencies through contracts (Baker et al. 2005). This type of organizational structure results in inconsistent and inadequate delivery of services, perpetuating gaps in service delivery, service quality, and access. Thus, the existence and capacity of the public health agency affects the adequacy of services provided and the ability to effectively serve the communities. Furthermore, there is variation in the organization, structure, performance, and existence of public health agencies across the country.

However, improvements in public health organizational capacity and structure were recorded in the US following the 9/11 terrorist attacks, another momentous event in the history of the US that exposed the fragility of the public health system. Subsequent surveys conducted by NACCHO showed that local public health departments did not have the proper infrastructure to adequately provide apt and timely public health response (Baker et al. 2005). At the time of 9/11, not only were public health departments not well prepared, but they did not have comprehensive emergency response plans and lacked the needed resources to properly respond to inquiries (Baker et al. 2005). However, following the attacks, public health officials reported that their agencies' organizational capacity had improved, especially in their ability to respond to bioterrorism, but their capacity to respond to other threats and emergencies continued to be limited (Baker et al. 2005). This is one reason the COVID-19 pandemic had such a devastating effect on the nation's population.

US Public Health Workforce

The funding and policy foundation also affects the public health workforce. Due to funding cuts and reprioritization, the public health workforce has dwindled immensely. Over the thirty-year period from 1970 to 2000, the ratio of public health workforce to US residents fell from 1 in 457 to 1 in 635 (Baker et al. 2005). These numbers have continued to fall due to several reasons, including lack of funding to support hiring needed public health professionals, low salaries, increased rates of retirement/attrition, nonreplacement of vacated positions, hiring freezes, lack of qualified applicants, relocation requirements, and the absence of validated standards for positions required to carry out essential functions (Beck, Boulton, and Coronado 2014; Nganga-Good and McLaine 2017a; Resnick et al. 2019). These shortages affect the adequacy of the supply of the public health workforce and are further exacerbated by a lack of resources and opportunities available to train and certify such professionals.

A 1989 study estimated that only 44% of public health workers had any formal academic public health training and only 34% had advanced public health degrees (Baker et al. 2005). These numbers have increased since 1989, but the training of public health workers is still not commensurate with public health needs nationwide. The inadequate training and supply of public health workers involves all levels of the public health workforce, including its leadership, and areas of practice such as nursing, paraprofessionals, environmental health, and epidemiology. Not only is the adequacy of training of the next generation of public health professionals an issue, but the current practicing workforce are aging out or letting go of their jobs and not being replaced (Nganga-Good and McLaine 2017a). In Maine, reports showed that public health nurses are vital in serving the state's population, especially in gap areas like rural communities, by providing essential services such as administering immunizations, conducting screening and testing for infections such as tuberculosis, and conducting postpartum home visits for new mothers to help the transition to parenthood; however, their ability to provide such services has been compromised over time because of decreasing public health nursing staff, vacant positions not being filled, and workforce funding being diverted (Stone 2016). This decline is expected to continue, and the inadequacy in the public health workforce is detrimental to the ability of the US public health system to meet the routine needs of the population as well as respond to public health threats and emergencies.

US Public Health Infrastructure

The US public health system also contends with infrastructural challenges related to inconsistent application of information technology. While some public health systems are advanced in their use of information technology to support surveillance, data collection, reporting, records, and workflow, others do not have access to adequate or appropriate technology or use antiquated technology (DeSalvo et al. 2021). This means that in some areas of the nation public health systems function to their full capacity in using information technology, while in other areas public health services are hampered by insufficient information technological capacity. While the US healthcare system as a whole has benefited from vast technological advancements, as is evident in the evolution of testing equipment such as MRIs, surgical procedures, pharmaceutical developments, and use of electronic health records, the public health system is still lagging behind in the utilization of information technology to conduct essential public health services (DeSalvo et al. 2021). Due to limited funding and unconducive policy foundation, public health departments have to prioritize funding to basic needs such as staffing and service delivery. The use of the most up-to-date computer software for a public health department may be compared to reaching self-actualization in Maslow's theory, and takes a back seat to other, more pertinent needs.

Since the nation's healthcare needs have become more complex over time and the nation has been continuously faced by challenges such as public health emergencies, the decline in the public health workforce and infrastructure over time has resulted in a severe deterioration of the public health system and an inability to effectively respond to ongoing needs (Baker et al. 2005). Many public health departments face a variety of hardships, including limited funding; silo program–based funding that often does not holistically address pertinent public health and operations issues; staffing issues arising from lack of competitive salaries; poor working conditions, including old, poorly maintained buildings; and poor recognition of and respect for the expertise by policy-makers and legislators. A sound public health system that includes adequate infrastructure and workforce ensures the ability to execute core functions and deliver essential public health services efficiently. However, recent and continued cuts in federal and state funding counter the gains that have been achieved in the system and create uncertainty about the future of the system. Cuts to public health services make those services less accessible and cause reduction in hours for the workforce. Without funding to sustain certain public health programs or support the workforce who deliver the services, these services may become extinct (Kuehn 2011). To be able to effectively manage the public's health and respond to current and emerging threats, the public health system will require infrastructure support and strengthening efforts; however, the system faces numerous challenges that make attaining the ideal public health system unreachable (Baker et al. 2005).

Public Health COVID-19 Response

When COVID-19 was declared a pandemic in March 2020, the US public health system was already strained after years of poor funding allocation, funding cuts and rigid funding streams, institutional siloes, decreased staffing, and antiquated, fragmented data and information systems—concerns that had been raised by advocates for years (Baker et al. 2005; DeSalvo et al. 2021; Krisberg 2021; Kuehn 2011). Previous public health emergencies such as H1N1, SARS, and Zika demonstrated that our public health systems could be overwhelmed by similar future emergencies, and yet, almost ten years later, we had not heeded to the calls for action (Smith 2021). Many communities were already burdened with other health issues, such as the substance use disorder crisis, gaps in mental health care, infectious disease outbreaks, increase in chronic diseases rates, environmental hazards and disasters, health disparities, and social justice issues (TFAH 2019).

According to J. P. Leider, director of the Center for Public Health Workforce and Applied Practice at the University of Minnesota, public health, unlike other government sectors, never fully recovered from the Great Recession. He found that per capita public health spending, including maternal-child health, communicable disease control, and chronic disease prevention spending, was flat, or decreased, in every category other than injury prevention, which had a modest increase (Smith 2021). State and local health department spending had also dropped by over 16% since 2008, and less than 3% of their government funding was allocated to public health (Weber et al. 2020). The strained public health system also affected the workforce. Federal, state, tribal, and local public health had lost nearly a quarter of its workforce (50,000 positions) since the 2008 economic downturn (Krisberg 2020; Weber et al. 2020). Several studies prior to the pandemic indicated that more than a third to nearly half of the public health workforce was considering leaving their organizations (Halverson 2019; Beck, Boulton, and Coronado 2014). The pandemic also presented an opportunity for enhancements such as increased awareness of the need for a functioning and stable public health system in order to address the current and emerging health needs of the nation. The pandemic has also highlighted the crucial need to improve public health, including building a sustainable workforce and infrastructure.

Ramping up the COVID-19 response was no easy feat, and the response was marred by politics, economic woes, fear, mistrust, differences in opinion/beliefs/values, vaccine hesitancy, stigma, discrimination, and harassment and threats to public health staff. There were also many unknowns, myths, and conspiracy theories. Policies often had to be made rapidly based on the information available at the time; guidance changed over time, making risk communication difficult, and was often contradictory (intentionally and unintentionally); and COVID-19 mandates varied between jurisdictions. Sometimes the response at the federal, regional, state, and local jurisdiction differed, further exacerbating the overall response to the pandemic (DeSalvo et al. 2021).

The COVID-19 vaccine rollout also brought another complication to the national response. Vaccine hesitancy, conspiracy theories, and mixed information about COVID-19 intervention and the vaccines were common. This created divisions between those who were for vaccines and those that were against them, creating tensions in society. Vaccine mandates also resulted in numerous debates, differences of opinion, and protests. Vaccine mandates in the workplace led to staffing and legal challenges, including staff quitting their jobs over vaccine mandates ("Hospital Worker Quits" 2021; Cerullo 2021). Amidst all this was an understaffed but dedicated public health workforce that did what they do best in times of crisis.

Public Health Workforce

It is important to underscore the vital role of the public health workforce in the US during the pandemic, and the impact of inadequate staffing on the pandemic response. Existing public health staff were either reassigned or had the COVID-19 pandemic response added to their regular duties. Staff COVID-19 response duties included testing, lab services, contact tracing, vaccinations, health education and risk communication, data management and surveillance, policy development and implementation, mandates enforcement, program planning, implementation, monitoring and evaluation, fiscal and personnel management, supply chain and logistics management, and community planning and mobilization. Some jurisdictions were faster than others in launching a coordinated response, depending on the local emergency preparedness capacity and infrastructure capabilities. Many core public health functions were stalled for months after the country went into shutdown mode. Some services and functions resumed over a year later, and many staff continued to work from home. Once health departments returned to full operation, major catch-up with work activities was needed, and some programs may never be able to fully recover from the shutdown. How many school-aged children missed their immunizations, how many vulnerable women could not access family planning services, and how many people with chronic diseases skipped their medications because they could not access care in a timely fashion? As with many other industries in the US, the impact of the shutdown on the public health system and the nation's health may take years to fully comprehend and address.

Prior to the pandemic, many public health departments and jurisdictions were already operating on a shoestring budget and staffing capacity, especially after the 2008 financial crisis; consequently, additional funding and staff were needed to respond to the pandemic (DeSalvo et al. 2021). Many health departments' programs had been phased out or outsourced, leading to elimination of positions. Not only did the phasing out of programs affect the continuation of services, but agency historical knowledge and experienced staff were lost, which were critically needed during the pandemic. The public health workforce is also aging, and uncompetitive salaries make it difficult to recruit and retain staff (Baker et al. 2005).

Provisions mostly from state-of-emergency funds allowed for quick hiring and training of temporary staff, who were hired to assist with testing, contact tracing, and vaccinations, among other tasks. The federal COVID-19 response funding also had decent allocations for enhancing the public health workforce, which led to a substantial surge in the number of staff hired to respond to pandemic needs (Kilmarx, Long, and Reid 2021; DeSalvo et al. 2021; Weber et al. 2020). However, most of these funding streams were one-time emergency funds that cannot build a sustainable workforce in the long term (Kilmarx, Long, and Reid 2021). Strategies to expand and retain the public health workforce especially at the local, tribal, territorial, and state levels are needed as much as during the peak of the pandemic. These strategies could include ensuring competitive salaries, favorable professional development and advancement opportunities, loan repayment and tuition reimbursement programs, pipeline programs, and potentially the expansion of the US Public Health Service (Kilmarx, Long, and Reid 2021). Sustainable funding and intentional prioritization of public health will be critical in sustaining an adequate well-trained and diverse workforce and public health infrastructure. Furthermore, policy, structural, and system changes will be needed to ensure that the increased federal funding benefits the local and state health departments' workforce and infrastructure.

In addition to staffing shortages, the prolonged public health response resulted in negative physical and psychosocial effects in the workforce, such as burnout, anxiety, insomnia, depression, compassion fatigue, and emotional exhaustion (Stone et al. 2021). Not only did many have to deal with the fear of getting infected and/or transmitting the virus to their loved ones, but some did become infected, and many lost their loved ones and watched their colleagues and community members die. Others had to be separated from their loved ones for fear of transmitting the virus. Many worked hours on end without breaks or days off, sometimes working while they were not feeling well and feeling guilty when taking time off to recuperate (Weber et al. 2020). These physical and psychosocial effects may exacerbate staffing issues when they prematurely leave the workforce or are unable to perform to their fullest capacity due to poor health.

To make matters worse for the strained workforce, many health practitioners reported being threatened, harassed, bullied, and stigmatized (Stone et al. 2021). Then there were the political conflicts between health practitioners and legislators and threats to the public health authorities during the COVID-19 shutdown and COVID-19 mandates, mainly by legislators (Krisberg 2020; Narayan, Curran, and Foege 2021). This resulted in top officials and experienced staff resigning in the midst of a pandemic, causing leadership vacuums in a time crisis. All this resulted in undesirable effects on the workforce, including resignations, early retirements, increased use of alcohol and drugs, and difficulty dealing with issues due to poor coping skills. Well-planned and easily accessible provider resilience programs are needed to help providers cope with these stressors and psychosocial issues. Federal COVID-response funding included funding for provider resilience programs (Kilmarx, Long, and Reid 2021). Local resources are also needed to support and sustain these programs beyond the federal funding in order to have a healthy public health workforce capable of responding to current and future public health threats and emergencies.

Generally, hiring and operationalization of funding at most government agencies is a lengthy process that goes through several approval processes (Kilmarx, Long, and Reid 2021). This often results in delays in hiring, distribution of funding to programs and subcontractors, and implementing programs, which impacts the outcomes of the programs or initiatives. For example, it takes several months to recruit, interview, and hire staff or to execute a work subcontract. In the case of subcontracts, it may take months before vendors are paid for their services, which can be problematic for smaller community-based organizations that do not have a large pool of expendable resources even though they are often at the core of local community responses. Some COVID-19 response delays may have resulted from these complexities, but further delays were largely averted by the emergency protocols, which allowed for some flexibility in hiring, contracting, and procurement procedures. Future response plans should have mechanisms for quickly hiring and operationalizing funding while ensuring that public funds and resources are used for the intended purposes and have the intended outcomes. Governmental administrative barriers such as those in human resources, fiscal, and procurement departments need to be addressed and more favorable policies and procedures implemented to avoid implementation delays and bottlenecks that could be disastrous in responding to emergencies and delivering essential public health core services.

Data and Information Systems

As a result of years of working with limited resources, antiquated systems, and complicated government and administrative policies and procedures, many public health departments have honed their expertise in building coalitions and collaborating with various stakeholders, including hospitals, primary care providers, behavioral and other health providers, academia, and non–health sector organizations. During the COVID-19 pandemic, health departments collaborated with the private sector and academia to assist them in rapidly establishing dashboards and websites to track the data. For example, Louisiana's health department collaborated with Blue Cross Blue Shield to develop a COVID-19 Outbreak Tracker, the Washington state health department partnered with Microsoft to develop a data dashboard, and the Michigan health department partnered with academia to develop data dashboards and make model-based projections to aid decision-making (DeSalvo et al. 2021). The widespread closures resulted in most of the nonemergent health services being offered through virtual platforms such telehealth (DeSalvo et al. 2021). This enhanced the need for and use of technology that could be scaled up post-COVID-19 to increase health access, especially in rural and underserved areas, and improve overall health outcomes.

Furthermore, health departments usually work well with their local communities and grassroots organizations to address public health issues. Many members of the community view the health department as trusted source of information; it may be the only source of health services in some resource-limited areas (DeSalvo et al. 2021). Public health agencies have historically utilized community health workers and patient advocates to improve health outcomes and access to care, and to educate communities. These staff members are often members of the communities they work in and therefore have a good rapport with their communities. Leveraging their expertise and their established partnerships and relationships was advantageous during the COVID-19 pandemic and helped in coordinating the pandemic response. Enhancement and sustenance of these collaborations are critical in the delivery of public health services and in responding to public health emergencies.

The pandemic response was hampered by public health systems' insufficient information technology capacity. Many public health departments have antiquated data and information systems that are often in silo based on individual program use and not integrated to communicate with each other or share the data across entities (DeSalvo et al. 2021). Prior to the pandemic, program data had to be entered in various databases and could not be easily crossmatched, which can result in fragmentation of services and uncoordinated care. In fact, some departments still use paper records. This posed problems during the COVID-19 closures, which limited working from the office. Some had only old desktop computers, and their information systems were not secure enough to support virtual private networks or working from home. One example involved county public health offices in California. During the COVID-19 pandemic, biochemist Joe DeRisi and his team from the University of California, San Francisco, built a testing lab within eight days and offered to provide free COVID testing services and results in twenty-four hours to the county (Dickerson 2021). In one county, official results had to be sent by fax, so the lab had to buy a fax machine—and another one for the county public health office, whose ancient machine could not handle the volume of results the lab was sending, and the county did not have the budget to buy a new one itself (Dickerson 2021). To support seamless and comprehensive services and reporting, modernized and user-friendly data and information systems are needed.

Public health system infrastructure capacity related to information systems also impacted vaccinations. In the context of the COVID-19 response, health departments struggled with contact tracing due to challenges such as blocked or unanswered calls (DeSalvo et al. 2021). States ended up setting up a standard tag such as "MD COVID" for Maryland, to be used on their phones' call ID to help identify their calls and reduce the number of blocked or unanswered calls. Others established dedicated COVID-19 call centers to triage questions and keep their communities informed (DeSalvo et al. 2021). These enhancements can be sustained and replicated post-COVID-19 to facilitate public health responses in times of emergencies as well as provision of regular public health services.

Fragmented data and surveillance systems also posed challenges for a coordinated response. With people being tested or vaccinated by different entities that did not have data-sharing agreements, it was impossible to verify past testing and vaccination history except by relying on self-reporting. Further complicating data accuracy, there were reports of falsified test results and vaccination records. Contact tracing significantly helped with reducing transmissions, but not everyone adhered to the quarantine and isolation guidance, and some were not forthcoming with the information needed to adequately facilitate proper contact tracing (DeSalvo et al. 2021). Mistrust of the system and the government, coupled with fragmented data and information systems, may also have resulted in poor-quality, untimely, and inaccurate data to manage contact tracing.

On the other hand, COVID-19 may have forced health departments to scale up and enhance their data and information systems, such as use of text-messaging platforms for contact tracing, daily communication, and securing their information systems to allow staff to work from home where possible for continuity of services. Health departments and other government agencies used media, including social media, to communicate with the community and keep stakeholders informed. The use of social media by government agencies is a welcome change that can enhance public health systems' ability to respond to emergencies and deliver essential public health services. Sustainable funding and intentional commitment to modernizing data, surveillance, and information systems are needed to ensure that these system enhancements are well maintained and functional for day-to-day operations and to respond to emergencies.

LESSONS LEARNED AND RECOMMENDATIONS FOR FUTURE PRACTICE

The COVID-19 pandemic has taught us a lot of lessons. These include increased awareness of what is public health, what it does, how it works, and what is needed to ensure that the system is capable of responding to current and future public health threats and emergencies. Like previous major crises in the world, such as major wars and pandemics, which resulted in proactive collective action that facilitated the creation of progressive institutions such as the United Nations and the World Health Organization, COVID-19 has presented an opportunity to take proactive action to ensure that the world is better prepared for the next global public health emergency (Narayan, Curran, and Foege 2021). A well-prepared public health system must have an adequate, well-trained, and diverse public health workforce, as well as comprehensive well-coordinated data and information systems to execute the public health work. Efforts should be made to ensure that there are enough resources to hire, retain, and develop a diverse public health workforce—competitive salaries, favorable hiring and promotion processes, professional development and advancement opportunities, provider resilience and retention programs, recognition, and respect. For the staff and system to work efficiently, data and information systems need to be sophisticated enough to ensure the availability of accurate and comprehensive real-time data to help make data-informed decisions and that policies and procedures are in place to ensure smooth operations. Decisions should be quickly communicated and translated into policy and practice and disseminated appropriately to the different audiences. This will only be possible with adequate and sustainable public health funding that provides workforce and infrastructure support.

The other lessons learned include the need to address health and geographical disparities, social and structural determinants of health, and barriers at the individual, community, and system levels. The COVID-19 pandemic highlighted many disparities between the haves and have-nots in society. These crossed racial and socioeconomic lines and geographical areas, and sometimes the response differed based on the political affiliation of a jurisdiction. It is critical to have a unified response to widespread emergencies such as a pandemic while being careful to customize the response to what is happening at the local level. For example, the COVID-19 response in an urban area that is densely populated and resource-rich may not be translatable to a rural area. Similarly, the local cultural context should be factored into the response. In a community where multigenerational families live in the same household or where there has been generational mistrust of the system, attention should be paid when educating the community about the risks of COVID-19, how to isolate or quarantine in case of an exposure or illness, and the safety of the testing and treatment options.

Overall, there is a need for intentional prioritization of public health funding and widespread awareness that public health not only plays an important role in protecting, promoting, and maintaining the health of entire communities, it also affects everyone's daily life, from ensuring air, food, water, housing, and environmental safety to responding to and mitigating disease outbreaks. In alignment with the Healthy People 2030 Public Health Infrastructure objectives, a strong public health system should have high-performing health departments, workforce development and training, data and information systems, planning, and partnerships in order to respond to the nation's public health needs (DHHS 2020). Efforts to support public health improvements should include support for the current and new public health practitioners. Decision-makers and stakeholders need to make efforts to ensure adequate and sustainable funding in order to guarantee a diverse, skilled, and competent workforce and to build and maintain a strong organizational infrastructure including efficient, up-to-date data, surveillance, and information systems so that the US public health system can better respond to emergencies and public health threats.

DISCUSSION QUESTION

- How can the US proactively ensure that its public health system is adequately prepared to provide health security and respond to the next public health threat or emergency?

REFERENCES

Baker, Edward L., Margaret A. Potter, Deborah L. Jones, Shawna L. Mercer, Joan P. Cioffi, Lawrence W. Green, Paul K. Halverson, et al. 2005. "The Public Health Infrastructure and Our Nation's Health." *Annual Review of Public Health* 26, no. 1: 303–18. https://doi.org/10.1146/annurev.publhealth.26.021304.144647.

Beck, A. J., M. L. Boulton, and F. Coronado. 2014. "Enumeration of the Governmental Public Health Workforce, 2014." *American Journal of Preventive Medicine* 47, no. 5 (November): S306–13. https://doi.org/10.1016/j.amepre.2014.07.018.

Butler, S., and C. Diaz. 2017. *Nurses as Intermediaries in the Promotion of Community Health: Exploring Their Roles and Challenges.* Washington, DC: Brookings Institution. https://www.brookings.edu/wp-content/uploads/2017/09/es_20170921_nurses_as_intermediaries.pdf.

Cerullo, Megan. 2021. "Can You Be Fired for Refusing to Get Vaccinated against COVID-19?" *Moneywatch,* CBS News, August 31, 2021. https://www.cbsnews.com/news/covid-vaccine-mandate-refusal-employment-firing/.

Ciotti, Marco, Massimo Ciccozzi, Alessandro Terrinoni, Wen-Can Jiang, Cheng-Bin Wang, and Sergio Bernardini. 2020. "The COVID-19 Pandemic." *Critical Reviews in Clinical Laboratory Sciences* 57, no. 6: 365–88. https://doi.org/10.1080/10408363.2020.1783198.

DeSalvo, Karen, Bob Hughes, Mary Bassett, Georges Benjamin, Michael Fraser, Sandro Galea, J. Nadine Gracia, and Jeffrey Howard. 2021. "Public Health COVID-19 Impact Assessment: Lessons Learned and Compelling Needs." *NAM Perspectives,* April 7, 2021. https://doi.org/10.31478/202104c.

DHHS (US Department of Health and Human Services). 2020. "Healthy People 2030." US Department of Health and Human Services—Office of Disease Prevention and Health Promotion. https://health.gov/healthypeople/objectives-and-data/browse-objectives/public-health-infrastructure.

Dickerson, John. 2021. "Doctors, Scientists Who Warned Officials about Oncoming Pandemic Focus of New Michael Lewis Book." *60 Minutes,* May 5, 2021. https://www.cbsnews.com/news/michael-lewis-premonition-60-minutes-2021-05-02/.

Fairchild, Amy L., David Rosner, James Colgrove, Ronald Bayer, and Linda P. Fried. 2010. "The EXODUS of Public Health: What History Can Tell Us about the Future." *American Journal of Public Health* 100, no. 1 (January): 54–63. https://doi.org/10.2105/AJPH.2009.163956.

Halverson, P. K. 2019. "Ensuring a Strong Public Health Workforce for the 21st Century: Reflections on PH WINS 2017." *Journal of Public Health Management and Practice* 25: S1–3. https://doi.org/10.1097/PHH.0000000000000967.

"Hospital Worker Quits as Maryland Vaccine Mandate Set to Take Effect." 2021. WJZ News (CBS News Baltimore), August 31, 2021. https://www.cbsnews.com/baltimore/news/hospital-worker-quits-as-maryland-vaccine-mandate-set-to-take-effect-baltimore-city-to-require-employee-vaccinations/.

Institute of Medicine. 2003. *The Future of the Public's Health in the 21st Century.* Washington, DC: National Academies Press. https://doi.org/10.17226/10548.

Kilmarx, Peter H., Theodore Long, and Michael J. A. Reid. 2021. "A National Public Health Workforce to Control COVID-19 and Address Health Disparities in the United States." *Open Forum Infectious Diseases* 8, no. 7: ofab304. https://doi.org/10.1093/ofid/ofab304.

Krisberg, Kim. 2020. "Already-Strained US Public Health Workforce Grapples with COVID-19: Despite Resource Gaps, Workers Fight On." *Nation's Health,* June 2020. https://www.thenationshealth.org/content/50/4/1.2.

Kuehn, B. M. 2011. "Public Health Cuts Threaten Preparedness, Preventive Health Services." *JAMA* 306, no. 18: 1965–66. https://doi.org/10.1001/jama.2011.1623.

Narayan, K. M. Venkat, James W. Curran, and William H. Foege. 2021. "The COVID-19 Pandemic as an Opportunity to Ensure a More Successful Future for Science and Public Health." *JAMA* 325, no. 6: 525. https://doi.org/10.1001/jama.2020.23479.

Nganga-Good, Carolyn, and Pat McLaine. 2017a. "Enumerating and Characterizing an Aging and Shrinking Workforce in Maryland: Public Health Nursing." Presented at the American Public Health Association Annual Meeting, Atlanta, GA. https://apha.confex.com/apha/2017/meetingapp.cgi/Paper/380720.

———. 2017b. "Unsung Heroes of Public Health: Public Health Nurses Leading the Charge to Healthier and More Equitable Communities." Presented at the American Public Health Association Annual Meeting, Atlanta, GA. https://apha.confex.com/apha/2017/meetingapp.cgi/Paper/381470.

PHNCI (Public Health National Center for Innovations) and De Beaumont Foundation. 2020, "10 Essential Public Health Services." Public Health Systems and Best Practices. https://www.cdc.gov/publichealthgateway/publichealthservices/essentialhealthservices.html.

Resnick, B. A., L. Morlock, M. Diener-West, E. A. Stuart, M. Spencer, and J. M. Sharfstein. 2019. "PH WINS and the Future of Public Health Education." *Journal of Public Health Management and Practice* 25: S10–12. https://doi.org/10.1097/PHH.0000000000000955.

Smith, Carl. 2021. "What Will It Take to Recruit and Retain Public Health Workers?" Governing: The Future of States and Localities, August 21, 2021. https://www.governing.com/work/what-will-it-take-to-recruit-and-retain-public-health-workers?_amp=true&__twitter_impression=true&s=09.

Stone, Kahler W., Kristina W. Kintziger, Meredith A. Jagger, and Jennifer A. Horney. 2021. "Public Health Workforce Burnout in the COVID-19 Response in the U.S." *International Journal of Environmental Research and Public Health* 18, no. 8: 4369. https://doi.org/10.3390/ijerph18084369.

Stone, M. 2016. "Maine Has Sliced the Ranks of Nurses Who Prevent Outbreaks, Help Drug-Affected Babies." *Maine Focus,* August 18, 2016. http://bangordailynews.com/2016/08/09/news/bangor/maine-has-sliced-the-ranks-of-nurses-who-prevent-outbreaks-help-drug-affected-babies/.

TFAH (Trust for America's Health). 2019. *The Impact of Chronic Underfunding of America's Public Health System: Trends, Risks, and Recommendations, 2019.* Washington, DC: Trust for America's Health. https://www.tfah.org/report-details/2019-funding-report/.

Weber, L., L. Ungar, M. R. Smith, H. Recht, and A. M. Barry-Jester. 2020. "Hollowed-Out Public Health System Faces More Cuts amid Virus." *Kaiser Family Foundation Health News,* July 1, 2020. https://khn.org/news/us-public-health-system-underfunded-under-threat-faces-more-cuts-amid-covid-pandemic/.

13

Public Health Leadership in the Times of COVID-19

A Tale of Three Countries

PABLO VILLALOBOS DINTRANS, CLAIRE CHAUMONT, AND JEFFREY GLENN

> It was the best of times, it was the worst of times, it was the age of
> wisdom, it was the age of foolishness, it was the epoch of belief, it was
> the epoch of incredulity, it was the season of Light, it was the season of
> Darkness, it was the spring of hope, it was the winter of despair, we had
> everything before us, we had nothing before us, we were all going direct
> to Heaven, we were all going direct the other way—in short, the period
> was so far like the present period, that some of its noisiest authorities
> insisted on its being received, for good or for evil, in the superlative
> degree of comparison only.
>
> —Charles Dickens, *A Tale of Two Cities*

The famous opening sentence of Charles Dickens's 1859 novel *A Tale of Two Cities* could describe the situation of many cities around the world during the COVID-19 pandemic. On December 31, 2019, Chinese authorities informed the World Health Organization (WHO) about an outbreak of an unknown respiratory disease. On January 30, 2020, the WHO declared the outbreak of COVID-19 a public health emergency of international concern. Cases extended quickly from the city of Wuhan to other parts of China and, since then, to the whole world (WHO 2020a). By August 6, 2020, there were almost 19 million cases confirmed in 216 countries, with more than 700,000 deaths (WHO 2020b). One year later, in August 2021, this number had shot to 212 million cases and 4.4 million deaths (WHO 2021).

Just as Dickens describes, we are living today in conflicted times. After advances in science and technology, huge improvements in life expectancy and health systems, and a relatively long period of global peace and political stability, COVID-19 emerged as an unexpected threat to many things we took for granted. It raised several questions, not only regarding the virus itself but also countries' responses to the pandemic. Looking back and thinking forward, we all ask whether something different could have been done to deal with the disease better.

In this context, there is a critical need for public leadership. Crises always present complex leadership challenges for people in positions of authority (Boin and 't Hart 2003). Public leaders are expected to play several roles, including understanding the problem, as well as planning and implementing solutions to restore normalcy; they are also expected to communicate with their people (Jong 2017). Effective communication is essential to ensuring that authorities are perceived as leaders as they act within their roles to manage the crisis.

The COVID-19 situation shared similarities with other types of crises, but it also differed in several important aspects. First, it was a public health crisis, which required a different type of specific technical knowledge and experience from many other recent crises (Deitchman 2013). In addition, while uncertainty is to be expected in any crisis, leaders can usually quickly gather data to make sense of the situation. Due to its novelty, the lack (or excess) of information, and the rise of new variants, COVID-19 presented an unusual level of uncertainty, making it an endless conundrum for decision-makers. This situation was neatly summarized by Netherlands prime minister Mark Rutte, who remarked early on in the pandemic that "in crises like this, you have to make 100 percent of the decisions with 50 percent of the knowledge, and bear the consequences" ("'Everyone Stay Home'" 2020). Second, it was different from other public health crises not just in terms of its consequences and countries' capacities to foresee the event, but in its scale (Hannah et al. 2009). As a global problem, COVID-19 posed the same (meta-)problem to different countries with different contexts. In addition, this situation added the feature of being a "creeping crisis" that arrived slowly and has been slow to leave (Boin, Lodge, and Luesing 2020). Finally, COVID-19 intermingled health, social and economic aspects on a scale rarely seen before during modern disease outbreaks, becoming a megacrisis (Boin, Lodge, and Luesing 2020).

Given this scenario, we consider where breakdowns in public leadership occurred during the COVID-19 response, whether public leadership could have played a different role in managing the crisis, and how we can encourage this type of leadership in the future. In particular, we consider what role public health leaders—individuals who have vision, influence, and competencies regarding public health issues (Yphantides, Escoboza, and Macchione 2015)—should play in public health crises.

Following Dickens's book, our tale of three places—Chile, France, and the United States—contains different stories about leadership during COVID-19. These countries cover different geographical areas, demographic profiles, and economic, social, and cultural differences. As table 13.1 shows, in terms of the COVID-19 situation, they also present interesting differences: the pandemic reached the United States and France almost a month before the first case was identified in Chile, and the countries exhibited different outcomes in terms of cases, although the three of them were among the most affected countries in the world during 2020 (Johns Hopkins University 2020). All these differences constitute an opportunity to analyze the evolution of politics, leadership, and public health under a single problem in different contexts.

TABLE 13.1. COVID-19 IMPACT IN SELECTED COUNTRIES

Indicator	Chile	France	United States
Population (millions)	19.1	65.3	331.0
COVID-19 starting date	March 3, 2020	January 24, 2020	January 20, 2020
By August 20, 2021			
Cumulative cases	1,630,831	6,362,616	36,924,023
Cases per 100,000 people	8,531.15	11,155.2	9,782.72
Cumulative deaths	36,456	111,476	618,468
Deaths per 100,000 people	190.71	186.85	171.81
% population fully vaccinated	70.2	56.5	52.3

Source: WHO (2021) and Johns Hopkins University (2021).

A TALE REVISITED: NEW SCENARIOS

Building on our previous analysis (Glenn, Chaumont, and Villalobos Dintrans 2020), we follow a similar strategy and framework to study the described situation. This update and extension are much needed because:

1. The previous analysis tells an incomplete story. It was written in the middle of 2020, when many uncertainties about the situation of the pandemic remained, particularly its evolution (e.g., duration, ability of countries to deal with it, arising of new variants) and full impact on the countries.

2. Revisiting the original analysis at a later date also allows us to analyze other key crisis-management tasks (termination and learning) that were not highlighted in the analysis of the first months of the pandemic in 2020.

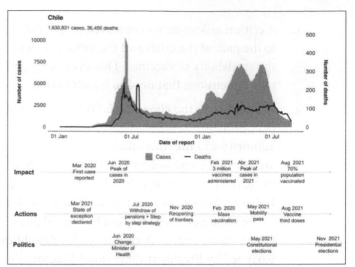

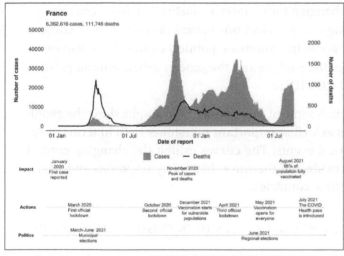

FIGURE 13.1. Time frame of COVID-19 and political events in Chile, France, and the United States (August 20, 2021).

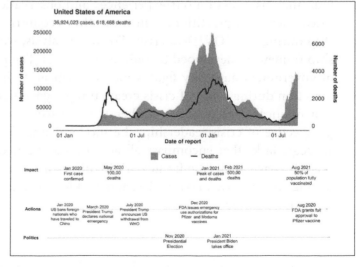

3. A critical milestone was observed at the global level that relates both to the path of the crisis and the influence of politics and leadership: the availability of vaccines. This event changed the analysis and posed new dimensions that need to be addressed.

4. In addition to the changing COVID-19 scenario, the political environments in the studied countries altered. Some changes in authority and the interrelation between these events and COVID-19 are relevant to include: the United States had a presidential election in November 2020, which led to a change of president, with Joe Biden replacing Donald Trump; France had municipal elections in the spring of 2020, marked by record abstention, the rise of the Green Party, and weak results for La Republique en Marche, the party led by President Emmanuel Macron. Finally, Chile started the process of changing the country's constitution and faced presidential and congressional elections toward the end of 2021. These important changes in the countries' political context were also expected to change the analysis and the general debate around politics, leadership, and COVID-19.

Figure 13.1 summarizes some of these issues. The graphs show the evolution of COVID-19 cases as well as important milestones both in terms of epidemiological and political events. The curves exhibit the changing context in which decisions are made and the ways that policy responses and health outcomes relate in the three countries.

A FRAMEWORK TO UNDERSTAND LEADERSHIP IN CRISIS: CRITICAL TASKS

Our analysis draws on our experiences and observations as public health researchers and practitioners in these three countries to explore leadership during the COVID-19 crisis. For our analysis, we use a crisis leadership framework developed by Boin et al. (2005). The public's expectations of government authority figures making critical decisions and providing direction during times of crisis create unique governance challenges with real political consequences. Rather than focusing on a person-centered perspective of crisis leadership, the model defines leadership as a set of strategic tasks that encompass all activities associated with the stages of crisis management. The framework identifies five core tasks of leadership during crises: sense-making, decision-making, meaning-making, termination, and learning.

Sense-making involves leaders' attempts to recognize that a crisis exists and to understand what is happening and why as events unfold in real time. This task presents several significant leadership challenges. Public organizations are usually ill-designed to quickly identify and respond to threats, and when they do, it is typical for crucial information to become subject to intra- and interorganizational politics (Boin et al. 2005, 20–22). Stress associated with professional (and personal) responsibilities is amplified during a crisis and may have serious consequences for the performance of decision-makers (29). Additional individual constraints, such as cognitive heuristics and biases, egocentric motives, and affiliations to particular groups or values, affect leaders' capacity for processing large amounts of data (31–33).

Decision-making involves evaluating alternatives, making critical choices, and coordinating the response network in the face of uncertainty and political risk. Group dynamics among the various stakeholders involved in a crisis response make this task inherently difficult; some groups tend toward excessive cordiality and conformity while other groups are paralyzed by conflict and politicking (46–48). Since critical decisions are often required across a range of policy-makers and small groups, factors such as decentralization, interorganizational relations, and improvisation are critical for the decision-making task (52–55). Rather than acting as all-powerful decision-makers, effective leaders should consider themselves designers and facilitators of a robust coordination process (64).

Meaning-making considers crisis management as political communication and involves leaders' attempts to influence the public's understanding of the situation. The challenge in this task comes from communicating a persuasive narrative in a context of overwhelming amounts of information and uncertainty, all while maintaining credibility and building trust (78). Leaders who succeed may find a greater degree of permissive consensus to enact their policies, while leaders who fail often fall into a vicious cycle of distrust, breeding lower credibility (81). Barriers to effective crisis communication include coordination of outgoing information between government entities, tension between political and administrative messengers, and communicating clearly in the context of mediated messages (77–78). Carefully framing messages, staying attentive to public "rituals," and avoiding unnecessary masking of facts are critical factors in maintaining leaders' credibility (81–87).

The leaders' efforts to return to normalcy and shift away from emergency operations are related to the termination task (93–98). This task represents a political challenge since political factors may lead some actors to seek a premature end to a crisis while others may seek to overextend it. Crisis termination may be considered in terms of both operational and political dimensions. The task of terminating a crisis also includes reconciling with the issue of accountability in order for governance to be restabilized (99–103). Leaders must often negotiate the challenges of accountability to maintain their legitimacy. Successful crisis termination depends largely on accountability processes perceived as legitimate by the population (102). While an honest, truth-telling process may promote systemic improvement that can aid in the management of future crises, heightened political tensions during this process often lead to political blame games (111–12).

Finally, learning involves drawing political and organizational lessons to plan and train for future crises. Whether crises lead to meaningful change depends on the capacity of leaders to learn and their capacity to reform (116). Despite the widespread belief that crises are opportunities for reform, Boin et al. (2005) argue that major changes are inherently difficult and that they can inhibit learning that may actually lead to better management of future crises. Successful reform is more likely if leaders can attribute the causes of the crisis to external factors if their political supporters favor reform, and if they operate in a centralized framework with high levels of authority (Boin et al. 2005, 127–30). One major challenge to learning and reform is that managing a crisis often requires a different type of leadership (i.e., command and control) than managing a learning and reform process (i.e., reflection and persuasion) (131–32).

Using these five core tasks, we extracted examples for each of the selected countries to illustrate how leadership was exercised regarding the management of COVID-19—particularly by public health leaders—but also by political and administrative leaders.

LEADERSHIP IN TIMES IN CRISIS: EXAMPLES FROM CHILE, FRANCE, AND THE UNITED STATES

As described above, several events regarding the COVID-19 pandemic and its management developed since the start of the crisis in 2020. The nature of the problem—including its duration, scale, uncertainty, and permanent change—became a challenge for each country. In addition, countries needed to address other non-COVID-19 issues in a complex political environment. This section explores these issues using the crisis-management framework proposed by Boin et al. (2005). Table 13.2 summarizes the main topics arising from the examples of Chile, France, and the United States, considering the five core leadership tasks proposed by Boin et al. (2005).

TABLE 13.2. SUMMARY OF CORE LEADERSHIP TASKS AND TOPICS

Leadership task	Topics from the case studies
Sense-making (how leaders acknowledge the existence of a crisis)	Creeping crisis means sense-making is continuous, not just at the start. Too much or too little information makes it hard to make sense of the crisis. Public leaders struggle to be seen as legitimate actors to make sense of the crisis. The nature of the crisis evolves: Is this a health crisis? An economic crisis? A civil liberties crisis?
Decision-making (ability to make adequate decisions)	Centralized or decentralized, both in terms of who makes the decisions and how they get applied Tension between politics and scientific experts Balance between health decisions and other decisions (education, freedom of movements, economy)
Meaning-making (political communication)	Credibility of authorities Rise of distrust of science
Terminating	Failed attempts to terminate the crisis in all countries end up extending it. Conflict between slow death of pandemics and need for clear-cut political narratives of success and failure.
Learning	Ability to make (structural) changes as a result of the lessons coming from the pandemic Changes focused on improving the response to crises

Source: Authors' elaboration.

SENSE-MAKING

As described above, sense-making relates to the way in which leaders acknowledge (or do not acknowledge) the existence of the crisis. Throughout the pandemic, we have seen this ability affected by many factors, including the ability of public figures to make sense of an uncertain "creeping" situation, their role in disseminating and making sense of information, their legitimacy in using it, and their ability to reframe or shape the scope of the crisis.

At the beginning of the pandemic in 2020, the initial recognition of the crisis differed in the three countries, with the United States reacting slowly and initially neglecting the real impact of the virus and leaders in both France and Chile quickly recognizing the risk but failing to understand its scale (Glenn, Chaumont, and Villalobos Dintrans 2020). Later on, the crisis duration and dynamics kept posing new challenges to decision-makers. The concept of a creeping crisis, defined as one that arrives slowly and keeps going on for a long time, is key in the discussion of the COVID-19 crisis management (Boin, Lodge, and Luesing 2020). In this case, after the initial crisis recognition, new questions that required sense-making continued to arise as the crisis changed. In the case of the vaccine, people started asking whether the crisis could be terminated by a mass vaccination campaign and, if so, what the real threat was (why keep implementing restrictive preventive measures?). With the rapid emergence of the more contagious and deadly Delta variant in the United States in July 2021, leaders were essentially forced to start the sense-making process over again to recognize the new form of the crisis and appropriately warn the public. Overall, the presidential administration of Joe Biden managed the Delta variant wave much more smoothly than the Trump administration had managed the initial emergence of the virus. Biden and his COVID task force spoke openly and often about the threat of the Delta variant and encouraged state officials and the public to use every means possible—in particular the vaccines—to prevent the spread (Shalal and Mason 2021; Shear, Stolberg, and Karni 2021). However, motivating action to stop the Delta wave was more difficult in many ways due to crisis fatigue and because the country already bore the political scars of more than a year of bitter partisanship and division surrounding COVID-19. Fewer government officials were willing to ask their constituents to make the necessary sacrifices to slow this wave of the pandemic, which proved to be a major barrier to enacting protective public policies. The arrival of the Delta variant also brought new questions; since it became the more prevalent variant in the country in 2021, people continued asking about what to expect of the evolution of the pandemic, the risk of contagion and death, and the effectiveness of the vaccines in this new scenario (Yáñez 2021).

Throughout the pandemic, information proved to be a key issue in making sense and managing the crisis. The lack of information (sometimes the excess of it) acted as a barrier throughout the whole period. New information kept adding entropy: while at the beginning of the pandemic in 2020 the main questions were whether COVID-19 was a real threat (justifying drastic measures), new questions arose as time passed: Can we eliminate COVID-19? What happens with the new variants? Is it dangerous for children? What about the adverse effects of vaccines?

Another important issue regarding the sense-making element evolved around the nature of the crisis. Was this a health crisis or something else? From the beginning of the crisis, an ongoing debate revolved around whether leaders should focus on health or the economy. While many experts correctly recognized the inherent inseparability of the health and economic issues, the false dichotomy that was initially widely accepted impeded efforts to make good public policy that could balance the health and economic needs of the country (Glenn, Chaumont, and Villalobos Dintrans 2020). In hindsight, many political leaders in the United States perceived that the initial lockdowns un-necessarily damaged economic livelihoods, which increased the reluctance of leaders across the political spectrum to enact COVID-19 control policies that had the potential to impede economic growth. In addition, while initially pub-lic debate focused on the divide between health and the economy, it slowly shifted to focusing on personal freedom and government control as stringent measures initially understood as temporary turned long term. In France, at the time of writing, many ongoing demonstrations to protest the government's new health pass (which required citizens to show their vaccine certificate or a recent negative PCR test to access cafés, restaurants, and malls using QR technology) include both anti-vax and anti-pass citizens, the latter protesting the curtail-ing of individual freedom and an increase in government control rather than vaccines per se (Rouquette 2021). In Chile, the local effect of the pandemic and the impact of COVID-19 on the global markets and the economy added to the shocks experienced by the economy during the social outbreak in October 2019. The president of the Central Bank pointed out that a key determinant for economic recovery in the short run is necessarily the flexibilization of the restrictions imposed by the health authorities (Marcel 2020). The debate about whether this was one (health) or two (health and economic) crises has not gone away, with health and economic measures seen as contradictory (Roa 2021).

DECISION-MAKING

In terms of the ability of governments to make adequate decisions, we have observed several tensions at play: centralized versus decentralized, scientific versus political, and health versus broader social considerations.

First, countries' decision-making around the implementation of lockdowns as well as the enforcement of preventive measures evolved substantially across time. Due to existing structures, the United States initially imposed state-level measures, while both Chile and France opted for centralized management of COVID-19 (Glenn, Chaumont, and Villalobos Dintrans 2020). France slowly evolved from a very centralized response, with a strict first lockdown in March 2020 imposed uniformly across the country, to a more nuanced response as the country started to reopen, with the establishment of local measures in regions more affected by the virus ("UPDATE" 2021). Regardless, decisions made by authorities remained concentrated at the national level, with local authorities holding little decision power. Similarly, in 2020 and 2021 in Chile, crisis man-agement was directly addressed by the president and the minister of health, with more authorities being included in the government team throughout the period (e.g., the Ministry of Science in charge of data management and the Ministry of Internal Affairs assuming responsibility for compliance of health measures) (Gobierno de Chile 2021a; Ministerio de Ciencias, Tecnología, Conocimiento e Innovación 2021). The authorities decided to stick to their initial strategy—the Step-by-Step Plan—where local restrictions were implemented from the central level, based on each region's epidemiological context. This strategy was updated to reduce restrictions on vaccinated people and allow the establishment of regional (instead of national) curfews, also based on vaccination coverage (Gobierno de Chile 2021b). Although these changes gave more flexibility to the application of COVID-19 restrictions, decision-making was still centralized; for example, the regional curfew was not in the hands of regional authorities but set by the central government (10 p.m. for regions with less than 80% of the population vaccinated and midnight for regions with more than 80% of the population vaccinated). The situation in the United States—where the decentralized federal system grants significant decision-making authority to individual states—continued to be marked by a wide range of responses between states. To give one example, while the CDC issued guidelines for which populations should be prioritized to receive the vaccine, states ended up with distinct guidelines depending on the decisions of state governors (e.g., some states included teachers in their initial prioritization groups while others did not).

A second key element in this process was the tension between politics and scientific experts in the decision-making process. In all countries, both parties played an important role during the first stage of the pandemic. Disagreement was observed in many cases, but politicians also used technical advisers to justify their actions. In the three countries, scientific committees and institutions were used to validate and communicate information and decisions (Glenn, Chaumont, and Villalobos Dintrans 2020). As COVID-19 progressed, the scientific evidence base available for decision-makers grew, but this did not necessarily lead to better policy decisions. As has been discussed in other research, the political climate in which decisions are made typically plays a bigger role than the evidence available to policy-makers (Greer et al. 2017; Hunter 2016). In the United States, many policy decisions to address the Delta wave were worse than those for the initial surge due to the politicization of the pandemic and to crisis fatigue over time. The political fights in various states over mask and vaccine mandates have received significant attention, but other issues for which sound scientific evidence exists (e.g., the call for improved ventilation in schools) have been largely ignored by many policy-makers. In some cases political leaders enacted policies to limit the decision-making authority of health officials, such as in Utah, where the state legislature passed a law banning local health officials from enacting school mask mandates without the approval of elected county commissions, many of which are highly partisan (Williams 2021). This issue was compounded by the fact that, due to uncertainty around many issues, scientists did not necessarily agree among themselves. This was exemplified by the Great Barrington Declaration, a statement put forward by three recognized academics criticizing lockdowns, and, in France, by the debacle around the efficacy of hydroxychloroquine against COVID, an antimalarial medicine, first hailed as "promising" by the government based on dubious studies led by a controversial doctor and then widely discredited by the scientific community (Gump 2020; Sayare 2020).

Finally, the acknowledgment that the crisis was not over after the initial decrease in cases considerably broadened the scope of decisions to be made by public leaders, including the need to weigh health considerations against other social factors. One of the persistent debates involved the opening of schools. In Chile, this issue turned into a battleground, generating a permanent debate on whether schools are prepared to reopen, their ability to implement effective strategies to education at distance, and the long-term effect of children's confinement in terms of their educational, social, and emotional outcomes (Ministerio de Educación 2020; Murillo and Duk 2020; UNICEF 2021). The decision was eventually put in the hands of schools and local authorities and included a (failed) attempt to impeach the minister of education in August 2021 (Garrido 2021). As mentioned in the preceding paragraph, the United States faced a similar challenge regarding whether primary and secondary schools should open and what, if anything, should be done to create a safer environment for these openings. France, after closing its borders to French nationals living abroad in February 2021, had to backtrack after its Conseil d'Etat, the equivalent of the US Supreme Court, deemed the measure "disproportionate" (Saint-Martin 2021). More mundane debates also revealed governments' difficulty in balancing health trade-offs with broader social and economic benefits. For example, many pointed to France's complex set of rules as to which essential services would remain open and which ones would close (hairdressers yes, but beauty parlors no, for example), or which criteria should be used to control individuals' mobility throughout its three lockdowns in 2020 and 2021 (Cohen 2021).

Finally, the decisions related to the vaccine rollout in each country also highlight the challenges in crisis decision-making. Chile opted for embracing the vaccine as the solution, starting a rapid mass vaccination campaign in 2021. By August 20, 2021, more than 80% of the target population of the country had already received two doses (Departamento de Estadísticas e Información en Salud 2021). The successful vaccine rollout also generated debate since the message sent by the authorities, that vaccination would reduce the crisis, was contrary to the prevention message; in fact, cases were rising while authorities were praising the success of the campaign (Castillo, Villalobos Dintrans, and Maddaleno 2021). The US vaccine rollout was initially relatively successful despite the failure of the Trump administration to leave the new Biden administration a detailed rollout plan. President Biden set and publicized an ambitious national goal of having 70% of adults receive at least one shot by July 4, but the goal was not achieved until a month later due to vaccine hesitancy among large proportions of the population (Smith-Schoenwalder 2021). France initially favored a cautious vaccine rollout, influenced by the failure of its H1N1 vaccination rollout in 2009, where vaccine orders had to be canceled or resold and millions of vaccines expired due to low demand (Davis 2011). However, the government eventually imposed a much stricter approach, including compulsory vaccinations for health workers and a forceful nudge through its health pass. Finally, as the Delta wave surged, health officials in all countries announced plans to make booster shots available despite criticism from the World Health Organization and others that its member states should prioritize vaccinations in lower-income countries before using additional vaccines in high-income countries for people who had already been fully vaccinated.

MEANING-MAKING

Communication proved to be crucial during the pandemic, especially considering the need to enforce measures during a long-term crisis. Trust issues and the political environment are closely linked to the way the leaders' messages resonate with the people (Glenn, Chaumont, and Villalobos Dintrans 2020). Determining who has legitimacy to disseminate and interpret data also came into question. In Chile, information and official figures proved to be a barrier during the first year of the pandemic, with people questioning information from the authorities (CNN-Chile 2020; Sepúlveda 2020); the change of minister of health in June 2020, and the call from several institutions—including the academia and the health sector—plus pandemic fatigue in the population, contributed to building the sense of a true crisis (Araya 2020; iCOVID-Chile 2021; Espacio Público 2021; Olave 2021). Although communication about the ongoing crisis improved in Chile, a permanent questioning of the rationale behind government authorities' decisions and the way they are communicated remained, which can be partially attributed to the social outbreak during 2019 and 2020 and the many elections held during 2021. For example, the decision to maintain curfews as health measures has been criticized, and is considered today more an instrument for controlling the population and preventing social protest (Vega 2021). In France, the rise to fame of an unknown young engineer who created widely used websites providing data visualization on COVID cases, then access to vaccine appointments, then vaccine coverage, and was later awarded the Legion d'Honneur revealed the failures of the government to properly inform its constituents in the midst of the crisis ("Guillaume Rozier" 2021).

In Chile, efforts were made to increase credibility after several problems related to information on COVID-19 in the country ("Encuesta" 2020; Ministerio de Ciencias, Tecnología, Conocimiento e Innovación 2021). After the resignation of the minister of health, Jaime Mañalich, in June 2020, the new minister, Enrique Paris, established a new way to interact with the press and communicate information and government decisions in an attempt to improve transparency and credibility (Román and Piérola 2020; Miranda and Borroni 2020). This new approach included routine press conferences held to report daily statistics, and a website with official figures and data published by the Ministry of Science. Maintaining credibility in the United States became increasingly difficult due to heightened politicization of COVID-19. An "us versus them" mentality developed as people on both sides of the political spectrum lost trust in leaders on the opposite side. This dynamic resulted in a lack of trust in science, particularly among Republicans, and a situation in which people tend to trust what they see on cable news or their social media feeds more than the information coming from health authorities or political leaders who communicate the messages of health authorities (Gollust 2021). There were even dozens of reports of threats and violence toward health workers and public health officials from people who were convinced those officials were corrupt and seeking their own interests (Larkin 2021; Mello et al. 2020). In all three countries, the rise of fake news, conspiracy theories and extremist views on the internet suggested such issues were likely to expand beyond the crisis (Sabbagh 2021).

TERMINATING

As described by Boin et al. (2005), terminating a crisis represents a political challenge since political factors may lead some actors to seek a premature end to the crisis. In addition, terminating a pandemic presents an additional challenge: as history shows, epidemics rarely end in a clean-cut narrative; rather, they end "once the diseases become accepted into people's daily lives and routines, becoming endemic—domestic—and accepted" (Charters and Heitman 2021). This slow death presents a challenge for public leaders, themselves driven by the need to promote short-term success to match election cycles.

In Chile, there were several attempts toward implementing termination strategies. However, the many turns in the COVID-19 situation, including the ups and downs in COVID-19 statistics and the rise of new variants, delayed completion of this task. The political environment at the time COVID-19 hit the country explains this situation: the social outbreak of October 2019 endangered the country's governability, as the administration faced COVID-19 with very low popularity figures (Bossert and Villalobos Dintrans 2020). In this environment, there was a political need to show results and success (crisis management and termination), particularly considering the complex political scenario for the ruling party. Termination attempts began during the first months of 2020, with the authorities announcing that the country had reached a plateau of cases in April 2020 ("Experta integrante" 2020a) and a call for a "new normalcy" and return to activities in May 2020 ("Mañalich no cede" 2020); soon, with the increase in cases during June–July 2020 (see figure 13.1), this effort was abandoned. The arrival of vaccines in 2021 and the successful vaccine rollout process reignited desires to end the crisis, which again had to be put on hold with the increase in new cases in mid-2021 (Ministerio de Salud 2021a). The need to finish the government period with successful management of the crisis forced the authorities to try and rush the termination task.

Similarly, in the United States there was a widespread feeling that the crisis was over once vaccinations became available to all adults. Many scientists and health officials continued to urge the public to maintain vigilance with protective measures such as social distancing and masking in public, but even the CDC guidelines changed to recommend masks in public only for the unvaccinated ("CDC Says" 2021). Unfortunately, although it was in the political interest of nearly all elected officials to terminate the crisis, the actions taken were insufficient to actually end the COVID-19 threat before the Delta wave became a reality. Vaccination rates remained too low, mass gatherings became the norm again, and few places had the political will to enact proof of vaccination that would limit the dangers the unvaccinated posed to the rest of the population. Rather than collaborating to make a final strong push toward the end, Republicans and Democrats fought over which side had mismanaged the situation more.

Finally, France got caught in its own narrative: after Macron in early 2020 emphasized the need to save lives "whatever it costs," it became hard to justify reopening the country unless the number of cases went down significantly ("'Quoi qu'il en coûte'" 2020). The government managed this situation by maintaining a constant story of absolute tenacity in the face of the crisis while quietly softening measures.

LEARNING

Learning should be inherent to crises, and the COVID-19 pandemic does not seem an exception. Learning, as described by Boin and colleagues, does not merely imply understanding past mistakes and correcting them but developing the ability to generate meaningful change and build capacity for better management of future crises.

In Chile, the process of addressing the crisis during the first months led to several adjustments in strategy that could be seen as part of a learning process. As stated above, one improvement was in the process of collecting, synthesizing, and communicating data. As these issues were key in explaining the resignation of the minister of health, the new minister emphasized this change of strategy as part of the lessons of the pandemic (Román and Piérola 2020; Miranda and Borroni 2020). Similarly, several changes were introduced to the Step-by-Step strategy throughout the period, including regional (instead of national) curfews, allowing time for physical exercise during lockdowns, and reducing mobility restrictions for people who were fully vaccinated (Ministerio de Salud 2021; Gobierno de Chile 2021b).

In the United States, congressional hearings and other formal investigations were held related to the pandemic, but they were largely attempts at scoring points in the blame game rather than true dialogue and inquiry to identify lessons that would help prevent future pandemics. As could be expected, some structural reforms were made (such as the establishment of the CDC Center for Forecasting and Outbreak Analytics) that will likely increase the capacity of the federal government to respond to disease outbreaks (CDC 2021). However, as mentioned above, some states also made structural reforms that limit the powers of health officials during public health emergencies and increase the likelihood that future public health threats will be subject to partisan rather than evidence-based decision-making (Williams 2021).

Finally, in France, the crisis revealed health system dysfunctions that had not been fully addressed or acknowledged, creating a window of opportunity for policy change. As early as May 2020, a broad consultation with healthcare actors led to salary increases for key healthcare staff and increased funding for hospitals and long-term care (Ministère des Solidarités et de la Santé 2020). In 2021, the government launched three expert missions to review public health policies and present recommendations for improvement (Ministère des Solidarités et de la Santé 2021). More broadly, the epidemic accelerated societal concerns with climate change and environmental damage, as politicians, the media, and the general public all underlined the link between emerging infectious diseases and wildlife and environmental damage (Ministère des Affaires étrangères 2020). The country (and the European Union) also increased their focus on global health governance, characterized by the Union's push to develop a new pandemic treaty at the international level.

Overall, the three countries' capacity to learn from the pandemic remained limited. This might be in part due to the sheer scope and unprecedented scale of the crisis, whose effects will ripple for decades to come. But it could also be because this crisis represented a change of paradigm in our approach to epidemiological risks and diseases. Our collective inability to imagine a different path for ourselves might just reveal how profound this shift is. As a quote that is often attributed to Einstein says, "The problems that face us cannot be solved at the same level of consciousness that created them. What we need is a shift in consciousness." This shift in consciousness is still in the making to prevent future pandemics and other public health crises.

CONCLUSIONS

Recommendations for Future Practices

Outbreak management and response—including contact tracing, quarantine, and treatment scale-up—is not a new field. But by its sheer scope, the COVID-19 pandemic crisis projected these routine public health tasks into a new dimension: public health was abruptly placed at the center of the public arena.

Key Lessons Learned for Public Health Experts

- Public health experts need to have a much more in-depth understanding of the policy process in order to better communicate with elected officials and influence decision-making.

- To increase the likelihood of their involvement in broader priority-setting discussions, public health experts should avoid a "health tyranny" approach, in which health is prioritized over every other issue without regard to cost-benefit discussions.

- In a crisis with such radical uncertainty, public health officials and other public leaders need to quickly collect accurate data, but also to communicate clearly with the public about limitations and gaps in knowledge.

- Public health experts need to help national leaders navigating global versus national discourse to emphasize our global connectedness and the risks (e.g., vaccine nationalism) presented by too narrow a focus on national interests.

- Public health experts need to initiate and fully participate in much more robust public discussions on conflicting values (e.g., human rights versus personal freedoms) in public health, considering current measures.

This new situation created unexpected challenges for both public leaders and public health professionals. On the one hand, policy-makers and public servants were suddenly forced to make complex public health decisions in a moment of heightened uncertainty, often with limited backgrounds in public health. For example, a study found that out of all US state legislators in 2018, only 0.3% had formal public health training, making them particularly ill-equipped to handle such a complex public health crisis (Jones et al. 2021). On the other hand, public health professionals were suddenly thrust from being actors within their own discipline into roles as leaders in a much broader context.

As shown by the three examples of Chile, France and the United States, this created many challenges. Public leaders struggled to balance economic, social, and public considerations when making decisions. Communication was patchy, contradictory, or even deceptive. Some political leaders instrumentalized the crisis for political gains, either on the national or international stage. Public leaders struggled to balance a natural societal desire to get back to normal, with the need to continue to protect vulnerable populations, often less vaccinated and potentially more exposed to the deadly Delta variant.

On the other end of the spectrum, public health professionals also struggled to provide or impose their leadership. Often these individuals had limited knowledge or experience of the systems that shape policymaking and implementation, including interest groups, partisanship, and the electoral process. In the case of COVID-19, they may also not have had sufficient knowledge of how to balance public health considerations with broader considerations such as the global economy or geopolitics. Finally, because public decision-making must often consider elements that go beyond science, public health leaders had to tread a thin line: if they chose to remove themselves from the politics, they could end up confined as "technical" experts, easily ignored by decision-makers, but if they got too involved in the political decision-making process, they could lose the scientific credibility that provided them authority in the first place (Greer et al. 2017; Hunter 2016).

Lessons Learned about Crisis Management

First, this unique moment highlights the importance of better understanding public leadership as a key for better crisis management (Crosby and Bryson

2018). We explored five dimensions of this relationship—sense-making, decision-making, meaning-making, termination, and learning—showing how they can be used to explain some of the observed outcomes. Beyond assessing what could have been done ex post, this framework helps us anticipate and design policy responses ex ante.

Second, it emphasized the role not just of public leaders but of public health leaders in managing COVID-19. In the future, our understanding of public health may need to be renegotiated. Health in All Policies approaches, which consider engagement with sectors outside the traditional healthcare sector that either directly impact or are impacted by public health phenomena as a key responsibility of public health professionals, may become more prominent in coming decades (Hahn 2019). Public health professionals themselves may also need to redefine their technical and political power and learn how to deal with the ambiguities that come with more political roles, while still promoting evidence-based decision-making (Deitchman 2013). The field of public health itself may take a more prominent role in the public eye (Gray 2009; Moodie 2016). Public health differs from medicine because it focuses on the population level rather than the individual level (Frenk 1993). Nevertheless, public health practitioners are regularly eclipsed by medical doctors without public health training in the media and in decision-making processes. An increased focus on public health could be a welcome benefit from this devastating crisis.

In Chile, France and the United States, the COVID-19 crisis placed public health leaders at the forefront of crisis management and public leaders at the helm of a public health emergency. Lessons about how to handle this particular situation are relevant not only as a scrutiny of the actions taken but as a guide for managing the remaining consequences of COVID-19 as well as other future global crises—starting with climate change, the "greatest threat to global public health" of our times (Nyenswah, Engineer, and Peters 2016; Atwoli et al. 2021).

QUESTIONS FOR DISCUSSION

- What role did public health professionals play in your country during the COVID-19 crisis?

- Do you think public health professionals have a duty to remain neutral or, to the contrary, to get involved in the public debate? Why or why not?

- How can public health professionals become public health leaders? What tools are missing today and how can you acquire them?

REFERENCES

Araya, Alex. 2020. "Grupo Epidemiológico y Matemático de la Universidad de Santiago estudia los datos de la pandemia." *USACH al día,* May 20, 2020. https://www.usach.cl/news/grupo-epidemiologico-y-matematico-la-universidad-santiago-estudia-los-datos-la-pandemia

Atwoli, Lukoye, Abdullah H. Baqui, Thomas Benfield, Raffaella Bosurgi, Fiona Godlee, Stephen Hancocks, Richard Horton, et al. 2021. "Call for Emergency Action to Limit Global Temperature Increases, Restore Biodiversity, and Protect Health." *New England Journal of Medicine* 385, no. 12:1134–37. https://doi.org/10.1056/nejme2113200.

Boin, Arjen, and Paul 't Hart. 2003. "Leadership in Times of Crisis: Mission Impossible?" *Public Administration Review* 63, no. 5 (September–October): 544–53. https://www.jstor.org/stable/3110097.

Boin, Arjen, Martin Lodge, and Marte Luesing. 2020. "Learning from the COVID-19 Crisis: An Initial Analysis of National Responses." *Policy Design and Practice* 3, no. 3: 189–204. https://doi.org/10.1080/25741292.2020.1823670.

Boin, Arjen, Paul 't Hart, Eric Stern, and Bengt Sundelius. 2005. *The Politics of Crisis Management: Public Leadership under Pressure.* Cambridge: Cambridge University Press.

Bossert, Thomas J., and Pablo Villalobos Dintrans. 2020. "Health Reform in the Midst of a Social and Political Crisis in Chile, 2019–2020." *Health Systems and Reform* 6, no. 1: e1789031. https://doi.org/10.1080/23288604.2020.1789031.

Castillo, Claudio, Pablo Villalobos Dintrans, and Matilde Maddaleno. 2021. "The Successful COVID-19 Vaccine Rollout in Chile: Factors and Challenges." *Vaccine: X* 9 (December): 100114. https://doi.org/10.1016/j.jvacx.2021.100114.

CDC (Centers for Disease Control and Prevention). 2021. "CDC Stands Up New Disease Forecasting Center." Centers for Disease Control and. Prevention August 18. https://www.cdc.gov/media/releases/2021/p0818-disease-forecasting-center.html.

"CDC Says Fully Vaccinated Americans Can Go without Masks Outdoors, Except in Crowded Settings." 2021. *Washington Post,* April 27, 2021. https://www.washingtonpost.com/health/2021/04/27/cdc-guidance-masks-outdoors/.

Charters, Erica, and Kristin Heitman. 2021. "How Epidemics End." *Centaurus* 63, no. 1: 210–24. https://doi.org/10.1111/1600-0498.12370.

CNN-Chile. 2020. "Los cuestionamientos que marcaron la renuncia del ahora ex ministro Mañalich." CNN-Chile, June 13, 2020. https://www.cnnchile.com/pais/los-cuestionamientos-que-marcaron-la-salida-de-jaime-manalich-del-ministerio-de-salud_20200613/.

Cohen, Roger. 2021. "The Entangling, Ever-Extending Labyrinth of French Lockdowns." *New York Times,* April 26, 2021. https://www.nytimes.com/2021/04/26/world/europe/france-covid-lockdowns.html.

Crosby, Barbara C., and John M. Bryson. 2018. "Why Leadership of Public Leadership Research Matters: And What to Do about It." *Public Management Review* 20, no. 9: 1265–86. https://doi.org/10.1080/14719037.2017.1348731.

Davis, Tony. 2011. "La France détruit ses vaccins contre la grippe A." *L'Express,* September 12, 2011. https://www.lexpress.fr/actualite/societe/sante/la-france-detruit-ses-vaccins-contre-la-grippe-a_1029142.html.

Deitchman, Scott. 2013. "Enhancing Crisis Leadership in Public Health Emergencies." *Disaster Medicine and Public Health Preparedness* 7, no. 5 (October): 534–40. https://doi.org/10.1017/dmp.2013.81.

Departamento de Estadísticas e Información en Salud. 2021. "Avance vacunación SARS-CoV-2." Ministerio de Salud. Accessed August 29, 2021. https://informesdeis.minsal.cl/SASVisualAnalytics/?reportUri=/reports/reports/9037e283-1278-422c-84c4-16e42a7026c8.

"Encuesta: Siete de cada diez chilenos no confían en la información del Gobierno sobre el Covid-19." 2020. *Cooperativa,* May 22, 2020. https://www.cooperativa.cl/noticias/sociedad/salud/coronavirus/encuesta-siete-de-cada-diez-chilenos-no-confian-en-la-informacion-del/2020-05-22/233159.html.

Espacio Público. 2021. "Reporte COVID-19 de Espacio Público. Inventario de Reportes." Espacio Público. Accessed August 26, 2021. https://espaciopublico.cl/nuestro_trabajo/espacio-publico-presenta-reportes-semanales-de-la-evolucion-del-contagio-y-fallecidos-por-covid-19-chile-y-resto-del-mundo-en-fechas-comparables/.

"'Everyone Stay Home' if Sick, Many Events Banned: Dutch Government Tightens Coronavirus Rules." 2020. *NL Times,* March 12, 2020. https://nltimes.nl/2020/03/12/everyone-stay-home-sick-many-events-banned-dutch-government-tightens-coronavirus-rules.

"Experta integrante del Consejo Asesor Covid-19 contradice a Mañalich: 'No estamos en una meseta.'" 2020. *El Mostrador,* April 30, 2020. https://www.elmostrador.cl/noticias/pais/2020/04/30/experta-integrante-del-consejo-asesor-covid-19-contradice-a-manalich-no-estamos-en-una-meseta/.

Frenk, J. 1993. "The New Public Health." *Annual Review of Public Health* 14:469–90. https://doi.org/10.1146/annurev.pu.14.050193.002345.

Garrido, Mónica. 2021. "Comisión revisora rechaza acusación constitucional contra ministro de Educación Raúl Figueroa." *La Tercera,* August 11, 2021. https://www.latercera.com/politica/noticia/comision-revisora-rechaza-acusacion-constitucional-contra-ministro-de-educacion-raul-figueroa/IOBDG6WOVFHGTB2UHSJYJMSEJ4/.

Glenn, Jeffrey, Claire Chaumont, and Pablo Villalobos Dintrans. 2020. "Public Health Leadership in the Times of COVID-19: A Comparative Case Study of Three Countries." *International Journal of Public Leadership* 17, no. 1: 81–94.

Gobierno de Chile. 2021a. "Mesa Social COVID-19." Gobierno de Chile. Accessed August 26, 2021. https://www.gob.cl/mesasocialcovid19/.

———. 2021b. "Paso a Paso nos cuidamos." Gobierno de Chile. Accessed August 26, 2021. https://www.gob.cl/coronavirus/pasoapaso/.

Gollust, Sarah E. 2021. "Partisan and Other Gaps in Support for COVID-19 Mitigation Strategies Require Substantial Attention." *American Journal of Public Health* 111, no. 5 (May): 765–67. https://doi.org/10.2105/AJPH.2021.306226.

Gray, Muir. 2009. "Public Health Leadership: Creating the Culture for the Twenty-First Century." *Journal of Public Health* 31, no. 2 (June): 208–9. https://doi.org/10.1093/pubmed/fdp034.

Greer, Scott L., Marleen Bekker, Evelyne de Leeuw, Matthias Wismar, Jan-Kees Helderman, Sofia Ribeiro, and David Stuckler. 2017. "Policy, Politics and

Public Health." *European Journal of Public Health* 27, no. S4: 40–43. https://doi
.org/10.1093/eurpub/ckx152.

"Guillaume Rozier, Covidtracker, Vitemadose et . . . l'ordre national
du Mérite." 2021. *Libération,* May 22, 2021. https://www.liberation.fr/societe
/sante/guillaume-rozier-covidtracker-vitemadose-et-lordre-national-du-merite
-20210522_5SR4KAAX7NBV5CVI4QAEXMOUOY/.

Gump, B. 2020. "The Great Barrington Declaration: When Arrogance Leads to
Recklessness." *US News,* November 6, 2020. https://www.usnews.com/news
/healthiest-communities/articles/2020-11-06/when-scientists-arrogance-leads
-to-recklessness-the-great-barrington-declaration.

Hahn, R. 2019. "Two Paths to Health in All Policies: The Traditional Public Health
Path and the Path of Social Determinants." *American Journal of Public Health*
109, no. 2 (February): 253–54. https://doi.org/10.2105/AJPH.2018.304884.

Hannah, Sean T., Mary Uhl-Bien, Bruce J. Avolio, and Fabrice L. Cavarretta. 2009.
"A Framework for Examining Leadership in Extreme Contexts." *Leadership
Quarterly* 20, no. 6 (December): 897–919. https://doi.org/10.1016/j.leaqua.2009
.09.006.

Helsloot, Ira, Arjen Boin, Brian Jacobs, and Louise K. Comfort, eds. 2012. *Mega-
Crises: Understanding the Prospects, Nature, Characteristics and the Effects of
Cataclysmic Events.* Springfield, IL: Charles C. Thomas.

Hunter, Edward L. 2016. "Politics and Public Health—Engaging the Third Rail."
Journal of Public Health Management and Practice 22, no. 5 (September):
436–41. https://doi.org/10.1097/PHH.0000000000000446.

iCOVID-Chile. 2021. "iCOVID-Chile: Inicio." iCOVID-Chile. Accessed August 26,
2021. https://www.icovidchile.cl/.

Johns Hopkins University. 2020. "Mortality Analyses." Johns Hopkins University and
Medicine. Accessed August 12, 2021. https://coronavirus.jhu.edu/data/mortality.

———. 2021. "Coronavirus Resource Center." Johns Hopkins University and Medicine. Accessed August 25, 2021. https://coronavirus.jhu.edu/.

Jones, David K., Paula Atkeson, Andrea Goodman, and Megan Houston. 2021.
"More Public Health Leaders Should Run for Office." *Journal of Public Health
Management and Practice* 27, no. 1 (January/February): 1–3. https://doi.org/10
.1097/phh.0000000000001131.

Jong, Wouter. 2017. "Meaning Making by Public Leaders in Times of Crisis: An
Assessment." *Public Relations Review* 43, no. 5 (December): 1025–35. https://doi
.org/10.1016/j.pubrev.2017.09.003.

Larkin, Howard. 2021. "Navigating Attacks against Health Care Workers in the
COVID-19 Era." *JAMA* 325, no. 18: 1822–24. https://doi.org/10.1001/jama.2021
.2701.

"Mañalich no cede: Ministro insiste en 'nueva normalidad' y casos de COVID-19
se disparan a nuevo peak de 4.895 casos." 2020. *El Mostrador,* May 25, 2020.
https://www.elmostrador.cl/noticias/pais/2020/05/25/manalich-no-cede
-ministro-insiste-en-nueva-normalidad-y-casos-de-covid-19-se-disparan-a
-nuevo-peak-de-4-895-casos/.

Marcel, Mario. 2020. "La economía chilena frente a la pandemia del COVID-19:
Fortalezas, desafíos y riesgos." Banco Central de Chile, December 18, 2020.

https://www.bcentral.cl/documents/33528/133214/mmc18122020.pdf/83f103c6
-53c9-4c96-9190-7b0314a4574d?t=1608295798437#:~:text=El%20impacto%20de
%20la%20crisis%20del%20COVID%2D19%20se%20concentr%C3%B3,fuerte
%20heterogeneidad%20a%20su%20interior.

Mello, Michelle M., Jeremy A. Greene, and Joshua M. Sharfstein. 2020. "Attacks on
Public Health Officials during COVID-19." *JAMA* 324, no. 8: 741–42. https://
doi.org/10.1001/jama.2020.14423.

Ministère des Affaires étrangères. 2020. "Evènement du 12/11. Renforcement
de l'architecture multilatérale de santé: Lancement du Conseil d'experts de
haut niveau 'One Health.'" *France Diplomatie,* November 12, 2020. https://
www.diplomatie.gouv.fr/fr/politique-etrangere-de-la-france/societe-civile
-et-volontariat/evenements-incluant-la-societe-civile/forum-de-paris-sur-la
-paix/precedentes-editions/article/evenement-du-12-11-renforcement-de-l
-architecture-multilaterale-de-sante.

Ministère des Solidarités et de la Santé. 2020. "Ségur de la santé: Les conclusions,
26 July, 2021." Ministère des Solidarités et de la Santé. Accessed November 19,
2021. https://solidarites-sante.gouv.fr/systeme-de-sante-et-medico-social/segur
-de-la-sante/article/segur-de-la-sante-les-conclusions.

———. 2021. "Communiqué de presse: Olivier Véran lance trois missions dédiées à la
santé publique française, 10 June 2021." Ministère des Solidarités et de la Santé.
Accessed November 19, 2021. https://solidarites-sante.gouv.fr/actualites/presse
/communiques-de-presse/article/olivier-veran-lance-trois-missions-dediees-a
-la-sante-publique-francaise.

Ministerio de Ciencias, Tecnología, Conocimiento e Innovación. 2021. "Base
de Datos COVID-19." Ministerio de Ciencias, Tecnología, Conocimiento e Innovación. Accessed August 26, 2021. https://www.minciencia.gob.cl/covid19/.

Ministerio de Educación. 2020. "Impacto del COVID-19 en los resultados de
aprendizaje y escolaridad en Chile." Ministerio de Educación de Chile. Accessed August 29, 2021. https://www.mineduc.cl/wp-content/uploads/sites/19
/2020/08/EstudioMineduc_bancomundial.pdf.

Ministerio de Salud. 2021a. "COVID-19: Casos nuevos disminuyen 20% en los úl-
timos siete días." Ministerio de Salud, July 1, 2021. https://www.minsal.cl/covid
-19-casos-nuevos-disminuyen-20-en-los-ultimos-siete-dias/.

———. 2021b. "Presidente Piñera presenta actualización del 'Plan Paso a Paso' 'El
objetivo es compatibilizar mejor la protección de la salud y la vida con may-
ores niveles de libertad y movilidad.'" Ministerio de Salud, July 8, 2021. https://
www.minsal.cl/presidente-pinera-presenta-actualizacion-del-plan-paso-a-paso
-el-objetivo-es-compatibilizar-mejor-la-proteccion-de-la-salud-y-la-vida-con
-mayores-niveles-de-libertad-y-movilidad/.

Miranda, Cristóbal, and Enzo Borroni. 2020. "Expertos destacan el cambio en
el estilo comunicacional de Paris con respecto a Mañalich." USACH al día,
June 19, 2020. https://www.usach.cl/news/expertos-destacan-cambio-estilo
-comunicacional-paris-respecto-manalich.

Moodie, Rob. 2016. "Learning about Self: Leadership Skills for Public Health." *Journal of Public Health Research* 5, no. 1: 679. https://doi.org/10.4081/jphr.2016.679.

Murillo, F. Javier, and Cynthia Duk. 2020. "El Covid-19 y las Brechas Educativas." *Revista Latinoamericana de Educación Inclusiva* 14, no. 1 (June): 11–13. http://dx.doi.org/10.4067/S0718-73782020000100011.

Nyenswah, Tolbert, Cyrus Y. Engineer, and David H. Peters. 2016. "Leadership in Times of Crisis: The Example of Ebola Virus Disease in Liberia." *Health Systems and Reform* 2, no. 3: 194–207. https://doi.org/10.1080/23288604.2016.1222793.

Olave, Ricardo. 2021. "La cuenta que entrega cifras en tiempo real del Covid-19 en Chile." *La Tercera,* June 7, 2021. https://laboratorio.latercera.com/laboratorio/noticia/covid-19-en-chile/1018136/.

"'Quoi qu'il en coûte': Emmanuel Macron lance un appel général à la mobilisation contre le coronavirus." 2020. *Franceinfo,* March 12, 2020. https://www.francetvinfo.fr/sante/maladie/coronavirus/quoi-qu-il-en-coute-emmanuel-macron-lance-un-appel-general-a-la-mobilisation-contre-le-coronavirus_3863731.html.

Roa, Tomás Pablo. 2021. "La apertura de la actividad económica en Chile se acerca al 100% del PIB." *El Economista,* August 30, 2021. https://www.eleconomista.es/actualidad/noticias/11373002/08/21/La-apertura-de-la-actividad-economica-en-Chile-se-acerca-al-100-del-PIB.html.

Román, Cecilia, and Gladys Piérola. 2020. "Cómo se ideó en La Moneda la estrategia de vocerías con un 'panel de expertos.'" *Pauta,* June 17, 2020. https://www.pauta.cl/politica/covid-nueva-estrategia-panel-de-expertos-ministerio-de-salud-vocerias-paris.

Rouquette, Pauline. 2021. "Les anti pass-sanitaire ont-ils une couleur politique?" *Europe 1,* August 14, 2021. https://www.europe1.fr/societe/anti-passantivax-comme-les-gilets-jaunes-cest-un-mouvement-extremement-bigarre-et-contradictoire-4062121.

Sabbagh, Dam. 2021. "Pandemic Has Spurred Engagement in Online Extremism, Say Experts." *Guardian,* October 19, 2021. https://www.theguardian.com/world/2021/oct/19/covid-pandemic-spurred-engagement-online-extremism.

Saint-Martin, Emmanuel. 2021. "Le Conseil d'Etat suspend la fermeture des frontières pour les Français de l'étranger." *French Morning,* March 12, 2021. https://frenchmorning.com/le-conseil-detat-suspend-la-fermeture-des-frontieres-pour-les-francais-de-letranger/.

Sayare, S. 2020. "He Was a Science Star. Then He Promoted a Questionable Cure for COVID-19." *New York Times,* May 12, 2020. https://www.nytimes.com/2020/05/12/magazine/didier-raoult-hydroxychloroquine.html.

Sepúlveda, Nicolás. 2020. "Minsal reporta a la OMS una cifra de fallecidos más alta que la informada a diario en Chile." *Ciper-Chile,* June 13, 2020. https://ciperchile.cl/2020/06/13/minsal-reporta-a-la-oms-una-cifra-de-fallecidos-mas-alta-que-la-informada-a-diario-en-chile/.

Shalal, Andrea, and Jeff Mason. 2021. "Biden Zeroes in on Delta Variant as U.S. Nears 160 Million Fully Vaccinated." Reuters, July 6, 2021.

Shear, Michael D., Sheryl Gay Stolberg, and Annie Karni. 2021. "Biden Rekindles Vaccination Push with New Orders." *New York Times,* July 30, 2021.

Smith-Schoenwalder, Cecelia. 2021. "Biden Reaches Goal of 70% of Adults Par-
    tially Vaccinated against COVID-19 a Month Late." *US News,* August 2, 2021.
    https://www.usnews.com/news/health-news/articles/2021-08-02/biden-reaches
    -goal-of-70-of-adults-partially-vaccinated-against-covid-19-a-month-late.
UNICEF. 2021. "Los niños no pueden permitirse otro año sin escuela." UNICEF,
    January 12, 2021. https://www.unicef.org/es/comunicados-prensa/ninos-no
    -pueden-permitirse-otro-ano-sin-escuela.
"UPDATE: The Parts of France That Have Enforced Extra Local Covid Restric-
    tions." 2021. *Local France,* July 16, 2021. https://www.thelocal.fr/20210716/area
    -breakdown-extra-local-covid-restrictions-in-france/.
Vega, Jeanette. 2021. "¿Debemos mantener el toque de queda?" *La Tercera,* May 14, 2021.
    https://www.latercera.com/la-tercera-sabado/noticia/columna-de-jeanette-vega
    -debemos-mantener-el-toque-de-queda/HL2WFC4QR5E2LCSYHHOQYJDKOY/.
WHO (World Health Organization). 2020a. "Rolling Updates on Coronavirus Disease
    (COVID-19)." World Health Organization. Accessed August 12, 2021. https://www
    .who.int/emergencies/diseases/novel-coronavirus-2019/events-as-they-happen.
———. 2020b. "Coronavirus Disease Pandemic." World Health Organization.
    Accessed August 12, 2021. https://www.who.int/emergencies/diseases/novel
    -coronavirus-2019.
———. 2021. "COVID-19 Explorer." World Health Organization. Accessed Au-
    gust 20, 2021. https://worldhealthorg.shinyapps.io/covid/.
Williams, Jordan. 2021. "Utah Legislature Passes Prohibition on Mask Mandates in
    Schools." Hill, May 19, 2021. https://thehill.com/policy/healthcare/554476-utah
    -legislature-passes-prohibition-on-mask-mandates-in-schools.
Yáñez, Cecilia. 2021. "¿Qué tan letal está siendo la variante Delta en
    Chile?" *La Tercera,* September 30, 2021. https://www.latercera.com
    /que-pasa/noticia/que-tan-letal-esta-siendo-la-variante-delta-en-chile
    /VQS42ARKK5AJVEE6F3MPCMWUTY/.
Yphantides, Nick, Steven Escoboza, and Nick Macchione. 2015. "Leadership in
    Public Health: New Competencies for the Future." *Frontiers in Public Health*
    3:24. https://doi.org/10.3389/fpubh.2015.00024.

Contributors

VASHTI ADAMS, MSW, is a PhD student at the University of Maryland, Baltimore, School of Social Work. She earned her MSW from Columbia University and is an emerging public health social work researcher. Her research interests include antioppressive, weight-inclusive approaches to health promotion and eating disorder prevention among Black adolescent and young adult populations.

ADANNA AGBO, DrPH, is chief of the Advanced Nursing Education Branch at the Health Resources and Services Administration, where she oversees a team that supports innovative nursing workforce programs that advance public health, with an investment of over $102M annually. She has over twenty years' experience as a nurse and nurse educator.

KOBI V. AJAYI, PhD, is a health system and health policy scientist with experience in conducting culturally and gendered appropriate research to achieve timely and quality access to care. Dr. Ajayi, a nonprofit organization leader, leads and conducts research and public health initiatives to improve maternal and neonatal well-being in Nigeria.

ADAEZE AROH, DrPH, is a health policy management scientist and digital health transformation strategist with over fifteen years of global public health, financial services, health services research, information technology, and project management expertise. She has extensive experience using community-based participatory research methodologies to reduce disparities and improve outcomes in underserved communities.

UGONWA AROH, PhD, is a researcher with the Peterloo Institute in Manchester, United Kingdom. She has a keen interest in using education to achieve ultimate well-being and sustainable development goals. Her research interests are the well-being of defined populations and sustainable development.

EMMA BIEGACKI, MPH, is program manager of the Yale Program in Addiction Medicine and coordinator of the Collaborative Addiction Medicine and Behavioral Health in Primary Care (CHAMP) training program at Yale School of Medicine. Her work focuses broadly on substance use, addiction, and advancement of evidence-based treatments and harm reduction.

OBASANJO AFOLABI BOLARINWA, MSc, is a senior lecturer at the Department of Public Health and Well-being, Faculty of Health and Social Care, University of Chester, United Kingdom. He possesses vast research and applied knowledge in reducing inequalities in adverse sexual and reproductive health outcomes among adolescent girls and young women in Africa.

CLAIRE CHAUMONT, DrPH, is a global health systems and policy expert with extensive experience in global health governance, health systems strengthening, and evidence-based policymaking. A Fulbright Scholar, Chaumont holds a DrPH from Harvard, a master's in health policy, planning, and financing from the London School of Hygiene and Tropical Medicine, and a master's in international business from Sciences Po Paris.

JAIH CRADDOCK, PhD, is an assistant professor at the University of California, Irvine, in the Department of Family Medicine. She is a public health social work scientist committed to understanding the impacts of digital technologies on human development and social interaction. Dr. Craddock's principal scholarship leverages social networks and network dynamics to decrease new HIV incidences among at-risk populations.

MARQUITTA DORSEY, PhD, is an assistant professor at Loyola University Chicago, School of Social Work. Her research uses intersectionality to examine health equity for Black adolescent and young adult females as they interact within and across family, healthcare, education, child welfare, and carceral systems.

GHANEM ELHERSH, PhD, is an assistant professor of mass communication at Stephen F. Austin State University. Elhersh researches the entertainment industry, storytelling, stereotypes, and digital media using computational social science methods.

KRISTEN GARCIA, MPH, is a research specialist at Texas A&M University, School of Public Health. Garcia leads community-based program planning and evaluation efforts on a variety of local, state, and nationally funded projects. Garcia also has experience in leading community-based coalitions and other on-the-ground public health and health education efforts.

WHITNEY GARNEY, PhD, is an associate professor in the Department of Health Behavior at Texas A&M University and the principal investigator of the Laboratory for Community Health Evaluation and Systems Science. Her expertise is in community-based research and evaluation, with an emphasis in ecological and systems approaches to public health.

TIMNIT BERHANE GHEBRETINSAE, MPH, supports research projects at the Institute for Health Equity Research based on core concepts of community involvement and engagement. With a passion for addressing health dispari-ties and promoting equity in minoritized and vulnerable communities, Ghe-bretinsae previously worked as a research consultant, specifically addressing disparities in chronic diseases and substance abuse, among other areas.

JEFFREY GLENN, DrPH, is an assistant professor of public health at Brigham Young University. He holds an MPA from the University of Southern Califor-nia and a DrPH from Harvard. His research focuses on public health leader-ship and systems thinking approaches to public health problems.

F. TODD GRAY, MDiv, is a pastor of Fifth Street Baptist Church in Richmond, Virginia. He has developed innovative ministries and led several churches to significant growth. Additionally, he is the co-chairman of the City's Commis-sion on African American Males, chairman of the City-Wide Men's Revival, and chairman of Virginia Churches of the National Baptist Convention.

RUDENE HAYNES, JD, is a partner at Hunton Andrews Kurth and co-leader of the servicer advance financing practice. She was recognized as a Nation's Best Honoree and featured in the National Black Lawyers Top 100 List. Com-mitted to ending health disparities, she co-founded "Facts and Faith Fridays" to educate the Black faith community about COVID-19.

ROBERT HEIMER, PhD, is a professor of epidemiology at the Yale School of Public Health and of pharmacology at the Yale School of Medicine. His major research efforts have included scientific investigation of mortality and mor-bidity associated with illicit drug use and evaluation of interventions to re-duce related medical complications. His current work focuses on the opioid overdose crisis.

TASMIM HOQUE, BS, born in Bangladesh and raised in New York City, is a CUNY Macaulay Honors College graduate with a bachelor's degree in interdepartmental anthropology and health education. Passionate about dismantling poverty-related barriers to healthcare and education, she collaborates with volunteer organizations, education nonprofits, and research initiatives to effect change.

IMAN IKRAM, MBA, is a visiting assistant professor at the School of Communication Studies, Ohio University. She practiced dentistry and healthcare administration for over seven years. Ikram received the Ohio University Women's Leadership award for her contribution to the university community. She was awarded the top panel from CSCA health communication division.

LAEEQ KHAN, PhD, is an associate professor and director of SMART Lab at Ohio University and specializes in social media and data analytics. Khan's work focuses on technology's role in addressing global challenges and has been acknowledged by The Hill, the *Tribune Chronicle,* and NPR. He also brings a decade of industry experience in mentoring future media and business scholars.

CAROLINE KINGORI, PhD, is an associate dean for faculty affairs and associate professor at Ohio University. She has led the OHIO Reproductive and Sexual Health Initiative, mentoring students and supporting junior faculty. Her research in health behavior is dedicated to addressing global, national, and local reproductive and sexual health issues. Active in the American Public Health Association, Kingori has held multiple leadership roles.

KUJANG LAKI, MA, is an assistant professor in communication studies at Ohio Northern University and a doctoral candidate at Ohio University. She has previously worked at Ohio University, UNICEF South Sudan, and the American Red Cross. Kujang received her BA from Central State University and MA degrees from Ohio University and DePaul University.

JESSICA GOKEE LAROSE, PhD, is a tenured associate professor (Sociobehavioral Sciences Department) at Virginia Commonwealth University. Her program of research focuses on understanding the interplay of behavioral, psychological, and environmental determinants of obesity and chronic disease risk and developing novel and sustainable interventions to promote physical and psychological health among underserved populations.

RACHEL LUDEKE, PhD, is a postdoctoral research fellow at Thomas Jefferson University, Department of Family and Community Medicine, Sidney Kimmel Medical College. Her research examines the role of personal support networks in mental health help-seeking behaviors of young adults with foster care experience.

DEVIN MADDEN, MPH, has over a decade of experience in community-centered public health work. Currently, she manages community- and workforce-facing health and gender equity programming. In their role with the newly established Institute for Health Equity Research, Madden supports community-engaged projects addressing New Yorkers' needs.

TYRA MONTOUR, MPH, is a PhD student in the Department of Health Behavior at Texas A&M University. Her research focuses on health communications, telehealth, and socioeconomic factors that influence health literacy, knowledge, and awareness in vulnerable or immigrant populations. She is interested in mental health and health behaviors within communities.

KENNETH MORFORD, MD, is assistant professor in the Department of Internal Medicine at Yale School of Medicine. He is board-certified in internal medicine and addiction medicine. His clinical and scholarly work focuses on interprofessional addiction education and integrating substance use treatment in general medical settings.

MICHELE MORRONE, PhD, MS, is a professor of environmental health at Ohio University. She has authored numerous papers on environmental topics, including environmental health disparities in Appalachia and environmental justice. She has published six books, including *Ailing in Place: Environmental Inequities* and *Health Disparities in Appalachia.*

MAGHBOEBA MOSAVEL, PhD, is a professor (Health Behavior and Policy Department) at Virginia Commonwealth University. Her program of research focuses broadly on cancer prevention and control, community-engaged interventions, oral health disparities, and genomic biobanking. Her research is focused in urban and rural communities within the United States and South Africa.

CAROLYN NGANGA-GOOD, DrPH, is a branch chief at the Division of Practitioner Data Bank at the Health Resources and Services Administration, where she oversees the Policy and Disputes Branch. She has over twenty years of public health, nursing, and leadership experience and is a published author.

JERRY OKAL, PhD, is a social and behavioral scientist focused on designing and implementing research around social determinants of health in low- and middle-income countries. He leads the Population Council's Key Populations (KP) Project, focused on providing technical assistance to implementing partners in evaluating new ways to provide combination prevention to KPs.

AGGREY WILLIS OTIENO, PhD, is an assistant professor in the Journalism and Communication Department, Utah State University. His academic interests are around the intersections of big data, emerging media technology, and behavior change communication. He has won several international awards, such as the Excellence in Global Leadership Award and the African Children Hero Award, and was the Rolex Laureate recipient from 2012 to 2014.

SONYA PANJWANI, PhD, is a public health scientist with experience in community-based research, program evaluation, and systems science approaches to addressing complex public health challenges. Her research interests include health systems strengthening, maternal and child health, and the impact of policy-related and systemic factors on immigrant and refugee health outcomes.

ELIZABETH PROM-WORMLEY, PhD, is an associate professor (Family Medicine and Population Health Department) at Virginia Commonwealth University. Her work has focused on detailing the genetic and environmental factors that influence mental health and substance use to support community partners who alleviate the burden of chronic medical and mental health conditions in Richmond, Virginia.

TREMAYNE ROBERTSON, PhD, is the director for Diversity, Equity, and Inclusion at Virginia Commonwealth University Massey Comprehensive Cancer Center. His research is grounded in Black masculinity studies and in men and masculinity studies. He has led and supported DEI initiatives in higher education and K–12 schools to advance DEI in policy, practice, procedure, personnel, and patient care.

KATIE SCHENK, PhD, is an epidemiologist and public health informatics specialist focused on implementing community-based measures to control infectious disease. She served as senior epidemiologist on the front lines of the COVID-19 response for US government health departments. Previously, Dr. Schenk led a portfolio of sociobehavioral research focused on mitigating the effects of HIV on children and families in sub-Saharan Africa for the nonprofit Population Council.

VANESSA B. SHEPPARD, PhD, is the inaugural founding dean of the School of Population Health at Virginia Commonwealth University and director for Community Outreach, Engagement, at the Massey Comprehensive Cancer Center. Her research focuses on minoritized racial/ethnic groups and engages these groups to address health disparities, health-related outcomes, and barriers to care.

GRACE OFORIWA SIKAPOKOO, MBA, is an assistant professor of communication and Basic Course director at Northern Illinois University. She is also a health communication doctoral candidate at Ohio University. Sikapokoo was awarded the Claude Kantner Award for her dissertation at Ohio University and was the 2022 CSCA Cooper Award recipient for teaching excellence.

ARNETHEA L. SUTTON, PhD, is an assistant professor (Kinesiology and Health Sciences Department) at Virginia Commonwealth University. Her focus is on cancer disparities in breast cancer survivorship. Her current research focuses on examining causes of racial disparities in treatment-related cardiovascular toxicities in breast cancer survivors.

MARIA THOMSON, PhD, is an associate professor (Health Behavior and Policy Department) at Virginia Commonwealth University. Her work focuses on promoting informed and shared decision-making through effective communication and measuring and evaluating sociocultural and health disparities that influence cancer survivors and family caregivers' information needs, knowledge, attitudes, and behaviors.

KATHERINE Y. TOSSAS, PhD, is an assistant professor (Sociobehavioral Sciences Department) at Virginia Commonwealth University. Her research focuses on health equity and explores how individual and aggregate community experiences impact cancer outcomes for minoritized populations. She is currently investigating the microbiome's influence on HPV-related cancer outcome disparities.

NITA VANGEEPURAM, MD, is a pediatrician and clinical researcher in general pediatrics. Her research focuses on childhood asthma, obesity, and prevention of related conditions in urban minority youth. She has received funding from various organizations to develop programs using innovative methods such as peer education and mobile health technologies. She is a member of several nationwide and local committees dedicated to addressing health disparities.

PABLO VILLALOBOS DINTRANS, DrPH, is a researcher at the Universidad de Santiago, Chile. He holds a master's in economics and public policy from the Pontificia Universidad Católica de Chile, an MA in economics from Boston University, and a DrPH from Harvard. He has published in areas related to health policy and systems, population aging, and long-term care.

ELIZABETH WACHIRA, PhD, is an associate professor at Texas A&M University–Commerce. Her research aims to understand the often covert pathways of oppression and injustices that marginalized populations face. She aims to inform and expand authentic, lived-experienced knowledge on health vulnerabilities as determinants of health among marginalized individuals.

ROBERT A. WINN, MD, serves as the director of Virginia Commonwealth University Massey Comprehensive Cancer Center, a cancer center designated by the National Cancer Institute that provides advanced cancer care and conducts groundbreaking research. He is committed to community-engaged research centered on eliminating health disparities and is principal investigator on several community-based and basic cancer research projects.

RAFEEK YUSUF, PhD, is a health management and policy scientist, epidemiologist, informatician, and physician. He is a versatile health services researcher published in several national and international journals. He has twenty-plus years combined epidemiology, informatics, and clinical practice in hospitals, academic medical centers, long-term care facilities, state and local public health departments, biopharmaceutical, and medical device start-up companies.

ZENAB YUSUF, MD, is a physician-scientist and epidemiologist. She has over ten years of experience in clinical trials and clinical research project management in oncology and infectious diseases. She has authored several publications and has presented her work at multiple international and national conferences.

Index

Page numbers followed by an *f* indicate figures. Page numbers followed by a *t* indicate tables.

Printed and bound by CPI Group (UK) Ltd, Croydon, CR0 4YY

27/10/2024

14580329-0001